PUBLICATIONS OF THE NEWTON INSTITUTE

Epidemic Models:
Their Structure and Relation to Data

T0276128

Publications of the Newton Institute

Edited by J. Wright

Deputy Director, Isaac Newton Institute for Mathematical Sciences

The Isaac Newton Institute of Mathematical Sciences of the University of Cambridge exists to stimulate research in all branches of the mathematical sciences, including pure mathematics, statistics, applied mathematics, theoretical physics, theoretical computer science, mathematical biology and economics. The four six-month long research programmes it runs each year bring together leading mathematical scientists from all over the world to exchange ideas through seminars, teaching and informal interaction.

Associated with the programmes are two types of publication. The first contains lecture courses, aimed at making the latest developments accessible to a wider audience and providing an entry to the area. The second contains proceedings of workshops and conferences focusing on the most topical aspects of the subjects.

EPIDEMIC MODELS

Their Structure and Relation to Data

edited by

Denis Mollison

Heriot-Watt University

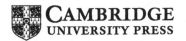

CAMBRIDGE UNIVERSITY PRESS
Cambridge, New York, Melbourne, Madrid, Cape Town, Singapore, São Paulo

Cambridge University Press
The Edinburgh Building, Cambridge CB2 8RU, UK

Published in the United States of America by Cambridge University Press, New York

www.cambridge.org
Information on this title: www.cambridge.org/9780521475365

First published 1995
This digitally printed version 2008

A catalogue record for this publication is available from the British Library

ISBN 978-0-521-47536-5 hardback
ISBN 978-0-521-06728-7 paperback

CONTENTS

PART 4: HETEROGENEITY IN HUMAN DISEASES

PART 5: DATA ANALYSIS: ESTIMATION AND PREDICTION

Preface

The problems of understanding and controlling disease present a range of mathematical challenges, from broad theoretical issues to specific practical ones. This exciting and rapidly developing field is surveyed here by individuals with a wide range of mathematical expertise (including applied probability, deterministic modelling, and data analysis) and with close involvement in applied fields across the social, medical and biological sciences. Their collaboration originates from a NATO Advanced Research Workshop which marked the opening of a six month research programme on Epidemic Models at the Newton Institute in Cambridge in 1993.

The book is divided into five parts, covering the conceptual framework, three major problem areas (space, nonlinearity, heterogeneity), and the direct relation of models to data. A wide range of methodological issues are discussed, for instance comparing different approaches to the modelling of heterogeneity and relations between different types of model; and different data analytic approaches, together with the availability and quality of the data they require.

Two related volumes, based on the same research programme at the Newton Institute, tackle more specific topics. The spatial spread and persistence of animal and plant diseases is reviewed in Grenfell and Dobson (1995); while infectious human diseases, including AIDS and other sexually transmitted diseases, are discussed in Isham and Medley (1995).

In all three books it has been our aim to provide a view of the broad spectrum of current research on the dynamics of infectious diseases, and to identify major issues and outstanding problems. We have also kept in mind the importance of reporting to the public health community and decision makers on the state of the art in epidemic modelling, and requirements for further progress, whether in developing new models or in improved data collection and analysis.

Acknowledgements

Thanks are due to NATO for funding the workshop on whose proceedings this book is based, and to the Newton Institute and its staff for hosting the *Epidemic Models* research programme of which the workshop was the opening event. I should also like to thank all the authors for their conscientious work which greatly facilitated the editing, all those who helped referee their papers, and all the participants in the workshop for their contribution to its success.

Introduction

Denis Mollison

Infectious diseases have played a major role in evolution, of which their influence on human history is just the most recent and best documented example (McNeill 1976, Crosby 1986). The spectacular success of humans in dominating the world's ecology has meant that they — and their domestic animals and crops — provide an unprecedentedly rich resource for parasites. Not surprisingly, parasites have evolved, and continue to evolve, to exploit this resource. Meanwhile the earth's remaining natural ecosystems, often weakened by human influence, are in relative terms even more threatened by the spread of infectious diseases.

Until fairly recently it was possible to look back on over 100 years of fairly steady progress in the control of disease — including the introduction of antibiotics, and vaccination programmes leading to great reductions of the main 'childhood diseases' in developed countries, and to the worldwide eradication of smallpox — and to extrapolate to a future in which infectious disease had been conquered. The rise of AIDS and of vaccine-resistant strains of a number of the diseases thought to be no longer a threat has demonstrated that such simple optimism is unjustified. The war against disease is going to be a long one, in which lasting success can only be won through better understanding.

Epidemics involve processes at all scales, from the global population, through the individual level, right down to the behaviour of the immune system. The resulting dynamical systems are characteristically highly nonlinear, stochastic and subject to natural selection. The corresponding mathematical problems concern both the structure of models that are needed to describe this dynamical diversity, and also the modelling and statistical methods required to deal with heterogeneity, in space, time, social contact and so on. A third, vital and complementary area of work is the adaptation of developments in these areas to particular applied problems.

Much current work is driven by the great concern centred on the AIDS epidemic. This has raised many stimulating technical questions: AIDS is particularly difficult to model because of the complex heterogeneity of the relevant contact structures, and difficulties in collecting and analysing data which are enhanced by its long incubation period and by the social sensitivity associated with sexually transmitted diseases. Nevertheless, similar problems arise for all diseases, and any solutions or improvements in methodology will be of wider applicability.

As well as AIDS, the areas of application include: epidemics of other sexually transmitted diseases; childhood diseases like measles or polio and the question of appropriate vaccination policies; strategies for disease control in animals; the problems involved in the spatial spread of disease (e.g. rabies); and so on.

Improved computer technology has provided better data bases, and opened up new possibilities for the use of computationally-intensive methods in the analysis of data. It has also allowed the simulation of more realistic models; however this increases the need to improve our understanding of how a relatively few key components can drive the dynamics of such models.

1   The conceptual framework

The present volume opens with a review by Dietz of some of the basic concepts and problems of epidemic modelling; and of a wide range of questions related to vaccination strategies which should in principle be amenable to mathematical analysis.

This is followed by a chapter on the structure of epidemic models. We cannot begin to make use of models until we understand how their dynamics depend on basic components, and how sensitive they are to the way in which they are incorporated into the model; this is especially important where we extrapolate on the basis of a model, for instance for prediction and control.

Stochastic epidemic models, although generally more realistic than deterministic ones, have often been seen as too complex for analysis because of the level of detail they require, for instance relating to the probability that an individual with the disease will infect a particular subset of the population. However, in recent years it has been realised that this micro-structure can be turned to considerable advantage, especially when comparing one model with another, by the simple and elegant technique of *coupling*. Ball reviews this technique in the epidemic context, while Lefèvre and Picard use similar stochastic methods to generalise the classic Reed-Frost model for an epidemic in a closed population.

Nåsell discusses how the concept of an epidemic threshold should be extended to stochastic models, where the question of whether an outbreak can be regarded as 'large' is not as clearcut as in the simplified deterministic case. De Jong, Diekmann and Heesterbeek consider the transmission rate of infection, arguing from both theory and data in favour of the 'true mass-action' assumption, namely that the rate should rise with population *density* but not depend on the overall population size.

Part 1 concludes with a wide-ranging survey by Diekmann, Heesterbeek and Metz of the various possible types of disease dynamics, with special emphasis on the influence of heterogeneity and on how the appropriate modelling approach depends on the population and time scales of interest.

2   Spatial models

Recent developments in spatial stochastic processes and differential equations have applications to animal and plant diseases, where key questions concern long-distance contacts, endemic patterns, and the effectiveness of control zones.

Cliff reviews mapping methods for identifying the spatial corridors used by diseases, and the importance of different components in their spread. This is illustrated by analysis of the spread of measles and influenza over a wide range of population densities and spatial scales. Metz and van den Bosch present a very general framework in which the velocity of spread of epidemics and populations can be calculated from information at the individual level, and illustrate this with applications to a wide variety of cases, mainly of plant and animal diseases.

The breadth of applicability of Metz's approach is achieved at the expense of some loss of accuracy, particularly in neglecting stochastic effects. Durrett shows how significant progress is now being made in analysing the more accurate but relatively intractable stochastic models for the spatial spread of epidemics.

This part concludes with two more specialised papers. Daniels shows, for nonlinear deterministic models, how an elegant perturbation approach can be used to calculate the detailed shape of epidemic wavefronts. Billard *et al.* generalise classical logistic models for the rate of increase of infected tissue in epidemic plant diseases, so as to incorporate randomness and additional infections from the surrounding environment, and show how they can be fitted to experimental data on the spread of *anthracnose* in *Stylosanthes scabra*.

3   Nonlinear time and space-time dynamics

Data on recurrent epidemics of human 'childhood' diseases, especially measles, have played a key part in discussions of the role of nonlinearity and chaos in biological population dynamics. Ellner *et al.* review methods for the detection of nonlinearity and chaos, and apply them to a collection of data sets for four different diseases. Their broad conclusion is that evidence for chaos is generally lacking in these data sets, though measles may be close to it.

Grenfell *et al.* look at measles modelling in more detail: seasonal forcing has a destabilising effect on the dynamics, while the introduction of a realistic age structure to the model promotes stability. They also discuss the more problematic effects of spatial heterogeneity and of variations in the birth rate, in the light of data from a number of major cities of the developed world.

4   Heterogeneity in human diseases

It is vital for successful modelling to take appropriate account of both *population heterogeneity*, i.e. variations between individuals in parameters such as their contact rate or susceptibility (especially important for AIDS and other STDs); and *heterogeneity of mixing*, i.e. how the pattern of contacts depends on spatial location or on the connectivity of social networks. The development of satisfactory models for the contact structures of human diseases offers a challenging opportunity for collaborative research between workers with expertise ranging from random graphs to sociology.

Here, Levin gives an elegant analysis of the general mixing problem which is basic to the modelling of pairing in a heterogeneous population, and discusses the dynamics of formation and dissolution of pairs. Jacquez *et al.* analyse the relation between the epidemic threshold for a population composed of differing subgroups and the threshold of the individual subgroups.

Morris offers a very different approach to the same problem area, showing how log-linear models can provide a framework for estimation of mixing parameters from available sociological data, and for inference on the resulting patterns of transmission. This is illustrated from sexual preference data, and the implications for the spread of sexually transmitted diseases are discussed.

Gupta *et al.* consider a quite different kind of heterogeneity, in the disease agent, showing how this can make a substantial difference to estimates of the basic reproductive ratio in the case of malaria.

5   Data analysis: estimation and prediction

Even for relatively simple epidemic situations, statistical inference faces difficulties including identifiability problems, very complicated likelihood functions, multiple sources of errors, difficulties with the interpretation of 'parameters', and the need to make predictions for the epidemic from which the data are gathered. Becker reviews and illustrates methods to overcome such difficulties, including the use of effective simplifying assumptions, addressing estimation problems in a more specific context, and the use of martingale methods.

For many diseases, complex models are required to aid our understanding of the mechanics of transmission and evaluation of potential control strategies, but the crudeness of data makes the use of relatively simple models the only sensible approach to model fitting and projection. Cairns discusses how these two conflicting requirements may be reconciled through the identification of a minimal set of Primary Components, that is, functions of the basic parameters which dictate epidemic dynamics; illustrating the technique through reference to some simple models for the spread of AIDS.

The World Health Organisation's Onchocerciasis Control Programme in West Africa provides a large scale example of the use of epidemic modelling in disease control. Onchocerciasis (river blindness) is a complex disease – its dynamics depend on the interaction of three populations, the parasites, the human hosts and the vectors – which affects an estimated 18 million people, mainly in west and central Africa. Remme *et al.* describe how epidemic models have been used in the planning, implementation, evaluation and timely adjustment of control strategies.

A major problem in disease control is that vaccines may fail to confer immunity, or may only confer partial immunity. Longini *et al.* review the use of statistical methods to estimate vaccine efficiency both for single outbreaks and endemic conditions.

Norman Bailey, noted for his pioneering work in epidemic modelling (Bailey 1957, 1975), rounds off this final section of the book with a discussion of the vital practical issues involved in integrating modelling with public health decision-making and planning, illustrated from his recent work on the spread and control of HIV/AIDS.

Future work

During the NATO workshop on *Epidemic Models* there were discussions to identify key problem areas: the conclusions of these sessions are given as an Appendix, under the headings 'Model structure', 'Heterogeneity' and 'Data analysis and prediction'. A further review, in part based on these discussions, is given in Mollison, Isham and Grenfell (1994).

Many theoretical challenges remain, for instance to expand the scope of epidemic modelling to deal with the co-evolution of diseases and the species they affect (see e.g. Hamilton and Howard 1994). On the practical side, we need to use our understanding to achieve greater success in the war against disease. It seems ironic, when there is rightly much concern over the number of species disappearing from the earth as an incidental consequence of human activities, that it should be so hard to eliminate a species deliberately, with the smallpox virus still our only complete success.

References for Preface and Introduction

Bailey, N.T.J. (1957) *The Mathematical Theory of Epidemics*, Griffin, London.

Bailey, N.T.J. (1975) *The Mathematical Theory of Infectious Diseases and its Applications*, Griffin, London.

Crosby, A.W. (1986) *Ecological Imperialism: the biological expansion of Europe, 900–1900*, Cambridge University Press, Cambridge.

Grenfell, B.T. and Dobson, A. (eds.) (1995) *Ecology of Infectious Diseases in Natural Populations*, Cambridge University Press, Cambridge.

Hamilton, W.D. and Howard, J.C. (eds.) (1994) *Infection, Polymorphism and Evolution, Phil. Trans. R. Soc. Lond. B*, to appear.

Isham, V. and Medley, G. (eds.) (1995) *Models for Infectious Human Diseases: their Structure and Relation to Data*, Cambridge University Press, Cambridge.

Mollison, D., Isham, V. and Grenfell, B.T. (1994) 'Epidemics: models and data' (with Discussion), *J. R. Statist. Soc. A* **157**, 115–149.

McNeill, William H. (1976) *Plagues and Peoples*, Doubleday, New York.

CONTRIBUTORS

For email addresses of first authors, see p. xvii.

Soumbey Alley, Onchocerciasis Control Programme in West Africa, B.P. 549, Ouagadougou, Burkina Faso

Roy M. Anderson, Parasite Epidemiology Research Group, Department of Zoology, Oxford, OX1 3PS, UK

Norman Bailey, Chalet Chrine, Fang, 3782 Lauenen, Switzerland

Frank Ball, Department of Mathematics, Nottingham University, University Park, Nottingham, NG7 2RD, UK

Niels Becker, Department of Statistics, La Trobe University, Bundoora 3083, Australia

Lynne Billard, Department of Mathematics, University of Georgia, Athens, GA 30602-1952, USA

Ben Bolker, Department of Ecology and Evolutionary Biology, Princeton University, Princeton NJ 08544-1003, USA

Frank van den Bosch, Department of Mathematics, Agricultural University, Dreijenlaan 4, 6703 HA Wageningen, The Netherlands

Andrew Cairns, Department of Actuarial Mathematics and Statistics, Heriot-Watt University, Riccarton, Edinburgh, EH14 4AS, Scotland

Andrew Cliff, Department of Geography, University of Cambridge, Downing Place, Cambridge, CB2 3EN, UK

Martin J. Cox, Molecular Epidemiology Research Group, Imperial College, London, SW7 2BB, UK

Henry Daniels, Statistical Laboratory, 16 Mill Lane, Cambridge, CB2 1SB, UK

P.W.A. Dayananda, School of Applied Mathematics and Statistics, Griffith University, Nathan, Queensland 4111, Australia

Karen P. Day, Molecular Epidemiology Research Group, Imperial College, London, SW7 2BB, UK

Odo Diekmann, Institute of Evolutionary and Ecological Sciences PO Box 9516, 2300 RA Leiden, The Netherlands, and CWI, Kruislaan 413, 1098 SJ Amsterdam, The Netherlands

Klaus Dietz, Institut für Medizinische Biometrie, Universität Tübingen, Westbahnhofstrasse 55, D-72070 Tübingen, Germany

Richard Durrett, Cornell University, Department of Mathematics, Ithaca, NY 14853, USA

Stephen Ellner, Biomathematics Graduate Program, Department of Statistics, North Carolina State University, Raleigh, NC 27695-8203, USA

A. Ronald Gallant, Department of Economics, University of North Carolina, Chapel Hill NC 27533-3305, USA

Bryan Grenfell, Zoology Department, Cambridge University, Downing St, Cambridge, CB2 3EJ, UK

Sunetra Gupta, Parasite Epidemiology Research Group, Department of Zoology, Oxford, OX1 3PS, UK

Michael Haber, Division of Biostatistics, Emory University, School of Public Health, Atlanta, GA 30322, USA

Elizabeth Halloran, Division of Biostatistics, Emory University, School of Public Health, Atlanta, GA 30322, USA

J.A.P. (Hans) Heesterbeek Agricultural Mathematics Group (GLW-DLO), PO Box 100, 6700 AC Wageningen, The Netherlands

John Jacquez, Department of Physiology and Biostatistics, University of Michigan, Ann Arbor, MI 48109, USA

Mart (M.C.M.) de Jong, Department of Pathobiology and Epidemiology, Institute for Animal Science and Health (ID-DLO), 8200 AB Lelystad, The Netherlands

Adam Kleczkowski, Department of Plant Sciences, Cambridge University, Downing Street, Cambridge CB2 3EA, UK

James Koopman, Department of Epidemiology, University of Michigan, Ann Arbor, Michigan 48109, USA

Claude Lefèvre, Université Libre de Bruxelles, Institut de Statistique, CP 210, Boulevard du Triomphe, B-1050 Bruxelles, Belgium

Simon Levin, Department of Ecology and Evolutionary Biology, Princeton University, Princeton, NJ 08544, USA

Ira Longini, Division of Biostatistics, Emory University, School of Public Health, Atlanta, GA 30322, USA

Hans (J.A.J.) Metz, Institute of Evolutionary and Ecological Sciences, Theoretical Biology Section, Kaiserstraat 63, PO Box 9516, 2300 RA Leiden, The Netherlands

Denis Mollison, Department of Actuarial Mathematics and Statistics, Heriot-Watt University, Riccarton, Edinburgh, EH14 4AS, Scotland

Martina Morris, Department of Sociology, Columbia University, 538 West 120th St., New York, NY 10027, USA

Ingemar Nåsell, Department of Mathematics, The Royal Institute of Technology, S-10044 Stockholm, Sweden

Philippe Picard, Université de Lyon 1, Mathématiques Appliquées, 43 Boulevard du 11 Novembre 1918, F-69622 Villeurbanne, France

Anton Plaisier, Erasmus University, P.O.Box 1738, 3000 DR Rotterdam, The Netherlands

Hans Remme, WHO, 2- Av. Appia, CH-1211 Geneva 27, Switzerland

Carl Simon, Departments of Mathematics, Economics and Public Policy, University of Michigan, Ann Arbor, Michigan 48109, USA

James Theiler, Santa Fe Institute, 1660 Old Pecos Trail, Santa Fe NM 87501, USA

Katharine Trenholme, Molecular Epidemiology Research Group, Imperial College, London, SW7 2BB, UK *and* Papua New Guinea Institute of Medical Research, PO Box 378, Madang, Papua New Guinea *and* Walter and Eliza Hall Institute of Medical Research, Parkville 13050, Victoria, Australia

Zhen Zhao, Department of Mathematics, University of Georgia, Athens, GA 30602–1952, USA

E-mail addresses of first authors

Frank Ball		fgb@maths.nott.ac.uk
Niels Becker		n.becker@latrobe.edu.au
Lynne Billard		lynne@rolf.stat.uga.edu
Andrew Cairns		andrewc@ma.hw.ac.uk
Henry Daniels	c/o	secretary@statslab.cam.ac.uk
Mart De Jong		m.c.m.de.jong@id.agro.nl
Odo Diekmann		o.diekmann@cwi.nl
Rick Durrett		durrett@math.cornell.edu
Steve Ellner		ellner@stat.ncsu.edu
Bryan Grenfell		bryan@zoo.cam.ac.uk
Sunetra Gupta		sunetra.gupta@zoo.ox.ac.uk
John Jacquez		john.jacquez@um.cc.umich.edu
Claude Lefèvre		clefevre@ulb.ac.be
Simon Levin		simon@eno.princeton.edu
Ira Longini		longini@fox.sph.emory.edu
Hans Metz		metz@rulsfb.leidenuniv.nl
Denis Mollison		denis@ma.hw.ac.uk
Martina Morris		morris@columbia.edu
Ingemar Nåsell		ingemar@math.kth.se
Hans Remme		remmej@who.ch

Part 1
The Conceptual Framework

Some Problems in the Theory of Infectious Disease Transmission and Control

Klaus Dietz

Summary

The paper presents a personal selection of research problems in the theory of infectious disease transmission and control.

1 Introduction

The following contribution to these proceedings is based on a talk which opened the Workshop on 'Epidemic Models: Their Structure and Relation to Data', the beginning of the half-year research programme on Epidemic Models at the Isaac Newton Institute. It was given on 4 January 1993, i.e. on the 350th anniversary of Newton's birthday in the Gregorian calendar already in use on the Continent (but not in England where, according to the Julian calendar still in force, Newton was born on Christmas Day 1642).

Two associations between Newton and epidemics or epidemiologists, respectively, are to be mentioned. The first one is his stay at Woolsthorpe, his place of birth in Lincolnshire, from the summer of 1665 to the spring of 1667 which was forced upon him by the closure of Cambridge University because of a plague epidemic. During these *anni mirabiles* he laid the foundations for his epochal work (Westfall 1993). The second one is his friendship with his doctor Richard Mead (1673–1754), 'the leading medical practitioner in London' (Winslow 1980). Newton's personal library (Harrison 1978) includes two editions (presumably given to him by the author) of Mead's book on plague and its prevention (Mead (1721)), about which Winslow writes: 'His *Discourse on Plague* has won for him a permanent place in the little group who through the ages have been classed as the fathers of epidemiology.' (Winslow 1980)

The series of three Cambridge workshops (this volume, Grenfell and Dobson 1995, Isham and Medley 1995) in 1993 represent the culmination of a sequence of conferences which started with the Moscow Meeting in 1971 (see Table 1).

Place	Dates	Title	Organiser(s)
Moscow	23–27 November 1970	WHO Symposium on Quantitative Epidemiology[a]	N.T.J.Bailey
Alta, Utah	8–12 July 1974	SIMS Conference on Epidemiology[b]	D.Ludwig, D.L.Thomsen
Berlin	14–19 March 1982	Dahlem Workshop on Population Biology of Infectious Disease Agents[c]	R.M.Anderson, R.M.May
Luminy	23–29 October 1988	Stochastic Processes in Epidemic Theory[d]	J-P.Gabriel, C.Lefèvre, P.Picard
Oberwolfach	5–11 February 1989	Mathematical Models for Infectious Diseases[e]	K.Dietz, H.Hethcote, K.P.Hadeler
Skokloster	8–12 August 1990	Spread of Epidemics: Stochastic Modelling and Data Analysis[f]	D.Mollison, G.Scalia-Tomba
Luminy	4–8 November 1991	Stochastic Modelling for Infectious Diseases[g]	J.-P.Gabriel, C.Lefèvre, P.Picard

[a]Anonymous (1971)
[b]Ludwig and Cooke (1975)
[c]Anderson and May (1982)
[d]Gabriel *et al.* (1990)
[e]Kretzschmar (1989)
[f]Mollison *et al.* (1991)
[g]Gabriel *et al.* (1993)

Table 1.   Conferences on Epidemic Theory.

The increasing incidence of these meetings is a testimony to the impressive progress which the theory of epidemics has made during these last twenty years. The important rôle of mathematics in this field is more and more widely recognized. The potential that mathematics offers for the scientific study of epidemics was already recognized more than 100 years ago. In his Inaugural Address entitled 'Aids to epidemiological knowledge' George Buchanan opened the session 1881–82 of the Epidemiological Society of London with the following words:

> ...; we want, too, help from mathematics, from chemistry and physics, from meteorology, botany and zoology: ... I propose in meeting you at the commencement of our new session to speak of one or two ways in which we as epidemiologists are called upon to make applications of this wider knowledge .... The first idea that must occur to anyone who hears me is the place which among all such subjects we shall gratefully assign to mathematical science. (Buchanan 1881)

The following paper will present a personal selection of problems which are considered relevant for the *applications* of the theory of infectious disease transmission and control. According to a quote attributed (Hand 1992) to John Tukey 'It is better to have an approximate answer to the right question than a right answer to the wrong question'.

2 Vaccination strategies

The evaluation of vaccination strategies is one of the most important motivations for the development of epidemiological models for infectious diseases. There is no methodological alternative but to use modelling approaches because the likely outcome of a selected strategy depends in a nonlinear way on the alternative actions, and randomised control trials with whole nations as experimental units are impossible.

The oldest example is Daniel Bernoulli's calculation of the increase in life expectancy if smallpox could be eradicated by the method of inoculation (Bernoulli 1760). In modern terminology, he assumed an endemic situation with a constant force of infection. He correctly took into account that an infection causes immunity in the survivors of the infection so that only susceptible individuals are at risk of infection and subsequent death. Bernoulli calculated the age-specific proportion of susceptibles from which one gets the age-specific prevalence of past infection by the following modified catalytic curve, where λ is the force of infection, a is the age of an individual, and q is the probability of dying due to the infection:

$$\frac{(1 - e^{-\lambda a})(1 - q)}{1 - q(1 - e^{-\lambda a})}.$$

For $q = 0$ one obtains the 'simple catalytic curve' of Muench (1959). For positive q, the age-specific prevalence among the survivors is lower compared to the situation without mortality. In estimating the force of infection from age-specific prevalence data, one usually ignores the infection-induced mortality. This leads to an underestimate of the force of infection and hence of the minimum proportion $\bar{p}$ to be vaccinated successfully as a function of the basic reproduction number R_0 (see next section) in order to achieve elimination of an infection:

$$\bar{p} \geq 1 - \frac{1}{R_0}.$$

This lower bound was identified for the first time by Gordon Smith (Smith 1964).

In practice, vaccination may not produce lifelong immunity and therefore revaccination may be necessary from time to time. This raises the problem of determining an age-specific pattern of vaccination taking into account the underlying transmission dynamics and the rate of loss of immunity. During the conference at Alta, Utah, in 1974, I presented the following mathematical formulation of the vaccination problem (Dietz 1975a):

$$\frac{du}{da} = -\kappa\left[\int_0^\infty v(s)\mu e^{-\mu s}ds\right]u(a) - \pi(a)u(a) + \delta p(a), \qquad (2.1)$$

$$\frac{dv}{da} = \kappa\left[\int_0^\infty v(s)\mu e^{-\mu s}ds\right]u(a) - \gamma v(a), \qquad (2.2)$$

$$\frac{dp}{da} = \pi(a)u(a) - \delta p(a), \qquad (2.3)$$

$$\frac{dw}{da} = \gamma v(a). \qquad (2.4)$$

This system of equations describes the age-dependent proportion of susceptibles u, infectives v, vaccinated immunes p and naturally immunes w. The age-dependent vaccination rate is denoted by π, the natural death-rate by μ, the effective contact rate by κ, the rate of progression to natural immunity by γ, and the loss-rate of vaccine immunity by δ. The general problem would be to minimise an integral of a functional f which depends on the age-specific probability of disease given infection $m(a)$ (which for many infections increases with age) and the vaccination rate π.

$$\text{Min} \int_0^\infty f(v(a)m(a), \pi(a))\mu e^{-\mu a} \, da.$$

In this generality the problem has not been addressed since its publication. In Katzmann and Dietz (1984) the problem is simplified in the sense that the age-specific morbidity function is assumed to be constant and the vaccination rate is concentrated on two particular values. On the other hand the model is made more realistic by the inclusion of maternal antibodies. The paper calculates, for given values of the rate of loss of vaccine immunity and given ages at vaccination and for given vaccination coverage, the maximum basic reproduction numbers which could be accessible to elimination. Appendix B of the book by Anderson and May (1991) also contains a general formulation of the vaccination problem involving an age-dependent death-rate $\mu(a)$. The first mathematical proof that, without loss of vaccine immunity, vaccination at either one, or at most two, ages is optimal has been provided by Hadeler and Müller (1995).

During my stay at the Centers for Disease Control in the summer of 1991, Robert Chen of the Division of Immunization provided a list of problems which are relevant for vaccination strategies and which are considered amenable to mathematical analysis. He agreed that this list be brought to the attention of mathematical epidemiologists (see Appendix). The bewildering variety of the problems given is testimony to the fact that much remains to be done to bring the mathematical theory of infectious diseases closer to real-life applications.

1952	Macdonald (1952)		
1956			Bharucha-Reid (1956)
1964	Smith (1964)		Neyman and Scott (1964)
1969			Bartoszyński (1969)
1975	Dietz (1975a, 1975b)	Hethcote (1975)	Becker (1975)
1982		Anderson and May (1982)	
1990		Diekmann *et al.* (1990)	
1992		Heesterbeek (1992)	

Table 2.   Genealogy of R_0 in Epidemiology.

3   The basic reproduction number R_0

The basic reproduction number R_0 is the number of secondary cases which one case could generate during the infectious period if introduced into a completely susceptible population. See Dietz (1993) for a recent survey of the concept and estimation procedures in different contexts. In that paper reference is made to the contribution of Richard Böckh, the Director of the Statistical Office of Berlin, who published in 1886 for the first time a calculation of what he called the total reproduction ('totale Fortpflanzung') based on the life table for 1879 (Böckh (1886)). According to these calculations, the number of female births to one female throughout her reproductive life was 2.172. The credit of this concept to Böckh is acknowledged in writings by Lotka who developed it further and introduced the notation R_0 (Dublin and Lotka 1925). The index zero is explained by the following notation:

$$R_n = \int_0^\infty a^n p(a)\beta(a)\, da,$$

where $p(a)$ denotes the survival probability and $\beta(a)$ the age-specific birthrate.

Table 2 shows the genealogy of R_0 in epidemiology. The notion was first introduced into epidemiology by Macdonald in the context of malaria. This work was followed up by Gordon Smith who applied it to the transmission of arboviruses. There is a parallel sequence of papers started by Bharucha-Reid in 1956 which approximates the spread of infectious diseases in large populations by branching processes. In 1975 four papers were published which all documented the importance of this concept. The Dahlem Workshop organised by Anderson and May in 1982 helped tremendously to popularize this notion and the seminal paper by Diekmann *et al.* provided a mathematically rigorous framework for its definition. The dissertation of Heesterbeek is exclusively devoted to R_0 and gives further conceptual background.

The classical definition of R_0 has to be modified for the models introduced by Dietz and Hadeler (1988) which allow explicitly for the formation and dissolution of pairs. In these models it is possible to describe multiple contacts per partner. There is a certain rate ρ according to which new partners are contacted and a rate β which describes the rate of contacts between two partners during a partnership. Dietz and Tudor (1992) generalise these models to handle the possibility of up to two concurrent partnerships. For models with partnerships one has to start with a *typical* newly infected individual which by definition already has an infected partner such that the subsequent contacts with that partner will not generate new infective cases. Thus one cannot calculate R_0 with only *one* initial infective. The papers by Diekmann *et al.* (1991) and Dietz *et al.* (1993) provide a framework according to which such calculations can be performed.

The problem of multiple contacts per person does not only arise in the context of sexually transmitted diseases but also for infection transmission within and between households. One has to take into account that fraction of the contacts of a newly infected individual which take place with already infected individuals in the same household. There is a large literature on the spread of epidemics within households (Bailey 1975) and the estimation of infection parameters using household data (Becker 1989). A key concept for the estimation of household transmission is the secondary attack rate which is defined as the proportion of contacts who get a communicable disease as a consequence of contact with a case (Last 1988). It is intuitively clear that the secondary attack rate is positively correlated with R_0 but it is not clear how R_0 can be estimated on the basis of the data on secondary attack rates. The missing parameter is the transmission probability *between* households. These remarks show that there is a need to bring together into a consistent picture the models for the spread within very small mixing units like pairs and households and large populations being composed of such mixing units.

A further step would be the inclusion of a dynamic age structure into such models. During this century a major reduction in the birth-rate in developed countries has occurred which affects the size and age composition of households. The demographic theory of households is still in its early stages of development (Bongaarts *et al.* 1987). The demographic changes in household structure have so far not yet been incorporated into models to explain the oscillations of measles in large cities. It is conjectured that observed periods of one or two years may partly be explained by differences in household size and age distribution of children in households.

In spite of all the impressive theoretical progress, the practical application of R_0 is still at its beginning. So far it has mainly been defined for diseases where superinfection can be ignored. For those, Anderson and May (1991) have introduced the term 'microparasitic infections'. For helminthic infections (also called 'macroparasitic infections' (Anderson and May 1991) it is obvious that one has to take into account superinfections. So far it is not clear how the concept of R_0 can be modified for such situations.

4 Critical community size

Bartlett (1960) defined the critical community size for measles as the size of the population for which the mean time to fade out after a major epidemic is about two years. This shows that this concept can only be discussed in a stochastic framework where it makes sense to describe the distribution of the random variable 'time to extinction'. Schenzle and Dietz (1987) provide a survey of the problem of determining the critical community size for infectious diseases depending on the following epidemiological parameters: duration of the infectious period D, life expectancy of an individual L, proportion of the population successfully immunized $\bar{p}$ and a function which describes how the contact rate κ depends on the population size N. They point out that for large populations the contact rate is virtually independent of the population size. Using this assumption, one arrives at the following heuristic formula for the critical community size:

$$N^* = \frac{I^* L}{\left(1 - \bar{p} - \frac{1}{R_0}\right) D}.$$

Here I^* denotes an equilibrium number of infectives which corresponds to a chosen level for the time to fade out. The definition of the critical community size involves a certain degree of ambiguity because one has to choose a critical time to fade out. Extinction of the number of infectives is expected with probabilty one without the introduction of new infectives from outside for any population size. Both the expected time to extinction and the number of infectives increase with population size. The general problem therefore is really to determine how the time to extinction depends on population size. For the specific case of poliomyelitis, Eichner *et al.* (1995) describe the results of extensive simulations showing how the time to extinction depends on the parameters mentioned above. As one can also infer from the formula given above the major influence on the critical community size is exerted by the life-expectancy because this enters linearly. Changes in R_0 are less important. One can use the equation above in order to study the effect of finite population size on the minimum proportion to be immunized which is necessary for eradicating an infection:

$$\bar{p} = 1 - \frac{1}{R_0} - \frac{I^* L}{ND}.$$

This expression shows that for finite populations the minimum immunization coverage is reduced depending on the four parameters L, D, I^* and N. Previously Katzmann and Dietz (1982) had approached this problem using the (wrong) heuristic formula

$$\bar{p} = 1 - \frac{1}{R_0\left(1 - \frac{I \cdot L}{ND}\right)}.$$

The table which Katzmann and Dietz provide has been reproduced in Anderson and May (1991, page 97).

In spite of the fact that this problem of determining the critical community size in terms of the relevant epidemiological parameters has now been around for more than 30 years there is still no satisfactory solution. One method of approach may be the application of diffusion approximations for discrete stochastic processes following the methods proposed by Kurtz (1981). Another method might be the application of the dynamics of metapopulations which has recently undergone a major development (Mangel and Tier, 1993).

The concept of critical community sizes becomes extremely important in the context of global eradication projects like the one for poliomyelitis aiming to be finished by the year 2000 where the question arises as to whether the virus can persist unnoticed for a long time in a subpopulation which for some reason or another escaped vaccination.

5   Concluding remarks

In a stimulating review of mathematical models of infectious diseases Black and Singer (1987) express the opinion '... theoretical work in model building has outrun experimental verification'. One reaction to this might be the claim that models developed so far are at present sufficient and the plea that further model development should be stopped until more and better data become available. The problems listed in this paper were intended to show that there is not only a great need for practical work with very specific public health problems but also for more theoretical advances.

Acknowledgements

During his stay at the Isaac Newton Institute in Cambridge the author held a Prudential Fellowship. The University of Tübingen granted leave of absence.

References

Anderson, R.M. and May, R.M. (eds.) (1982) *Population Biology of Infectious Diseases: Dahlem Konferenzen*, Springer-Verlag.

Anderson, R.M. and May, R.M. (1991) *Infectious Diseases of Humans: Dynamics and Control*, Oxford University Press.

Anonymous (1971) 'WHO Symposium on Quantitative Epidemiology' (Abstracts only), *Adv. Appl. Prob.* **3**, 193–228.

Bailey, N.T.J. (1975) *The Mathematical Theory of Infectious Diseases and its Applications*, second edition, Griffin, London.

Bartlett, M.S. (1960) 'The critical community size of measles in the United States', *J. R. Statist. Soc. A* **123**, 37–44.

Bartoszyński, R. (1969) *Branching Processes and Models of Epidemics*, (Dissertationes Mathematicae), Panstwowe Wydawnictwo Naukowe, Warsaw.

Becker, N.G. (1975) 'The use of mathematical models in determining vaccination policies', *Bull. Int. Statist. Inst.* **46**, 478–490.

Becker, N.G. (1989) *Analysis of Infectious Disease Data*, Chapman and Hall, London.

Bernoulli, D. (1760) 'Essai d'une nouvelle analyse de la mortalité causée par la petite vérole et des avantages de l'inoculation pour la prévenir', *Mém. Math., Phys. Acad. Roy. Sci., Paris*, 1–45.

Bharucha-Reid, A.T. (1956) 'On the stochastic theory of epidemics'. In *Proceedings of the Third Berkeley Symposium on Mathematical Statistics and Probability. Volume IV: Biology and Problems of Health.*, J. Neyman (ed.) University of California Press, Berkeley, 111–119.

Black, F.L. and Singer, B. (1987) 'Elaboration versus simplification in refining mathematical models of infectious diseases', *Ann. Rev. Microbiol.* **41**, 677–701.

Bongaarts, J., Burch, T. and Wachter, K. (1987) *Family Demography: Methods and their Application*, Clarendon Press, Oxford.

Buchanan, G. (1881–82) 'Aids to epidemiological knowledge', *Trans. Epidemiol. Soc. Lond. (New Series)* **1**, 1–14.

Böckh, R. (1886) *Statistisches Jahrbuch der Stadt Berlin, Zwölfter Jahrgang. Statistik des Jahres 1884*, P. Stankiewicz, Berlin, 30–31.

Diekmann, O., Dietz, K. and Heesterbeek, J.A.P. (1991) 'The basic reproduction ratio for sexually transmitted diseases, Part 1. Theoretical considerations', *Math. Biosci.* **107**, 325–339.

Diekmann, O., Heesterbeek, J.A.P. and Metz, J.A.J. (1990) 'On the definition and the computation of the basic reproduction ratio R_0 in models for infectious diseases in heterogeneous populations', *J. Math. Biol.* **28** 365–382.

Dietz, K. and Hadeler, K.P. (1988) 'Epidemiological models for sexually transmitted diseases', *J. Math. Biol.* **26**, 1–26.

Dietz, K. and Tudor, D. (1992) 'Triangles in heterosexual HIV transmission'. In *AIDS epidemiology: methodological issues*, N.P. Jewell, K. Dietz and V.T. Farewell (eds.) 143–155.

Dietz, K., Heesterbeek, J.A.P. and Tudor, D.W. (1993) 'The basic reproduction ratio for sexually transmitted diseases, Part 2. Effects of variable HIV infectivity', *Math. Biosci.* **117**, 35–47.

Dietz, K. (1975) 'Models for parasitic disease control', *Bull. Int. Statist. Inst.* **46**, 531–544.

Dietz, K. (1975) 'Transmission and control of arboviruses'. In *Epidemiology: Proceedings of a SIMS Conference*, D. Ludwig and K.L. Cooke (eds.), SIAM, Philadelphia, 104–121.

Dietz, K. (1993) 'The estimation of the basic reproduction number for infectious diseases', *Statist. Meth. Med. Res.* **2**, 23–41.

Dublin, L.I. and Lotka, A.J. (1925) 'On the true rate of natural increase as exemplified by the population of the United States, 1920', *J. Amer. Statist. Assoc.* **20**, 305–339.

Eichner, M., Hadeler K.P. and Dietz, K. (1995) 'Stochastic models for the eradication of poliomyelitis: minimum population size for polio virus persistence'. In *Models for Infectious Diseases: their Structure and Relation to Data* V. Isham and G. Medley (eds.), Cambridge University Press, Cambridge, to appear.

Gabriel, J-P., Lefèvre, C. and Picard, P. (eds.) (1990) *Stochastic Processes in Epidemic Theory: Proceedings (Lecture Notes in Biomathematics)* **86**, Springer-Verlag.

Gabriel, J-P., Lefèvre, C., Picard, P. and Jacquez, J. (eds.) (1993) 'Stochastic Modelling for Infectious Diseases', *Math. Biosci.* **117**, 1–300.

Grenfell, B.T. and Dobson, A. (eds.) (1995) *Ecology of Infectious Diseases in Natural Populations*, Cambridge University Press, Cambridge, to appear

Hadeler, K. P. and Müller, J. (1995) 'Vaccination in age-structured populations II: Optimal strategies.' In *Models for Infectious Human Diseases: their Structure and Relation to Data*, V. Isham and G. Medley (eds.), Cambridge University Press, Cambridge, to appear

Hand, D.J. (1992) 'The first step in statistical consultancy'. In *Proceedings of Invited papers of the 1992 (XVIth) International Biometric Conference, 7–11 December, Hamilton, New Zealand*, 221–228.

Harrison, J. (1978) *The Library of Isaac Newton*, Cambridge University Press, Cambridge.

Heesterbeek, J.A.P. (1992) R_0. Centrum voor Wiskunde en Informatica, Amsterdam.

Hethcote, H.W. (1975) 'Mathematical models for the spread of infectious diseases.' In *Epidemiology: Proceedings of a SIMS Conference*, D. Ludwig and K.L. Cooke (eds.), SIAM, Philadelphia, 122–131.

Isham, V. and Medley, G. (eds.) (1995) *Models for Infectious Human Diseases: their Structure and Relation to Data.* Cambridge University Press, Cambridge, tp appear.

Katzmann, W, and Dietz, K. (1982) 'Evaluation of eradication strategies for virus infections'. In *Proceedings of the Second World Conference on Mathematics at the Service of Man, 28 June - 3 July 1982* A. Ballester, D. Cardús and E. Trillas (eds.), Universidad Politecnica de Las Palmas, Las Palmas, 378–383.

Katzmann, W. and Dietz, K. (1984) 'Evaluation of age-specific vaccination strategies', *Theor. Pop. Biol.* **25**, 125–137.

Kretzschmar, M. (1989) *Tagungsbericht 6/1989: Mathematical Models for Infectious Diseases* (Abstracts only). Mathematisches Forschungsinstitut Oberwolfach.

Kurtz, T.G. (1981) *Approximation of Population Processes*, SIAM, Philadelphia.

Last, J.M. (1988) *A Dictionary of Epidemiology*, second edition, Oxford University Press, Oxford.

Ludwig, L. and Cooke, K. L. (eds.) 1975 *Epidemiology: Proceedings of a SIMS Conference*, SIAM, Philadelphia.

Macdonald, G. (1952) 'The analysis of equilibrium in malaria', *Trop. Diseases Bull.* **49**, 813–829.

Mangel, M. and Tier, Ch. (1993) 'Dynamics of metapopulations with demographic stochasticity and environmental catastrophes', *Theor. Pop. Biol.* **44**, 1–31.

Mead, R.A. (1721) *A short discourse concerning pestilential contagion, and the methods to be used to prevent it*, second edition, George Grierson, Dublin.

Mollison, D., Scalia-Tomba, G. and Jacquez, J. (eds.) (1991) 'Spread of Epidemics: Stochastic Modelling and Data Analysis', *Math. Biosci.* **107**, 149–562.

Mollison, D. (ed.) (1995) *Epidemic Models: their Structure and Relation to Data.* Cambridge University Press, Cambridge, to appear .

Muench, H. (1959) *Catalytic Models in Epidemiology*, Harvard University Press, Cambridge, MA.

Neyman, J. and Scott, E.L. (1964) 'A stochastic model of epidemics.' In *Stochastic Models in Medicine and Biology*, J. Gurland (ed.), University of Wisconsin Press, Madison, 45–83.

Schenzle, D. and Dietz, K. (1987) 'Critical population sizes for endemic virus transmission'. In *Räumliche Persistenz und Diffusion von Krankheiten* W. Fricke and E. Hinz (eds.), Heidelberger Geographische Arbeiten, Heft 83, pp. 31–42.

Smith, C.E.G. (1964) 'Factors in the transmission of virus infections from animals to man', *Scientific Basis of Medicine. Ann. Rev.*, 125–150.

Westfall, R.S. (1993) *The Life of Isaac Newton*, Cambridge University Press, Cambridge.

Winslow, C-E.A. (1980) *The Conquest of Epidemic Disease: a Chapter in the History of Ideas*, University of Wisconsin Press, Madison.

Appendix: Vaccine-preventable disease issues amenable to mathematical modelling

Compiled by R.T. Chen (Division of Immunization, CDC, Atlanta)

Developed Countries

- Measles

    - effects of waning vaccine-induced immunity

- effects of shorter duration of maternal immunity in vaccinated populations
- impact of lowering age of 1st dose routinely to 12 or 9 months
- effect of two dose schedule in urban and 1 dose schedule in rural settings
- effect of two dose schedule, but with poor compliance in certain urban setting until primary school entry
- efficacy of mass immunization campaigns in response to outbreaks
- marginal increase in immunity needed to stop transmission during low season in urban settings
- impact of vaccine that can be administered earlier (e.g. 6 months) but with a higher rate of waning immunity
- impact of loss of boosting of immunity from wild virus circulation in vaccinated populations
- role of certain risk groups in sustaining measles transmission (e.g. medical personnel, religious objectors, delayed/non-vaccinated, primary vaccine failures)
- strategies necessary to eliminate measles in US by year 2000

- Varicella

  - short and long term impact of immunization of age-specific morbidity and mortality taking into account variables such as:
  - rate of seroconversion post-vaccination
  - vaccine efficacy in sucessfully vaccinated persons (rate of 'break-through' infections currently reported as 2%/year)
  - persistence of immunity
  - infectiousness of vaccinated vs unvaccinated cases
  - complication and mortality rates of vaccinated vs unvaccinated cases

- Pertussis

  - impact of routine adult boosters with acellular vaccine
  - does vaccination with whole cell vaccine decrease circulation of the bacterium (i.e. is there herd immunity against pertussis infection)
  - is school-based silent transmission important for sustainimg pertussis transmission vs other countries without pre-school dose

- Polio

  - impact of combined IPV/OPV schedule vs IPV alone vs OPV alone

- Rubella

- effect of having pockets of unvaccinated persons, eg. Amish in the Midwest or Latin immigrants in the West, who may also not have been exposed to natural disease (since rubella is less infectious than diseases like measles or varicella)
- effect of low rate of reinfection

- Diphtheria

  - feasibility of eradication

Developing Countries

- Measles

  - maximum reduction in morbidity and mortality possible with following schedules: 1 dose, 2 dose, 1 dose rural + 2 dose urban
  - marginal increase in immunity needed to stop transmission in low season in urban settings, in rural settings
  - impact of periodic school-based catch-up immunizations
  - minimum coverage which must be acheived with EZ vaccine 'at 6 months' (let say: before 7 months) to be equivalent to/better than Schwarz vaccine 'at 9 months'
  - feasibility of elimination in island populations
  - strategies for elimination in other populations

- Polio

  - feasibility of eradication taken into account:
  - sanitation
  - population density
  - seasonality
  - impact of using combined IPV/OPV schedule
  - effect of so-called 'outbreak containment' strategies, under various assumptions of time after the first case; area covered; pre-existing immunity levels; sanitation; etc.
  - mass campaigns during low season vs. routine service delivery

- Rubella

  - impact of using combined measles-rubella vaccine

General

- assessing whether a vaccine produces Model 1 or Model 2 immunity
- impact of multiple antigen 'magic bullet' vaccines

Cost-Benefit

- Influenza

  - cost-effectiveness of vaccination in high-risk vs general elderly population

- Measles

  - cost/benefit of targetting certain risk groups for special vaccination campaign relative to their role in sustaining measles transmission (*e.g.* medical personnel, religious objectors, delayed/non-vaccinated, primary vaccine failures)

The Structure of Epidemic Models

Denis Mollison

Summary

This paper reviews the basic components of epidemic models, and discusses some of the different ways of combining them, and relations between the resulting models. The fundamental aim is to help understanding of the relation between assumptions and the resulting dynamics: because without such understanding even a model which fits data perfectly can be of no scientific value.

Analysis of the structure of epidemic models is vital because of (1) the scarcity of good data and (2) the sensitive dependence of results on assumptions. In evaluating model dynamics, we need to look carefully at their dependence, not only on parameters, but also on the structure of the model: for instance, whether the population is treated as stochastic or deterministic, discrete or continuous, and how the timing and distribution of infectious contacts within the population is modelled. The practical target is to identify those parts of models that have most effect on dynamics: a few key parameters can drive a model (see e.g. Mollison 1984, 1985, Cairns, this volume).

The approach taken here is to analyse models in terms of their elements: expressing them in terms of simple key parameters that reflect individual life-histories, flows between states, and contact relationships. Basic definitions must be in terms of what one individual does to another; this implies that discrete models are basic, and that the stochastic aspect is usually important, if only in formulating and interpreting models.

Although more complex, stochastic models can have advantages in showing structure more clearly, as for instance in the technique of *coupling* which allows elegant comparisons of related models (see Ball, this volume).

Some results can be very sensitive to model assumptions, including hidden assumptions implicit in seemingly innocent parts of our model structure. Other results are so robust that they can be derived by 'pre-model' arguments, that is, by considering relations between basic components without choosing a specific model. As an illustration of this approach, the final section (Section 3) tries to express some basic results on epidemic models in their simplest and most general form, so as to analyse the range and limits of their applicability.

17

1   Introduction

1.1   Reasons for caring about structure

The aim of epidemic modelling is to understand and if possible control the spread of disease. To do this, it tries to relate disease dynamics at the population level to basic properties of the host and pathogen populations and of the infection process. Epidemic models thus express scientific hypotheses. Like other scientific models, if they are to be of value they need to be falsifiable; and if they are falsified, we need to know which part of the model has been disproved. There are two basic reasons why this is seldom easy.

The first is the nature of the data available for validating and testing models. The scope for experimental investigation of disease dynamics is severely limited, for both practical and ethical reasons. Data therefore are usually incomplete, and often complicated by many factors not of direct interest.

The second is that the dependence of modelling conclusions on assumptions is seldom straightforward. Some conclusions – for instance the existence of an epidemic threshold – are so robust that virtually any model will fit the data. Others may depend very sensitively on parameter values or, more insidiously, on assumptions implicit in the type of model chosen, for instance on the way in which it represents units of the population and contacts between them.

For both these reasons, it is essential to analyse the structure of epidemic models, and the relation between this structure and the resulting dynamics. To facilitate this, it is important to keep models clear and simple as far as possible. Thus we aim to find a small set of model components that determine the dynamics, and to describe these as far as possible in terms of simple parameters with clear ecological interpretations, such as the *basic reproductive ratio* (or *number*), R_0, and the *mean generation gap*, τ, of the disease. [R_0 is the mean number of infectious contacts made by an infective in a wholly susceptible population (see Dietz, this volume, Section 3); the generation gap is the time interval between an individual being infected and its infecting others.]

This approach should help us to see the similarities between many of the bewildering number of apparently different models in the literature; and thus allow comparison and synthesis of results on individual specific models into more general understanding. It can also clarify what data are needed to fit and to test a model.

1.2   Epidemic stages

It is generally helpful to distinguish three main epidemic stages: *Establishment, Spread* and *Persistence*. To these we might add *Arrival*, the question of how infection reaches the population under consideration; however, for an existing disease, this can be considered, on a larger spatial scale, as part of the process of spread (see e.g. Cliff, this volume). Also, *Evolution* is required to explain the first arrival of any disease, and can play a key role in long term persistence, though this is an aspect in which diseases vary widely, from the evolutionary stability of smallpox or measles to the instability of myxomatosis (Fenner and Myers 1978) or influenza (Cliff *et al.* 1986); see also Hamilton and Howard (1994).

Given that an infection arrives in a population, the first question is that of *Establishment*, that is whether it has a chance to infect a sizeable proportion of the host population, rather than just a few individuals. In the establishment stage, it is common to ignore any overlap between infections by different individuals, so that growth is governed by a branching process, or by linear equations; in either case, the threshold condition for establishment to be possible is $R_0 > 1$ (see e.g. Diekmann *et al.*, Ball, Jacquez *et al.*, all in this volume; also Nåsell, this volume, regarding the definition of the threshold for stochastic models). However, where mixing is heterogeneous, and particularly in the case where individuals interact only with their spatial neighbours, the linear approximation can be poor, and the threshold value of R_0 may be appreciably greater than unity (Mollison 1991).

For cases where the infection has initial success, we then require to model its *Spread* through the population. This may be expected to depend both on heterogeneity between individuals: for instance, the spread of a sexually transmitted disease may be restricted largely within a 'core' group, at least initially; and on heterogeneity of mixing: for instance where contacts are spatially local we may expect spread in a regular wave-like manner at a steady velocity (see Metz and van den Bosch, this volume). Note that in the case of spatial waves the number of infectives grows only linearly with time (and the cumulative total quadratically), in contrast to the simpler cases where a linear or branching process model is a reasonable initial approximation, when numbers of infected accordingly grow exponentially. Intermediate rates of growth may be expected in intermediate situations, such as where the population is divided into a hierarchy of mixing groups, but this is an area where useful theoretical results have so far proved hard to develop.

Finally, the conditions for long term *Persistence* of an infection, whether at a steady level or as a sequence of outbreaks, may be expected to involve other factors. Bartlett (1957) introduced the idea of a *critical community size* for a given disease, below which an isolated population cannot sustain the disease long term. This critical community size, N_c, will depend primarily on the relation between the timescale of the infection itself and that of the regrowth of susceptible numbers (see §3.1). For diseases such as measles with a mean generation gap of 10-14 days, N_c is around 250,000, which explains why such diseases first became persistent in the human population in the Middle East four to five thousand years ago with the development of the earliest large cities there (McNeill 1976, Cliff *et al.* 1993). Measles persists similarly today through reservoirs of infection in large cities, from which occasional epidemics are sparked off in rural and island communities (Cliff *et al.* 1993).

In populations of a more constant density, as in the case of many animals and plants, a disease may persist through wandering patches (see e.g. Mollison and Levin 1995) without any one population being continuously infected. The population size required for persistence depends on the spatial structure and connectivity of the population as well as on the parameters of the infection itself. Geographical connectivity is also important for human diseases. For instance the relatively one-dimensional connectivity of the Japanese population may at least partly explain why numerous epidemics of measles, 36 from the 11th to 19th centuries, failed to make it persist, even though Japan's population (30 million by 1868) was well over the Bartlett threshold (Cliff *et al.* 1993).

2 Building epidemic models

2.1 Components of models

Perhaps the most basic modelling components are those describing the time history of an individual infective. From the point of view of the individual, the course of the disease is best described in terms of the times at which it starts and ceases to feel ill; but from the epidemiological viewpoint, the essential element is the distribution over time and among the population of the infectious contacts made by the individual, relative to its own time and location of infection. This can be handled quite generally using a kernel describing the numbers of such contacts over time and location (see Metz and van den Bosch, this volume, Mollison 1991).

One convenient simplification is to assume constant transition rates from the incubating to the infectious and from the infectious to the removed or recovered state; the mathematical motivation for this assumption is to obtain a Markov process or differential equation model. An alternative simplification, the discrete time equivalent of this, is to assume a fixed incubation period and instantaneous infectious period, thus giving a constant generation gap.

Such simplifying assumptions will make little or no difference to some aspects of model behaviour: as we shall see below (Section 3), there are a number of basic formulae where only the mean of the generation gap or the infectious period is required. Other aspects, however, such as the stability of endemic conditions, may depend sensitively on the distribution of the generation gap (Mollison 1984, 1985).

Turning now to the contacts made by an individual, the simplest case is homogeneous mixing, where victims are selected from the whole population independently and with equal probabilities. Heterogeneous mixing can be through preference for some type of individual (e.g. 'high activity', or opposite sex), or from within some neighbourhood, whether defined socially (see e.g. Morris, Jacquez *et al.*, both in this volume) or by geography (see e.g. Durrett, and Metz and van den Bosch, both in this volume, or Mollison and Levin 1995). The definition of geographic neighbours needs to take into account frequency of communication, not simply distance (see Cliff, this volume, Sattenspiel and Powell 1993).

In modelling, variability in the number of contacts made by an individual, and correlation between the locations of the victims, is often ignored. Where the numbers of infectives are large, this may often be justified; indeed, for linear models, and for nonlinear spatial models where the 'linear conjecture' applies (see next subsection), only the expected numbers matter, and so variability and correlation have no effect. However, they can in practice be very significant at the beginning of an outbreak. [Cliff *et al.* 1993 give many interesting examples relating to measles, for instance how it was introduced to Fiji and most effectively spread, along with the news of the islands' new colonial status, by their king in 1875.] And for stochastic models, not only do these details matter; taking them into account can actually be theoretically advantageous (see next section).

Careful consideration of the probabilities of contact with different possible victims is of particular importance where the population is divided into groups. Where there is wide variation in contact rates, perhaps both within and between groups as in the case of sexually transmitted diseases, the outcome of the epidemic may depend sensitively on the contact structure (see Morris, this volume). Where the population is divided into a large number of broadly similar groups, as for instance in the spread of airborne infections among households, it may be possible to develop hierarchical models, in which the groups are treated as individuals at the higher level of the model (Becker and Dietz 1994, Ball *et al.* 1994).

An alternative approach to modelling the infectious process is to look from the susceptible's rather than the infective's viewpoint, working in terms of the infectious pressure to which a susceptible is subject. This approach may be forced on us, for instance if the probability of infection depends only on there being some infectives and not on their number, as in the Greenwood model (see e.g. Bailey 1975); it also has some advantages of analytical convenience, for instance in the consideration of equilibrium conditions (see Anderson and May 1991). However, the loss of the idea of a link between infective and susceptible removes a major avenue for structural analysis of the model.

Most deterministic models use the approximation of treating populations as continuous. This has considerable advantages of simplicity and generality, but we need to be aware of circumstances where this approximation is not good enough, notably where numbers oscillate, sometimes reaching low levels, or where mixing is heterogeneous with each individual interacting with only a small proportion of the population: an example combining both these factors is the differential equation model of Murray *et al.* (1986), which relies for its repeated waves of spread on minute fractions of an infectious individual – the 'atto-foxes' of Mollison (1991). Note that it may be the treating of the population as continuous, rather than determinism *per se*, that is the main problem here (Mollison 1991, Durrett and Levin 1994).

There has only been space here to scratch the surface of the wide subject of model choice. But I hope enough has been said to indicate the need to be aware of the process of model-building: while we must simplify, it is essential to understand the likely limits of our simplifications. The more easily we can interpret our model components – and compare them to available data – the easier it will be to understand how the structure of our model relates to reality, and its limitations. Thus, for example, it is traditional in many basic models to use a transmission rate parameter, β; but its units are 'time^{-1} population^{-1}', which make it difficult to interpret. Reinterpretation in terms of the more easily understood parameter R_0 greatly facilitates analysis of the various assumptions commonly made concerning β (see de Jong *et al.*, this volume, Mollison 1985).

2.2   Using the structure of models

The realistic detail of a stochastic model, specifying such things as the probability that one individual will infect another at a particular time and place, has long been recognised as a strength from the point of view of understanding and fitting models, but has generally been regarded as a grave handicap when it comes to analysis; even stochastic analyses have traditionally dealt whenever possible with massed variables such as the total number of infectives.

However, in recent years there has been an increasing recognition that the 'unnecessary' detail of a stochastic model framed in terms of individuals and their interactions can in many cases allow insights not possible from a 'higher level' stochastic or deterministic model.

A simple example of this is the use of the basic undirected random graph $G(n, p)$ as an internal description of the Reed-Frost chain-binomial epidemic in a homogeneous population (Barbour and Mollison 1989). The 'unnecessary' detail here is that we identify each infection by one individual of another (represented by a link in the graph), rather than just dealing in the total numbers of susceptibles, infectives and removed cases. This is particularly simple because of the independence we can allow in the random graph model between different infections made by an individual, and the symmetric relation between individuals; these allow us to represent the possibility that either *a* will infect *b*, or that *b* will infect *a*, by the same link in an undirected graph.

This idea of representing the relation between an infective and its victim by a link in a graph can be generalised to re-frame most of the common models for epidemics in a fixed population, though in general we must use a *directed* graph. We can then look at the question of who becomes infected in the course of the epidemic separately from the time structure: it only depends on the 'lists' of potential contacts of each individual, each such contact being represented by a link in the directed graph ('$a \to b$' meaning that *b* is on *a*'s list of contacts). The strength of this approach is well illustrated by the beautiful theorem of Cox and Durrett (1988) on the existence of velocities for spatial epidemics with removal: although such a result clearly deals with the epidemic's development in time, much of the hardest part of the proof is accomplished through consideration of the graph structure of who may infect whom, without any explicit consideration of time.

The representation of contact structures by a random graph can be generalised to allow correlated links (see Lefèvre and Picard, this volume), and to compare two or more models (see next subsection).

Another stochastic technique, which exploits the structure of the model in a quite different but equally elegant way, is the use of martingales to estimate parameters (see Section 3 of Becker, this volume; note that his θ is our R_0).

There is typically less structure to exploit in the case of deterministic models. An interesting illustration of this is the proof of a monotonicity result by Kendall and Saunders (1983; see Ball, this volume) for the total number infected by two competing epidemics. This monotonicity seems 'intuitively obvious' for the deterministic model, but the proof requires exploitation of the structure of a corresponding stochastic model.

Nevertheless, monotonicity arguments, and similar comparisons of a model with variants, are often possible for deterministic models. An important, if only partly rigorous, example is the 'linear conjecture' for deterministic spatial epidemic models, which in turn leads to the possibility of analysing such models through a single structural element, the reproduction and dispersal kernel (see Metz and van den Bosch, this volume).

2.3   Relations between models

We here discuss briefly ways in which stochastic models can be related to each other, and to deterministic models. Though important for understanding, these could be considered rather theoretical aspects; we also discuss the crucial practical question of the relations between simple and complex models.

Stochastic models that include detailed 'internal descriptions', as described in the preceding subsection, can be used in a variety of ways to make precise comparisons between different models. The basic technique is that of *coupling* (see Ball, this volume), in which two or more different models are defined using the same probability space. Usually this representation is chosen so as to exploit the similarities between the different processes For instance, it may be possible to demonstrate a monotone relation between models where one process can be regarded as being the same as the other but for the addition of certain infections, or, more subtly, where the correlation between an individual's contacts is less in one model than in the other (see e.g. Kuulasmaa 1982).

Coupling can also be used to compare the outcome of the same process from different initial conditions, for instance showing that the 'contact process' (a spatial epidemic with recovery) is *additive* (see e.g. Mollison 1986).

Some aspects of relations between stochastic and deterministic models have already been touched on. Deterministic models are normally derived (explicitly or otherwise) by considering how the average numbers change in a stochastic model: because taking averages does not treat nonlinearities correctly, such a derivation will in general only give an exact relation for simple linear (branching process) models.

Nonlinearities are especially important where individuals interact only with a local group, whether defined socially or spatially. Thus, it is a defect of spatial continuous population models that they take little account of the spatial dimension, treating one and two dimensions very similarly (see Metz and van den Bosch, this volume), whereas in nonlinear discrete models, whether stochastic or deterministic, the very different nature of two dimensional space comes through (see e.g. Durrett, this volume, Fisch *et al.* 1991). Linear stochastic models also essentially ignore dimensionality, and it is mutual ignorance that allows them, in certain basic cases, to have an exact relation to well-known *nonlinear* differential equations (McKean 1975, Mollison and Daniels 1993).

It is possible to prove quite general results showing that 'as numbers get large' the behaviour of stochastic population processes tends to a deterministic limit, typically with diffusion process variability about that limit (Kurtz 1981). However, this could be considered to be the wrong way round, in that the use of deterministic models would be better justified if we could establish that a given stochastic process could be approximated as a limit of deterministic processes; therefore such results, though very useful, need to be treated with caution where the number with whom an individual interacts is small or where we wish to consider the process over a long time span (see §2.1 above).

Lastly, the relations between simple and complex models, though seldom mathematically elegant, are of great practical importance. From the applied point of view it may be natural to include many parameters when setting up a model, yet its dynamics will often be almost exactly the same as that of a model with only a few basic components. Cairns (this volume) discusses the identification and estimation of such basic components, with application to modelling variable infectiousness during HIV infection.

Multi-parameter simulation models provide other examples where the complexity involved in an attempt at realism can hide crude (and unrealistic) assumptions about such basic components. For instance, the detailed spatial simulation model of Voigt *et al.* (1985) for fox rabies includes over thirty parameters; one effect of this is that important components may be handled too crudely; because of the way they discretize time, their value for the mean generation gap τ seems to be mistakenly taken as 2.5 months instead of its intended value of less than 1 month. More seriously, their conclusions as to the effect of varying population density, whether by culling or vaccination, all depend on their implicit assumption that R_0 is simply proportional to population density. This is a vital applied point: modelling should bring such crucial and debatable (see Mollison 1985, de Jong *et al.*, this volume) assumptions to ecologists' attention, not hide them.

3   Some simple general relations

In this final section, we turn to some almost 'model-free' results concerning epidemic models, relating such basic model components (see §2.1 above) as the basic reproductive ratio R_0 and mean times spent by an individual in various states.

There are a number of relations between basic population and disease parameters that can be expressed very simply. For example, we have the following three expressions for R_0:

$$R_0 = \beta N \tau_I = N/S = L/A, \qquad (3.1)$$

where N is the population size (or in spatial models density), β the 'transmission parameter', τ_I the mean infectious period, S the equilibrium number of susceptibles, L the mean lifetime, and A the mean age of acquiring the disease. The first of these, $R_0 = \beta N \tau_I$, is the most general, being little more than a restatement of the definition of R_0 (see §3.1). The equivalence of the last two, $N/S = L/A$, relies on the disease being in endemic equilibrium (see §3.2); while their both being equal to R_0 relies on the assumption of homogeneous mixing (see §3.3).

Most of these simple relations can be found either as exact or approximate formulae in the literature. Dietz (1975) seems to have been the first to note that $R_0 \approx L/A$. More recently, many of these relations appear in Anderson and May (1991)'s comprehensive survey of deterministic epidemic models. However, they are there derived for the most part as approximations, and this is one part of their otherwise impressive survey that could be improved in terms of elegance and generality.

We shall derive a number of such relations here in as general a way as possible, discussing the assumptions they rely on. For some of these results, it does not seem to have been recognised previously that they hold *exactly* in quite general circumstances. This is probably because there are alternative definitions for some of the parameters involved; these typically differ only by amounts too small to be of practical importance, but can render the simple relations unrecognisable.

Where there are such alternatives, the advantage of the simple relations, beyond their explanatory appeal, is that they will usually be of greater generality, or will at least indicate how far results can be generalised.

As well as deriving some of these simple exact results, I shall give examples to show how effectively a slight change of definition can disguise their simplicity.

3.1   Formulae for R_0

Let us first consider a simple and quite general formula, in that it does not require equilibrium conditions, concerning the *basic reproductive ratio R_0*. If we assume that infectives make contacts at a fixed rate βN, where N is the population total or density, throughout an infectious period of mean length τ_I, then their mean total number of contacts is exactly given by

$$R_0 = \beta N \tau_I. \tag{3.2}$$

This result can easily be modified to cover various different and more general assumptions. For instance, we could replace βN by a constant independent of N, so that R_0 is independent of N rather than proportional to it (Mollison 1985, de Jong *et al*, this volume); we could let β vary over time, in which case $\beta \tau_I$ should be replaced by $\int \beta(t)dt$, or over both time and space, as in Metz and van den Bosch (this volume)'s γ of their equation (2.3).

This simple formula, $R_0 = \beta N \tau_I$, is often hidden because it is common not to use the exact mean infectious period for an infective, τ_I, but instead what may seem a simpler parameter, τ_0, defined as the mean infectious period in the absence of other effects such as natural mortality.

As an example, consider the non-fatal disease model described in Anderson and May (1991, §4.4) in which individuals at birth possess immunity, which they lose at rate d, and in which infected individuals pass through successive latent and infectious stages with respective forces of removal σ and v; let us take the case of 'Type II' mortality, *i.e.* with an age-independent rate μ of natural mortality. Then $\tau_0 = 1/v$; τ_I can be evaluated by multiplying the probability of an individual's surviving the latent period, $q_L = \sigma/(\sigma + \mu)$, by the mean time spent in the infectious state if it does so, $\tau'_I = 1/(v + \mu)$; thus $\tau_I = \sigma/[(\sigma + \mu)(v + \mu)]$. If we follow Anderson and May in excluding immune individuals from the effective population size, which is therefore $N' = Nd/(d + \mu)$, then '$R_0 = \beta N \tau_I$' gives exactly their equation (4.55):

$$R_0 = \frac{\beta N \sigma d}{(d + \mu)(\sigma + \mu)(v + \mu)}. \tag{3.3}$$

The approximation, $R_0 \approx \beta N \tau_0$, can of course be deduced from this equation, but the advantage of the present approach is to clarify how the error in this approximation arises, through the component approximations: $q_L \approx 1$, $\tau'_I \approx \tau_0$, $N' \approx N$: each of which can be critically examined in a specific application. [For the case of age-dependent mortality, see §3.3 below.]

3.2 Equilibrium formulae: the microcosm principle

A number of simple equalities follow immediately from what I shall call the *microcosm principle*, which says that, for a quite general population process in equilibrium, the proportion of the population π_i in each state i is proportional to the mean time τ_i an individual spends in that state, and hence

$$\pi_i = \tau_i/L \tag{3.4}$$

[This result can be generalised to the case of a population growing at a steady rate r, essentially by including r as a discount rate – an individual's proportional contribution to the population diminishes exponentially, $\propto \exp(-rt)$. Thus in the righthand side of the equation τ_i is replaced by $\int p_i(t)e^{-rt}dt$, and L by the sum of such terms, $G = \int p(t)e^{-rt}dt$; where $p_i(t)$ denotes the probability of being in state i at age t, $p(t)$ the overall probability of being alive at that age.]

Now suppose we have a disease for which individuals are susceptible from birth, but immune once they have had the disease. Let A be the mean age of catching the disease, or of death for individuals who never get the disease. In this case the mean time spent susceptible, τ_S, is simply A, so from the microcosm principle we immediately have that

$$\pi_S \equiv S/N = A/L. \tag{3.5}$$

Note that this result makes no assumption about the epidemic process; it applies wherever individuals with a mean lifetime L start in a special state (here susceptible) and cannot return to that state once they have left it. The result is easily generalised to cases where individuals do not start susceptible. For example, if individuals begin life with a period of mean M spent in an immune state we would have $\pi_S = (A - M)/L$. And it can again be adapted to the case of a growing population, along the lines mentioned above (see also Anderson and May 1991, §4.1 and §13.1.1).

Where an individual may visit a state i either less or more than once, the mean time spent in that state, τ_i, will not be the same as the mean time of a single sojourn, but often this can easily be allowed for. For instance, in the situation we are currently considering of the equilibrium state of a disease which can only be caught once, the mean time spent infectious will be $p_I \tau_I$, where p_I is the probability that an individual will become infectious at some time during their life. Hence

$$\pi_I = p_I \tau_I / L \tag{3.6}$$

For a typical human 'childhood disease' such as measles, L/τ_I is of the order of several thousand. This provides an elementary explanation of why the critical community size for such diseases is so large, of the order of 250,000 (Bartlett 1957). This size corresponds to an average number infected at any one time of around 100; in view of the seasonally oscillatory nature of measles it is not surprising that such a population size is necessary if the disease is not to die out through stochastic fluctuations.

As an illustration of equation 3.6, consider a measles model of Grenfell *et al.* (this volume), which is the same as the example of §3.1 above, except that it omits immunity at birth. In our notation, their equation (3.1) becomes

$$\pi_I = \frac{\mu \sigma}{(\mu + \sigma)(\mu + v)} - \frac{\mu}{\beta N}. \tag{3.7}$$

To identify this with our equation 3.6, first use $R_0 = \beta N \tau_I$ and note that $\tau_I = \sigma/[(\sigma + \mu)(v + \mu)]$ as in §3.1. We can then deduce that $p_I = 1 - 1/R_0$; or this can be derived independently, by noting first that $1 - p_I =$ Prob.{Susceptible at death}, which because mortality does not depend on age is simply = Prob.{Susceptible}, $= 1/R_0$ from equation 3.9 below.

3.3   Equilibrium under homogeneous mixing

We could allow the rate of contacts to depend on the number of infectives, which would imply that an infective's mean total number of contacts also does so, in which case we have to replace R_0 by $R(I) = \beta(I) N \tau_I$; the usual definition of R_0 identifies it with $R(1)$. [To be pedantic, '$R(1)$' may not be quite right here, as we should allow for the possibility that the infectious period of the first infective may overlap with those of some of its victims, but it will do to make the point.]

If we now assume that mixing is homogeneous as regards susceptibles, so that the probability that a potentially infectious contact is with a susceptible is simply π_S, then the mean number of successful contacts per infective is $R(I)\pi_S$. But if the process is in equilibrium this number must equal 1, which immediately tells us that in that case

$$R(I_*) = 1/\pi_S \qquad (3.8)$$

where I_* is the equilibrium number of infectives.

If we also assume that the mean total number of contacts per infective is independent of the number of infectives, then $R(I) = R_0$, and so we have

$$R_0 = 1/\pi_S (= N/S) \qquad (3.9)$$

Note that Anderson and May (1991, Equation 4.13) are wrong in claiming that this equation relies only on 'weak homogeneous mixing'; it is only the previous, rather less useful, equation $(R(I_*) = 1/\pi_S)$ that holds in that case. The general issue they point to, of how the number of contacts depends on the numbers of susceptibles and infectives, is nevertheless a crucial one – already raised in the contrasting Reed-Frost and Greenwood models of the 1930s. The answer is likely to depend on the mode of transmission, for instance physical contact as opposed to aerosol, and on the heterogeneous social structure of the population (see §2.1 above).

A more hair-splitting reservation concerning equation 3.9 arises if mortality is age-dependent, because that induces (in practice usually negligible) variation with age in the mean infectious period, and thus (through equation 3.2) in R_0. [In the simple homogeneous mixing case, the age distribution of infectives conditional on survival is exponential in equilibrium, whereas during initial spread it is uniform.] In specific cases, for instance where everyone lives to exactly age L (Anderson and May's 'Type I mortality'), it is possible to write down the probability that an infective will die of natural mortality,

$$p_e = \frac{\lambda(e^{-\lambda L} - e^{-vL})}{(v - \lambda)(1 - e^{-\lambda L})}, \qquad (3.10)$$

hence calculate τ_I, and thus derive exact expressions for $R(I_*)$ and π_I (for the latter, see Anderson and May 1991, equation (4.41)). However for endemic measles p_e is at most of order 10^{-3}, and p_I not much larger (for 'Type I mortality'), so that the errors in the approximate equations

$$R(I_*) \approx R_0 \approx \beta N \tau_0 \qquad \text{and} \qquad \pi_I \approx \tau_0/L \qquad (3.11)$$

are minute compared with the error in estimating (for instance) τ_0 or τ_I.

Another simple equilibrium formula relates the force of infection λ to parameters already introduced. Equating inward and outward flows of attempted infections gives $p_I R_0 = \lambda L$.

A rather less neat result, but of considerable interest, concerns the period of oscillations about equilibrium. For both continuous and discrete time simple endemic models, this period is approximately $2\pi\sqrt{\tau A/p_I}$; thus, as Anderson and May (1991) nicely remark, it is proportional to the geometric mean of the two basic time scales of the process: the typically short time scale of the infection, as represented by the mean generation gap τ, and the longer time scale for replenishment of susceptibles. Similar results for simple fatal disease models were found by Mollison (1985), who also showed that the stability of oscillations was sensitive to the difference between continuous and discrete time models (with less stability for the fixed delay feedback of the discrete time model, as one might expect).

3.4   Discussion

We have considered in this section a number of simple formulae that can be found over and again in models in the literature, usually disguised to a lesser or greater extent. Often the conclusions drawn from those models depend essentially on the validity of the relationships described by these simple formulae, or the way in which they are used. For instance, it is common to take β constant, which through equation 3.2 embodies the questionable assumption that $R_0 \propto N$ (see de Jong *et al.*, this volume, Mollison 1985).

The estimation of R_0 presents a key difficulty in epidemic modelling, and several of the simple formulae are relevant to this, especially $R_0 = 1/\pi_S$ or $R_0 = L/A$. If the aim is to estimate the proportion we need to vaccinate, p_V say, where homogeneous mixing theory suggests we need $p_V \geq 1 - 1/R_0$, we can in fact short-cut the argument, omitting the estimation of R_0 itself: it would seem that $p_V > 1 - \pi_S$ should suffice, not only in the homogeneous mixing case. However, this deduction relies on treating the susceptibles remaining after vaccination as being similarly distributed within the population to the susceptibles in the endemic state when there is no vaccination, and in a heterogeneous situation (whether age or space dependent) this assumption would need careful examination.

Some of the simple formulae are known to require major correction, or to be simply invalid, under certain types of heterogeneous mixing. For instance, for simple spatial endemic models for a fatal disease, Mollison and Kuulasmaa (1985) found that π_S and π_I were respectively much larger and much smaller than the values given by the homogeneous mixing model. [Though the formulae can be adjusted to explain this; for instance the increase in π_S is inversely proportional to the change in the frequency of {infective, susceptible} pairs relative to the homogeneous situation.]

Further, the homogeneous model's oscillations, although they carry over to differential equation models (Murray *et al.* 1986), do not occur in the stochastic models, a result confirmed by Durrett and Levin (1994)'s comparison of different types of model for spatial competition. The stochastic spatial models instead have patterns of wandering patches; by a nice irony, in the case of fox rabies these have a 'turnover period' numerically similar to the homogeneous mixing model's period of oscillations (Mollison 1986). Endemic patterns in human diseases are more complex, but here too there is some evidence that the spatial structure deters chaotic and oscillatory behaviour (Ellner *et al.*, Grenfell *et al.*, both in this volume).

Although they have such limitations, the simple formulae do have the cardinal virtue of clarity. Consideration of the basic relationships that these formulae describe can clarify the assumptions inherent in a model; in contrast, complex formulae give a spurious appearance of precision that may distract our attention from structural faults in the model. It is only if any shortcomings are recognised that we can correct for them, or at least make some allowance for the error involved: an approximate answer to the right question is better than a precise answer to the wrong question.

References

Anderson, R.M., and May, R.M. (1991) *Infectious Diseases of Humans: Dynamics and Control*, Oxford University Press, Oxford.

Bailey, N.T.J. (1975) *The Mathematical Theory of Infectious Diseases and its Applications*, Griffin, London.

Ball, Frank (1995) 'Coupling methods in epidemic theory' this volume.

Ball, F.G., Mollison, D. and Scalia-Tomba, G. (1994) 'Epidemics in populations divided into groups or households', in preparation.

Barbour, A.D. and Mollison, D. (1989) 'Epidemics and random graphs'. In *Stochastic Processes in Epidemic Theory*, J.P. Gabriel, C. Lefevre and Ph. Picard (eds.), *Lecture Notes in Biomathematics* **86**, 86–89.

Bartlett, M.S. (1957) 'Measles periodicity and community size', *J. Roy. Statist. Soc. A* **120**, 48–70.

Becker, Niels (1995) 'Statistical challenges of epidemic data', this volume.

Becker, N.G., and Dietz, K. (1994) 'The effect of the household distribution on transmission and control of highly infectious diseases', in preparation.

Cairns, Andrew (1995) 'Primary components of epidemic models', this volume.

Cliff, Andrew (1995) 'Incorporating spatial components into models of epidemic spread', this volume.

Cliff, A.D., Haggett, P. and Ord, J.K. (1986) *Spatial Aspects of Influenza Epidemics*, Blackwell, Oxford.

Cliff, A.D., Haggett, P. and Smallman-Raynor, M. (1993) *Measles: an Historical Geography*, Pion, London.

Cox, J.T., and Durrett, R. (1988) 'Limit theorems for the spread of epidemics and forest fires', *Stoch. Procs. Applics.* **30**, 171–191.

de Jong, M., Diekmann, O. and Heesterbeek, J.A.P. (1995) 'How does transmission of infection depend on population size?', this volume.

Diekmann, O., Metz, J.A.J. and Heesterbeek, J.A.P. (1995) 'The legacy of Kermack and McKendrick', this volume.

Dietz, K. (1975) 'Transmission and control of arbovirus diseases'. In *Epidemiology*, D. Ludwig and K.L. Cooke (eds.), SIAM, Philadelphia, 104–121.

Dietz, K. (1995) 'Some problems in the theory of infectious disease transmission and control', this volume.

Durrett, Richard (1995) 'Spatial epidemic models', this volume.

Durrett, R., and Levin, S.A. (1994) 'The importance of being discrete (and spatial)', *Theor. Pop. Biol.*, to appear.

Ellner, S., Gallant, R. and Theiler, J. (1995) 'Detecting nonlinearity and chaos in epidemic data', this volume.

Fenner, F., and Myers, K. (1978) 'Myxoma virus and myxomatosis in retrospect: the first quarter century of a new disease'. In *Viruses and the Environment*, E. Kurstak and K. Maramorosch (eds.), Academic Press, New York and London, 539–570.

Fisch, R., Gravner, J. and Griffeath, D. (1991) 'Threshold-range scaling of excitable cellular automata', *Statistics and Computing* 1, 23–39.

Grenfell, B.T., Bolker, B. and Kleczkowski, A. (1995) 'Seasonality, demography and the dynamics of measles in developed countries', this volume.

Hamilton, W.D. and Howard, J.C. (eds.) (1994) *Infection, Polymorphism and Evolution, Phil. Trans. R. Soc. Lond. B*, to appear.

Jacquez, J., Simon, C. andKoopman, J. (1995) 'Core groups and R_0s for subgroups in heterogeneous SIS and SI models', this volume.

Kendall, W.S. and Saunders, I.W. (1983) 'Epidemics in competition II: the general epidemic', *J.R. Stat. Soc. B* **45**, 238–244.

Kurtz, T.G. (1981) *Approximation of population processes*, SIAM, Philadelphia.

Kuulasmaa, Kari (1982) 'The spatial general epidemic and locally dependent random graphs', *J. Appl. Prob.* **19**, 745–758.

Lefèvre, C. and Picard, Ph. (1995) 'Collective Reed-Frost processes: a general modelling approach to the final outcome of SIR epidemics', this volume.

Longini, I., Halloran, E. and Haber, M. (1995) 'Some current trends in estimating vaccine efficacy', this volume.

McKean, H.P. (1975) 'Application of Brownian Motion to the equation of Kolmogorov-Petrovskii-Piscunov', *Comm. Pure. Appl. Maths.* **28**, 323–331.

McNeill, William H. (1976) *Plagues and Peoples*, Doubleday, New York.

Metz, J.A.J., and van den Bosch, F. (1995) 'Velocities of epidemic spread', this volume.

Mollison, Denis (1984) 'Simplifying simple epidemic models', *Nature* **310**, 224–225.

Mollison, Denis (1985) 'Sensitivity analysis of simple endemic models'. In *Population Dynamics of Rabies in Wildlife*, P.J. Bacon (ed.), Academic Press, London, 223–234.

Mollison, Denis (1986) 'Modelling biological invasions: chance, explanation, prediction', *Phil. Trans. R. Soc. Lond. B* **314**, 675–693.

Mollison, Denis (1991) 'Dependence of epidemic and population velocities on basic parameters', *Math. Biosci.* **107**, 255–287.

Mollison, D. and Daniels, H.E. (1993) 'The simple deterministic epidemic unmasked', *Math. Biosci.* **117**, 147–153.

Mollison, D. and Kuulasmaa, K. (1985) 'Spatial epidemic models: theory and simulations'. In *Population Dynamics of Rabies in Wildlife*, P.H. Bacon (ed.), Academic Press, London, 291–309.

Mollison, D., and Levin, S.A. (1995) 'Spatial dynamics of parasitism'. In *Ecology of Infectious Diseases in Natural Populations*, B.T. Grenfell and A. Dobson (eds.), Cambridge University Press, Cambridge, to appear.

Morris, Martina (1995) 'Data driven network models for the spread of disease', this volume.

Murray, J.D., Stanley, E.A. and Brown, D.L. (1986) 'On the spatial spread of rabies among foxes', *Proc. R. Soc. Lond. B* **229**, 111–150.

Nåsell, Ingemar (1995) 'The threshold concept in stochastic epidemic and endemic models', this volume.

Sattenspiel, L. and Powell, C. (1993) 'Geographic spread of measles on the island of Dominica, West Indies', *Human Biology* **65**, 107–129.

Voigt, D.R., Tinline, R.R. and Broekhoven, L.H. (1985) 'A spatial simulation model for rabies control'. In *Population Dynamics of Rabies in Wildlife*, P.H. Bacon (ed.), Academic Press, London, 311–349.

Coupling Methods in Epidemic Theory

Frank Ball

Summary

An introduction to the use of coupling methods in epidemic theory is provided by illustrating a variety of contexts in which they can be used. The setting for most of the paper is a single closed population SIR stochastic epidemic with an arbitrary but specified distribution for the infectious period. Coupling methods are used to (i) derive the final size distribution, (ii) prove stochastic comparisons and investigate the consequences of variability in susceptibility, and (iii) prove strong convergence to a branching process as the initial number of susceptibles tends to infinity. Extensions to models incorporating variable infectiousness during the infectious period and heterogeneous populations are outlined. The use of coupling in analysing deterministic models is also described and some other applications of coupling in epidemic theory are briefly indicated.

1 Introduction

Stochastic models of epidemics are notorious for their high level of mathematical intractability. The classical approach to studying stochastic epidemics is to derive and analyse the forward equation for the model under consideration. Although in principle this provides a general method for determining the state transition probabilities for an epidemic, in practice the resulting differential equations are very difficult, if at all possible, to solve analytically. The only probabilistic structure utilised by the forward equation approach is the Markov property, hence its great generality. However, epidemic models possess a rich probabilistic structure and in the last decade important advances have been made by using techniques, such as embedding, martingales and coupling, which directly exploit that structure. As well as enhancing our understanding of stochastic epidemics, proofs using these techniques often admit straightforward generalisations to epidemics with non-exponential infectious periods, and also to multipopulation epidemics. The aim of this paper is to give an introduction to the use of coupling methods in epidemic models by illustrating a variety of situations in which they can be applied.

The paper is structured as follows. The coupling method is introduced in Section 2 by describing its application to a simple gambler's ruin problem.

In Section 3 the epidemic model that will form the basis for most of this paper is described. It is a single closed population SIR stochastic epidemic, see Lefèvre (1990) for a survey of this class of epidemic model. In Sections 4, 5 and 6 coupling methods are used to determine the final size distribution, to examine the effects of heterogeneity in susceptibility and to develop a threshold analysis for our epidemic model. In Section 7 we use an example of Kendall and Saunders (1983) to show how coupling methods can also be used to analyse deterministic models. The headings of Sections 4 to 7 are chosen to reflect some of the many different purposes for which coupling methods can be applied. In the concluding comments in Section 8 we describe briefly some other applications of coupling methods to epidemics and indicate how our methods can be extended to more general models.

2 What is coupling?

Coupling is a method of analysing stochastic models which involves defining realisations of two or more stochastic processes on the same probability space. The realisations will usually be highly related and the aim is to use the dependence structure to (a) answer questions about and (b) gain insight into the stochastic processes under consideration. A comprehensive account of the coupling method is given in Lindvall (1992), which both examines the method in depth and illustrates a broad range of applications. A good way of introducing the method is to give a very simple example of it in action. Our setting will be the standard gambler's ruin problem, see e.g. Grimmett and Stirzaker (1992, pages 17-18).

Suppose that an individual has a units of money but wishes to go on a holiday costing N units, where $N > a$. In an attempt to raise the extra capital he goes to a casino and plays a series of independent games, in each of which he wins one unit, with probability p, or loses one unit, with probability $1 - p$. He continues playing until either his capital reaches N and he takes his holiday, or he goes bankrupt. Let $P(p)$ be the probability that he takes his holiday and suppose we wish to prove that $P(p)$ is strictly increasing in p. One approach is to determine $P(p)$ by standard methods (see e.g. Karlin and Taylor 1975, pages 92-94) and then show that its derivative is strictly positive. An alternative coupling approach goes as follows.

Let $U_1, U_2, \ldots$ be independent and identically distributed (i.i.d.) random variables, each uniformly distributed on the interval $(0,1)$. For $p \in (0,1)$ let

$$X_i(p) = \begin{cases} +1 & \text{if} \quad U_i \leq p, \\ -1 & \text{if} \quad U_i > p, \end{cases} \quad (i = 1, 2, \ldots) \tag{2.1}$$

and

$$S_n(p) = a + \sum_{i=1}^{n} X_i(p), \quad (n = 1, 2, \ldots). \tag{2.2}$$

Now $\Pr(X_i(p) = 1) = \Pr(U_i \le p) = p$, so for fixed $p \in (0,1)$, $\{S_n(p)\} = \{S_n(p); n = 0, 1, \ldots\}$, where $S_0(p) = a$, is a realisation of the gambler's ruin problem with individual game success probability p, with the proviso that $\{S_n(p)\}$ stops as soon as it reaches 0 or N. Now suppose that $p > p'$ and construct $\{S_n(p)\}$ and $\{S_n(p')\}$ as above but from the same set $U_1, U_2, \ldots$ of uniform random variables. Then by construction, $X_i(p) \ge X_i(p')$ $(i = 1, 2, \ldots)$ so $S_n(p) \ge S_n(p')$ $(n = 1, 2, \ldots)$. It follows that if $\{S_n(p')\}$ reaches N before 0 then so does $\{S_n(p)\}$. Thus $P(p) \ge P(p')$. To prove that the inequality is strict, let $M = \max(a, N - a)$ and note from (2.1) that if $U_i \in (p', p)$ $(i = 1, 2, \ldots, M)$ then $X_i(p) = +1$ and $X_i(p') = -1$ $(i = 1, 2, \ldots, M)$. Thus $\{S_n(p)\}$ is absorbed at N and $\{S_n(p')\}$ is absorbed at 0. Finally, $\Pr(U_i \in (p', p), i = 1, 2, \ldots, M) = (p - p')^M > 0$, so $P(p) > P(p')$ as required.

Clearly the above example is rather trivial but it illustrates the basic concept of a coupling argument. That is an underlying probability space (in our case the sequence $U_1, U_2, \ldots$ of $U(0, 1)$ random variables) on which are defined realisations of two or more stochastic processes (in our case realisations $\{S_n(p)\}$ and $\{S_n(p')\}$ of gambler's ruin problems with success probabilities p and p', respectively) coupled to reflect the property of interest (in our case a monotonicity relationship). Notice that the coupling argument makes rigorous in a natural way the intuitively obvious fact that increasing the success probability of a single game decreases the probability of ruin. Notice also that the coupling argument is easily generalised to the situation in which the success probability varies from game to game. This is not the case for the approach that involves determining $P(p)$.

3   Closed population epidemic models

The most studied closed population epidemic model is the so-called general stochastic epidemic, see e.g. Bailey (1975, Chapter 6). It is a model for the spread of an epidemic amongst a closed homogeneously mixing population, consisting initially of a infectives and N susceptibles. For each $t \ge 0$, let $X(t)$, $Y(t)$ and $Z(t)$ be respectively the numbers of susceptible, infective and removed individuals at time t. An individual is considered removed once its infectious period has terminated. It is then immune to infection and plays no further part in the epidemic. The epidemic is completely described by the process $\{(X(t), Y(t)); t \ge 0\}$, because of the constraint $X(t) + Y(t) + Z(t) = N + a$. The epidemic is modelled by a continuous time Markov chain with infinitesimal transition probabilities

$$\Pr\left\{(X(t+\Delta t),Y(t+\Delta t)) = (x-1,y+1)) \mid (X(t),Y(t)) = (x,y)\right\} \quad (3.1)$$
$$= \beta xy\Delta t + o(\Delta t) \quad (3.2)$$

corresponding to an infection, and

$$\Pr\left\{(X(t+\Delta t),Y(t+\Delta t)) = (x,y-1)) \mid (X(t),Y(t)) = (x,y)\right\}$$
$$= \gamma y\Delta t + o(\Delta t) \quad (3.3)$$

corresponding to a removal, where β and γ are known as the infection and removal rates, respectively. The epidemic ceases as soon as there are no infectives present in the population. Note that the Markov nature of the model implies that the infectious period of a typical infective follows an exponential distribution with mean γ^{-1}. It is illuminating to write the infection term βxy in (3.2) as $(N\beta)(x/N)y$. We then have the interpretation that $N\beta$ is the rate a given infective makes contacts; contacts are chosen uniformly at random from the N initial susceptibles, so a proportion x/N of contacts are with current susceptibles and result in the spread of infection.

For $t \geq 0$ and suitable (x,y), let $p_{x,y}(t)$ be the probability that at time t there are x susceptibles and y infectives. The forward equations for $p_{x,y}(t)$ can be derived in the usual fashion, see Bailey (1975, page 89). However, their solution (Billard 1973; see also Kryscio 1975) is extremely complicated and does not readily lend itself to mathematical analysis. We shall use coupling methods to study the above epidemic but before doing so it is worthwhile to consider its assumptions more carefully.

The general stochastic epidemic makes several unreasonable assumptions. In particular, it assumes (a) that there is no latent period, i.e that freshly infected susceptibles are immediately able to infect other susceptibles, (b) that the infectious period follows an exponential distribution and (c) that the population is homogeneously mixing. None of these assumptions is likely to be even approximately true for any real-life epidemic. For the sake of clarity, we shall present our results within the context of a model in which only (b) is relaxed. However, as indicated in Section 8, the methods that we shall describe can all be generalised to cater for models in which (a) and (c) are relaxed. We close this section by describing the model that will form the basis of Sections 4 to 6.

We assume that initially there are a infectives (that have just become infected) and N susceptibles. The infectious periods of different infectives are independently and identically distributed according to a random variable T_I, having an arbitrary but specified distribution. Throughout its infectious period an infective makes contacts at the points of a Poisson process with rate $N\beta$. Succesive contacts are chosen independently and uniformly from the initial N susceptibles. If a contacted individual is still susceptible then it becomes infective and is immediately able to infect other susceptibles. If a contacted individual has previously been infected then nothing happens. The epidemic ceases as soon as there are no infectives present in the population. We shall denote the above epidemic model by $E_{N,a}(\beta, T_I)$. Note that the general stochastic epidemic is obtained by letting T_I follow an exponential distribution with mean γ^{-1}.

4   Coupling and exact results

In this section we use a coupling argument to determine the distribution of the total size of the epidemic $E_{N,a}(\beta, T_I)$. We shall require the following construction of our epidemic model, based on Sellke (1983). The key idea underlying the construction is that associated with each susceptible is a random critical level of exposure to infection, describing the total amount of infection there must be in the population before that susceptible becomes infected.

Label the initial infectives $-(a-1), -(a-2), \ldots, 0$ and the initial susceptibles $1, 2, \ldots, N$. Let $R_{-(a-1)}, R_{-(a-2)}, \ldots, R_N$ be i.i.d. random variables, each distributed according to T_I. Let $L_1, L_2, \ldots, L_N$ be an independent sequence of i.i.d. exponential random variables, each having mean β^{-1}. The epidemic is constructed as follows. For $i = -(a-1), -(a-2), \ldots, 0$, the initial infective labelled i remains infectious for a time R_i and is then removed. For $t \geq 0$, let $Y(t)$ be the number of infectives at time t and $A(t) = \int_0^t Y(u)\, du$ be the total amount of infection there has been in the epidemic by time t. For $i = 1, 2, \ldots, N$, susceptible i becomes infected when $A(t)$ reaches L_i. The jth susceptible infected by the epidemic remains infectious for a time R_j and is then removed. The epidemic ceases when the number of infectives becomes zero.

We should check that the above construction does yield the epidemic $E_{N,a}(\beta, T_I)$. Clearly the infectious periods follow the correct distribution and, if $Y(t) = y$ and i is still susceptible at time t, then the probability that i is infected during $(t, t+\Delta t)$ is $\beta y \Delta t + o(\Delta t)$ due to the lack-of-memory property of the exponential random variable L_i. This is consistent with $E_{N,a}(\beta, T_I)$ since in that epidemic contacts occur at an overall rate $\beta N y$, but only a proportion N^{-1} of them will be with susceptible i.

Let Z be the total number of initial susceptibles that are ultimately infected by the epidemic, and let $A = A(\infty) = \sum_{i=-(a-1)}^{Z} R_i$ be the total area under the trajectory of infectives (see Downton 1972). Following Picard and Lefevre (1990), we shall refer to A as the severity of the epidemic. Let $L_{(1)}, L_{(2)}, \ldots, L_{(N)}$ be the order statistics of $L_1, L_2, \ldots, L_N$, i.e. the sample

$L_1, L_2, \ldots, L_N$ arranged in increasing order. Then

$$Z = \min \{i : L_{(i+1)} > \sum_{j=-(a-1)}^{i} R_j\}, \qquad (4.1)$$

(where we have set $L_{(N+1)} = \infty$) since the epidemic stops when the total infection of the a initial infectives and the Z infected susceptibles is insufficient to infect any more susceptibles.

Let $\phi(\theta) = \mathrm{E}\left[\exp\left(-\theta T_I\right)\right]$ $(\theta \geq 0)$ be the moment generating function of T_I. We shall require the following Wald's identity for epidemics, proved in Ball (1986):

$$\mathrm{E}\left[\exp\left(-\theta A\right)/\phi(\theta)^{Z+a}\right] = 1 \quad (\theta \geq 0). \qquad (4.2)$$

We now require some more notation. Let ω be the set $\{1, 2, \ldots, \omega\}$ where $\omega = 1, 2, \ldots,$ and let $\mathbf{0}$ be the empty set. For $\omega = 0, 1, \ldots, N$, let $P_{\boldsymbol{\omega}}^N = \Pr\{T = \omega\}$ and P_ω^N be the probability that $E_{N,a}(\beta, T_I)$ infects precisely the initial susceptibles $1, 2, \ldots, \omega$, so, by symmetry, $P_\omega^N = \binom{N}{\omega} P_{\boldsymbol{\omega}}^N$. Now fix $0 \leq \omega \leq j \leq N$ and construct coupled versions of $E_{N,a}(\beta, T_I)$ and $E_{j,a}(\beta, T_I)$ by using the Sellke construction with the same sets of random variables $R_{-(a-1)}, R_{-(a-2)}, \ldots, R_N$ and $L_1, L_2, \ldots, L_N$ in both epidemics. (Thus $R_{j+1}, R_{j+2}, \ldots, R_N$ and $L_{j+1}, L_{j+2}, \ldots, L_N$ are not used in constructing $E_{j,a}(\beta, T_I)$.) The epidemic $E_{N,a}(\beta, T_I)$ infects precisely ω if and only if the epidemic $E_{j,a}(\beta, T_I)$ infects precisely ω and $L_i > A_j$ $(i = j+1, j+2, \ldots, N)$, where A_j is the severity of the epidemic $E_{j,a}(\beta, T_I)$. Now given A_j, $\Pr(L_i > A_j, i = j+1, j+2, \ldots, N) = \exp\left(-\beta(N-j)A_j\right)$, since $L_{j+1}, L_{j+2}, \ldots, L_N$ are independent exponential random variables, each having mean β^{-1}. It follows that

$$\begin{aligned} P_{\boldsymbol{\omega}}^N &= P_{\boldsymbol{\omega}}^j \, \mathrm{E}\left[\exp\left(-\beta(N-j)A_j\right) \mid E_{j,a}(\beta, T_I) \text{ infects precisely } \omega\right] \\ &= P_{\boldsymbol{\omega}}^j \, \mathrm{E}\left[\exp\left(-\beta(N-j)A_j\right) \mid Z_j = \omega\right], \end{aligned} \qquad (4.3)$$

by symmetry, where Z_j is the total size of $E_{j,a}(\beta, T_I)$.

Setting $N = j$ and $\theta = \beta(N - j)$ in (4.2) yields

$$\sum_{\omega=0}^{j} P_\omega^j \mathrm{E}\left[\exp\left(-\beta(N-j)A_j\right)/\phi(\beta(N-j))^{a+\omega}\right] = 1. \qquad (4.4)$$

Now $P_\omega^j = \binom{j}{\omega} P_{\boldsymbol{\omega}}^j$ and $P_\omega^N = \binom{N}{\omega} P_{\boldsymbol{\omega}}^N$, so after a little rearrangement we obtain

$$\sum_{\omega=0}^{j} \binom{N-\omega}{j-\omega} P_\omega^N / \phi(\beta(N-j))^{a+\omega} = \binom{N}{j} \quad (j = 0, 1, \ldots, N). \qquad (4.5)$$

The set of equations (4.5), which determine the total size distribution for the epidemic $E_{N,a}(\beta, T_I)$, was first obtained for the general stochastic epidemic by Whittle (1955), using an algebraic argument based on the forward equation. It has subsequently been derived by several authors for a variety of models, using a number of distinct methods; see e.g. Watson (1980), which uses a random time-scale transformation, and von Bahr and Martin-Löf (1980) and Picard and Lefèvre (1990), which use martingale arguments.

In principle, for given parameter values, the set of equations (4.5) can be solved numerically to yield the final size distribution. However, in practice rounding error problems can occur even for quite small values of N, say of the order $N = 100$. For the general stochastic epidemic, an alternative and numerically more stable algorithm for calculating the total size distribution is given in Bailey (1975, pages 93-94). Graphs of the total size distribution for the general stochastic epidemic are given in e.g. Bailey (1975, pages 98-99), and Nåsell (1995). They portray a threshold phenomenon, which can be loosely stated as follows. For small initial number of infectives a, if $R_0 = N\beta/\gamma \leq 1$ then only minor epidemics can occur, whilst if $R_0 > 1$ then both minor and major epidemics can occur. In Section 6 we make this threshold behaviour precise by letting $N \to \infty$. See Nåsell (1995) for a discussion of the threshold concept for stochastic SIR and SIS epidemic models.

The coupling methods of this section can be extended to obtain recurrence relations governing the moment generating functions of the total size, Z, and the severity, A, of the epidemic $E_{N,a}(\beta, T_I)$ (Ball (1986)). In a series of papers, Lefèvre and Picard have shown that a non-standard family of polynomials provides an elegant framework for analysing the total size and severity of closed population epidemic models (see e.g. Lefèvre 1995). Ball and Clancy (1992) provide a connection between the above coupling argument and their framework.

5   Coupling and stochastic comparisons

In this section we show how coupling can be used to prove stochastic comparisons for epidemic models. We first introduce some terminology. Let X and Y be real-valued random variables. Then X is stochastically larger than Y, written $X \overset{st}{\geq} Y$, if $\Pr(X \leq t) \leq \Pr(Y \leq t)$ for all $t \in \mathcal{R}$. If $X \overset{st}{\geq} Y$ then X and Y can be defined on the same probability space, (Ω, P) say, such that $X(\omega) \geq Y(\omega)$ for all $\omega \in \Omega$. Conversely, if X and Y are random variables defined on (Ω, P) such that $\Pr(\{\omega : X(\omega) \geq Y(\omega)\}) = 1$, then $X \overset{st}{\geq} Y$. A family of random variables, X_θ ($\theta \in \mathcal{R}$), is stochastically increasing in θ if $X_\theta \overset{st}{\geq} X_{\theta'}$ whenever $\theta > \theta'$. See Ross (1983, Chapter 8), for an elementary account of stochastic comparisons.

The Sellke construction described in Section 4 enables us to prove immediately that the total size of the epidemic $E_{N,a}(\beta, T_I)$ is stochastically increasing in N, a or β. Also, if we let Z and $\tilde{Z}$ be the total sizes of the epidemics $E_{N,a}(\beta, T_I)$ and $E_{N,a}(\beta, \tilde{T}_I)$, respectively, then $T_I \overset{st}{\geq} \tilde{T}_I$ implies that $Z \overset{st}{\geq} \tilde{Z}$. To prove the latter result, let (Ω, P) be a probability space on which are defined appropriately distributed random variables $L_1, L_2, \ldots, L_N, R_{-(a-1)}, R_{-(a-2)}, \ldots, R_N$ and $\tilde{R}_{-(a-1)}, \tilde{R}_{-(a-2)}, \ldots, \tilde{R}_N$ such that for all $\omega \in \Omega$, $R_i \geq \tilde{R}_i$ $(i = -(a-1), -(a-2), \ldots, N)$. Such a probability space exists since $T_I \overset{st}{\geq} \tilde{T}_I$. For each $\omega \in \Omega$, we construct realisations of $E_{N,a}(\beta, T_I)$ and $E_{N,a}(\beta, \tilde{T}_I)$ using $L_1, L_2, \ldots, L_N, R_{-(a-1)}, R_{-(a-2)}, \ldots, R_N$ and $L_1, L_2, \ldots, L_N, \tilde{R}_{-(a-1)}, \tilde{R}_{-(a-2)}, \ldots, \tilde{R}_N$, respectively. Note that the same set of critical exposures to infection, $L_1, L_2, \ldots, L_N$, is used in both epidemics. It follows from (4.1) that $Z \geq \tilde{Z}$ for all $\omega \in \Omega$, so $Z \overset{st}{\geq} \tilde{Z}$, as required. The above argument can be extended to time dependent comparisons. For example, we have in obvious notation that $T_I \overset{st}{\geq} \tilde{T}_I$ implies $X(t) \overset{st}{\leq} \tilde{X}(t)$ for all $t \geq 0$. Although the above results are all intuitively very obvious, they are difficult to establish formally without resorting to coupling. For example, it is not immediately clear how the total size comparisons would follow from (4.5), and the situation is far worse for time dependent results.

We now turn our attention to the effects of introducing heterogeneity into our model and, in particular, examine the consequences of variability in susceptibility. For $i = 1, 2, \ldots, N$, let β_i be the susceptibility of initial susceptible i, in the sense that if i is still susceptible and there are y infectives at time t, then the probability that i is infected in the time interval $(t, t + \Delta t)$ is $\beta_i y \Delta t + o(\Delta t)$. We denote the resulting epidemic model by $E_{N,a}(\boldsymbol{\beta}, T_I)$, where $\boldsymbol{\beta} = (\beta_1, \beta_2, \ldots, \beta_N)$ is termed the susceptibility vector. Note that $E_{N,a}(\boldsymbol{\beta}, T_I)$ can be constructed using the Sellke construction, but with $L_i \sim \mathrm{NE}(\beta_i)$ $(i = 1, 2, \ldots, N)$, i.e. L_i is exponentially distributed with mean β_i^{-1}.

In order to prove stochastic comparisons between epidemics with different susceptibility vectors, we shall require the following partial ordering. Let $\boldsymbol{\beta}$ and $\boldsymbol{\beta}'$ be two susceptibility vectors satisfying $\sum_{i=1}^N \beta_i = \sum_{i=1}^N \beta_i'$, then $\boldsymbol{\beta}$ majorises $\boldsymbol{\beta}'$, written $\boldsymbol{\beta} \succ \boldsymbol{\beta}'$, if $\sum_{i=1}^k \beta_{(i)} \leq \sum_{i=1}^k \beta_{(i)}'$ $(k = 1, 2, \ldots, N)$, where $\beta_{(1)}, \beta_{(2)}, \ldots, \beta_{(N)}$ are the order statistics of $\beta_1, \beta_2, \ldots, \beta_N$ and $\beta_{(1)}', \beta_{(2)}', \ldots, \beta_{(N)}'$ are defined similarly (see e.g. Marshall and Olkin 1979, Chapter 1). The partial ordering reflects the diversity of the individual susceptibilities. In particular, the constant vector $(\beta, \beta, \ldots, \beta)$ is majorised by any vector $\boldsymbol{\beta}$ with $\sum_{i=1}^N \beta_i = N\beta$. The following lemma, due to Proschan and Sethuraman (1976), enables us to make stochastic comparisons between epidemics with different susceptibility vectors.

Lemma 5.1 *Let $X_1, X_2, \ldots, X_N$ and $X_1', X_2', \ldots, X_N'$ be two sets of independent random variables, with $X_i \sim \mathrm{NE}(\beta_i)$ and $X_i' \sim \mathrm{NE}(\beta_i')$ $(i =$*

$1, 2, \ldots, N$), *where* $\boldsymbol{\beta} \succ \boldsymbol{\beta}'$. *Then there exists a probability space* (Ω, P), *on which are defined random variables* $Y_1, Y_2, \ldots, Y_N$ *and* $Y_1', Y_2', \ldots, Y_N'$ *such that*

(i)

$$(Y_1, Y_2, \ldots, Y_N) \stackrel{\mathrm{D}}{=} (X_{(1)}, X_{(2)}, \ldots, X_{(N)}),$$
$$(Y_1', Y_2', \ldots, Y_N') \stackrel{\mathrm{D}}{=} (X_{(1)}', X_{(2)}', \ldots, X_{(N)}'),$$

where $\stackrel{\mathrm{D}}{=}$ *denotes equal in distribution, and*

(ii) for all $\omega \in \Omega$, $Y_i(\omega) \geq Y_i'(\omega)$ $(i = 1, 2, \ldots, N)$, *with strict inequality for* $i = 2, 3, \ldots, N$ *if* $\boldsymbol{\beta} \neq \boldsymbol{\beta}'$.

We can compare the epidemics $E_{N,a}(\boldsymbol{\beta}, T_I)$ and $E_{N,a}(\boldsymbol{\beta}', T_I)$, where $\boldsymbol{\beta} \succ \boldsymbol{\beta}'$, by using the Sellke construction with a common set $R_{-(a-1)}$, $R_{-(a-2)}, \ldots, R_N$ of infectious periods and critical exposures to infection L_1, $L_2, \ldots, L_N$ and $L_1', L_2', \ldots, L_N'$, coupled by Lemma 5.1 so that $L_{(i)} \geq L_{(i)}'$ $(i = 1, 2, \ldots, N)$. It follows immediately that $Z \stackrel{\mathrm{st}}{\leq} Z'$, where Z and Z' are the total sizes of the two epidemics, since susceptibles have a greater resistance to infection in $E_{N,a}(\boldsymbol{\beta}, T_I)$ than in $E_{N,a}(\boldsymbol{\beta}', T_I)$. Again, time-dependent results are straightforward to obtain. In an obvious sense, $\boldsymbol{\beta} \succ \boldsymbol{\beta}'$ implies that the epidemic $E_{N,a}(\boldsymbol{\beta}, T_I)$ spreads slower than the epidemic $E_{N,a}(\boldsymbol{\beta}', T_I)$.

An important special case is when $\boldsymbol{\beta}' = (\beta, \beta, \ldots, \beta)$, which is majorised by any vector $\boldsymbol{\beta}$ with $\sum_{i=1}^{N} \beta_i = N\beta$. It follows that an epidemic with varying susceptibilities spreads stochastically slower than the corresponding model with uniform susceptibility (Ball 1985a). This phenomenon has a simple intuitive explanation. The epidemics are matched so that initially they have the same average susceptibility. However, in the model with varying susceptibility the more susceptible individuals are likely to be infected first. Thus the average susceptibility of the remaining susceptibles will fall below that of the homogeneous mixing epidemic, with the consequence that the heterogeneous epidemic will spread slower than the corresponding homogeneously mixing one.

Several authors have examined the effects of heterogeneities in epidemic models. For example, Becker (1973) and Lefèvre and Malice (1988) consider the consequences of varying infectivity and susceptibility in Weiss's (1965) carrier-borne epidemic model. Becker and Marschner (1990) and Marschner (1992) study heterogeneities in closed population epidemic models via a multitype branching process approximation. Finally, note that the methods of this section can be used to show that introducing varying infectivity into the general stochastic epidemic increases the spread of infection (Barbour *et al.* 1991).

6   Coupling and limit theorems

Consider the epidemic model $E_{N,a}(\beta, T_I)$ and focus attention on the process described by the number of infectives at time t ($t \geq 0$). If all contacts were to result in infection then this process would follow a Crump-Mode-Jagers branching process (see e.g. Jagers 1975, page 22), in which individuals give birth at the points of a homogeneous Poisson process with rate $N\beta$ during a lifetime that is distributed according to T_I. During the early stages of an epidemic in a large population it is unlikely that the same individual is contacted more than once, so the branching process will provide a good approximation to the process of infectives in the epidemic model. Such an approximation has a long history going back to Bartlett (1955, pages 147-148), and Kendall (1956). We shall use a coupling argument to make it exact in the limit as N tends to infinity. Our proof is based on Ball (1983), see also Metz (1978). Ball and Donnelly (1992, 1995) give a detailed treatment of the approximation of a wide class of epidemic models by branching processes. Ball and O'Neill (1994) consider approximating Markov epidemic processes, incorporating immigration and emigration, by birth and death processes.

Consider a sequence of epidemic processes $\{E_{N,a}(N^{-1}\beta, T_I); N = 1, 2, \ldots\}$, where the infection rate has been scaled so that the number of contacts made by an infective is independent of the initial susceptible population size N. Let $\{Y_N(t)\} = \{Y_N(t); t \geq 0\}$ be the process describing the number of infectives in $E_{N,a}(N^{-1}\beta, T_I)$ and let $\{Y(t)\}$ be the process describing the number of individuals alive at time t in the branching process, initiated by a ancestors, in which individuals give birth at rate β during a lifetime distributed according to T_I. We construct all the epidemic processes and the limiting branching process on the same probability space as follows.

Let (Ω, P) be a probability space on which is defined the branching process $\{Y(t)\}$ by realisations $\mathcal{H}_{-(a-1)}, \mathcal{H}_{-(a-2)}, \ldots$ of an individual life history $\mathcal{H} = (T_I, \eta)$ that are independent and identically distributed. Here, T_I is the lifetime of a typical individual and η is a Poisson process with rate β governing that individual's offspring times. The life histories can be pieced together in the obvious fashion, with $\mathcal{H}_{-(a-1)}, \mathcal{H}_{-(a-2)}, \ldots, \mathcal{H}_0$ being the life histories of the a initial ancestors and, for $i = 1, 2, \ldots, \mathcal{H}_i$ being the life history of the ith individual born into the branching process. Let $U_1, U_2, \ldots$ be an independent sequence of i.i.d. $U(0,1)$ random variables also defined on (Ω, P). For $N = 1, 2, \ldots$, a realisation of the epidemic $E_{N,a}(N^{-1}\beta, T_I)$ can be obtained as follows. Label the initial susceptibles $1, 2, \ldots, N$. The process of infectives $\{Y_N(t)\}$ follows the branching process $\{Y(t)\}$, with contacts occuring whenever a birth occurs in $\{Y(t)\}$. The individual contacted at the ith contact is $C_i = [NU_i] + 1$, where $[x]$ denotes the greatest integer $\leq x$. If C_i is still susceptible then it is infected in the epidemic, otherwise it and all of its descendants in the branching process are ignored in the epidemic process. Following Mollison (1977), we shall call individuals that exist in the branching process but not in the epidemic process *ghosts*. Note that the epidemics are coupled via the sequence $U_1, U_2, \ldots$ of uniform random variables.

The process of infectives $\{Y_N(t)\}$ in the Nth epidemic process and the branching process $\{Y(t)\}$ agree up until the time, τ_N say, of the first ghost. Thus we will examine the limiting behaviour of τ_N as $N \to \infty$. The uniform random variables $U_1, U_2, \ldots$ are distinct with probability one. The branching process $\{Y(t)\}$ will display one of two modes of behaviour; either it will go extinct or it will grow exponentially fast as $t \to \infty$ (see e.g. Jagers 1975, Chapter 6). In the former case, let Z be the total number of individuals born into $\{Y(t)\}$. Then $Z < \infty$ and, since $U_1, U_2, \ldots$ are distinct, $\epsilon = \min_{i,j=1,2,\ldots,Z(i \neq j)} |U_i - U_j| > 0$. Thus, for $N > \epsilon^{-1}$, $[NU_1] + 1, [NU_2] + 1, \ldots, [NU_Z] + 1$ will be distinct and no ghosts will appear in $E_{N,a}(N^{-1}\beta, T_I)$. Hence,

$$\Pr\left(\tau_N = \infty \text{ for all sufficiently large } N \mid \{Y(t)\} \text{ goes extinct}\right) = 1. \quad (6.1)$$

Suppose that the branching process does not go extinct and fix $t > 0$. Then the number of births during $[0, t]$ is finite with probability one, and a similar argument to the above shows that $\tau_N > t$ for all sufficiently large N. Thus

$$\Pr\left(\lim_{N \to \infty} \tau_N = \infty \mid \{Y(t)\} \text{ does not go extinct}\right) = 1, \quad (6.2)$$

which can be strengthened (Ball and Donnelly 1992, 1995) to

$$\Pr\left(\lim_{N \to \infty} \tau_N / \log N = (2\alpha)^{-1} \mid \{Y(t)\} \text{ does not go extinct}\right) = 1,$$

where α is the Malthusian parameter of the branching process $\{Y(t)\}$ (see e.g. Jagers 1975, page 10), which describes its asymptotic exponential rate of growth when extinction does not occur. Equations (6.1) and (6.2) imply that, with probablity one, if the branching process goes extinct then $E_{N,a}(N^{-1}\beta, T_I)$ and the branching process agree over $[0, \infty)$ for all sufficiently large N; if the branching process does not go extinct then they agree over any finite time interval $[0, t]$ for all sufficiently large N.

Let Z_N be the total size of the epidemic $E_{N,a}(N\beta^{-1}, T_I)$ $(N = 1, 2, \ldots)$ and Z be the total size of the branching process $\{Y(t)\}$, so that Z_N is always finite but Z may be infinite. Then (6.1) and (6.2) also imply that $\Pr(\lim_{N \to \infty} Z_N = Z) = 1$, which yields a threshold theorem for the stochastic epidemic $E_{N,a}(N^{-1}\beta, T_I)$. Following Williams (1971), we say that a major epidemic occurs if $Z_N \to \infty$ as $N \to \infty$. Then elementary branching process theory (see e.g. Jagers 1975) yields that a major epidemic can only occur if $R_0 = \beta E[T_I] > 1$, in which case the probability that a major epidemic occurs is $1 - p^a$, where p is the smallest root of $\phi(\beta(1 - s)) = s$. (Recall that ϕ is the moment generating function of the infectious period T_I.) See Ball (1983) for further details, and Whittle (1955) and Nåsell (1995) for alternative threshold theorems for stochastic epidemics. Kendall (1994) gives a coupling proof of a generalisation of Whittle's threshold theorem.

The above results do not yield any information concerning the size of a major epidemic for finite N. However, it can be shown that as $N \to \infty$ the total size of a major epidemic is asymptotically normally distributed about the size of the corresponding deterministic epidemic, see e.g. von Bahr and Martin-Löf (1980), Watson (1981), Scalia-Tomba (1985) and Martin-Löf (1986) for single population epidemics, and Scalia-Tomba (1986), Andersson (1993) and Ball and Clancy (1993) for multipopulation epidemics. The papers of Scalia-Tomba (1985) and Ball and Clancy (1993) use essentially the Sellke construction of Section 4.

The branching process $\{Y(t)\}$ can be used as an approximation to the epidemic process $E_{N,a}(N^{-1}\beta, T_I)$. Ball and Donnelly (1995) give bounds on the total variation distance (see e.g. Barbour *et al.* 1992, pages 253-4) between the two processes. The approximation is quite good for minor epidemics but it breaks down as soon as $N^{\frac{1}{2}}$ susceptibles have been infected in a major epidemic. In such circumstances the deterministic based approximations of Barbour (1974) and Kurtz (1970, or 1981, Chapter 9) take over, see Altmann (1993).

7 Coupling and deterministic models

Although coupling is primarily a method of analysing stochastic models, it can also be used in a deterministic setting, since a deterministic model can usually be obtained as a limit of an appropriate sequence of stochastic models (see e.g. Kurtz 1970, or 1981, Chapter 9). We shall illustrate the key idea, due to Kendall and Saunders (1983), by describing a main result of that paper. The methods we shall use are precisely those of Kendall and Saunders, though our construction and coupling of the epidemic processes are different. First we describe their model.

Consider a closed homogeneously mixing population that is exposed to two SIR epidemics that are in competition, in the sense that contracting either of the two diseases confers immunity to the other. For $t \geq 0$ and $k = 1, 2$, let $x(t), y_k(t)$ and $z_k(t)$ be respectively the numbers of susceptibles, infectives with disease k and removed cases with disease k at time t. The deterministic formulation is given by

$$
\begin{aligned}
\frac{dx}{dt} &= -(\beta_1 y_1 + \beta_2 y_2)x, \\
\frac{dy_k}{dt} &= \beta_k y_k x - \gamma_k y_k \quad (k = 1, 2),
\end{aligned} \tag{7.1}
$$

$$\frac{dz_k}{dt} = \gamma_k y_k \quad (k = 1, 2),$$

with initial condition

$$(x(0), y_1(0), z_1(0), y_2(0), z_2(0)) = (N - a_1 - a_2, a_1, a_2, 0, 0).$$

The principal problem that Kendall and Saunders addressed was to prove that if $a_1 + a_2$ is held fixed, say $a_1 + a_2 = a$, then the number of individuals removed with disease 2 at the end of the epidemic, $z_2(\infty)$, is increasing with a_2. This intuitively obvious fact has to date defied direct proof from (7.1).

Let $\{\mathbf{X}(t); t \geq 0\} = \{(X(t), Y_1(t), Z_1(t), Y_2(t), Z_2(t)); t \geq 0\}$ be the stochastic version of the above model, obtained by replacing the infinitesimal transition rates in (7.2) with infinitesimal transition probabilities. The stochastic model can be realised using a Sellke construction with for disease k ($k = 1, 2$), critical exposures to infection $L_{a+1}^{(k)}, L_{a+2}^{(k)}, \ldots, L_N^{(k)} \sim \mathrm{NE}(\beta_k)$ and infectious periods $R_1^{(k)}, R_2^{(k)}, \ldots, R_N^{(k)} \sim \mathrm{NE}(\gamma_k)$. The individuals are labelled $1, 2, \ldots, N$, with $1, 2, \ldots, a$ being the initial infectives and $a+1, a+2, \ldots, N$ being the initial susceptibles. The L's and R's have the same interpretation as in Section 4. Thus for $k = 1, 2$, $R_1^{(k)}, R_2^{(k)}, \ldots, R_{a_k}^{(k)}$ are the infectious periods of the initial disease k infectives, and $R_{a_k+j}^{(k)}$ is the infectious period of the jth susceptible to be infected with disease k $(j = 1, 2, \ldots, N - a_k)$. Further, susceptible i is infected with disease k as soon as $A_k(t)$ reaches $L_i^{(k)}$, where $A_k(t) = \int_0^t Y_k(u)\, du$, provided it has not previously been infected with the other disease.

Now construct two coupled competing epidemic processes, $\{\mathbf{X}(t); t \geq 0\}$ and $\{\tilde{\mathbf{X}}(t); t \geq 0\}$ say, using the same set of L's and R's but with initial numbers of infectives a_1, a_2 and $\tilde{a}_1, \tilde{a}_2$, respectively, where $a_1 + a_2 = \tilde{a}_1 + \tilde{a}_2 = a$ and $\tilde{a}_2 > a_2$. It follows immediately from our construction that for $t \geq 0$, $\tilde{A}_1(t) \overset{\mathrm{st}}{\leq} A_1(t)$ and $\tilde{A}_2(t) \overset{\mathrm{st}}{\geq} A_2(t)$, and hence that

$$Y_2(t) + Z_2(t) \overset{\mathrm{st}}{\leq} \tilde{Y}_2(t) + \tilde{Z}_2(t). \tag{7.2}$$

To prove that the same result holds for the deterministic model, let $\{\mathbf{X}^{(\nu)}(t); t \geq 0\}$ $(\nu = 1, 2, \ldots)$ be a sequence of competing stochastic epidemics, with $N^{(\nu)} = \nu N, a_k^{(\nu)} = \nu a_k, \beta_k^{(\nu)} = \nu^{-1}\beta_k, \gamma_k^{(\nu)} = \gamma_k$ $(k = 1, 2)$, and let $\{\tilde{\mathbf{X}}^{(\nu)}(t); t \geq 0\}$ $(\nu = 1, 2, \ldots)$ be a similar sequence, but with $\tilde{a}_k^{(\nu)} = \nu \tilde{a}_k$ $(k = 1, 2)$. Then by Kurtz (1970),

$$\lim_{\nu \to \infty} \nu^{-1} \mathrm{E}\left[Y_k^{(\nu)}(t) + Z_k^{(\nu)}(t)\right] = y_k(t) + z_k(t) \quad (t \geq 0; k = 1, 2), \tag{7.3}$$

see Kendall and Saunders (1983). From (7.2),

$$\mathrm{E}\left[Y_2^{(\nu)}(t) + Z_2^{(\nu)}(t)\right] \leq \mathrm{E}\left[\tilde{Y}_2^{(\nu)}(t) + \tilde{Z}_2^{(\nu)}(t)\right] \quad (t \geq 0; \nu = 1, 2, \ldots), \tag{7.4}$$

so applying (7.3) gives

$$y_2(t) + z_2(t) \leq \tilde{y}_2(t) + \tilde{z}_2(t) \quad (t \geq 0). \tag{7.5}$$

Letting $t \rightarrow \infty$ in (7.5) yields $z_2(\infty) \leq \tilde{z}_2(\infty)$, the result that so far has resisted direct proof.

The above argument can be extended so that the inequalities are strict and, for the deterministic model, the initial numbers of infectives, a_1 and a_2 etc., are non-integer (see Kendall and Saunders 1983). Note that the above method of deriving results for a deterministic model via an appropriate sequence of stochastic models is extremely versatile. For example, it can be used to extend all the comparisons of Section 5 to equivalent deterministic models.

8 Concluding comments

8.1 Other applications of coupling

We have described a number of different applications of coupling methods to epidemic models. There are of course other areas of epidemic models in which coupling methods have been applied and we shall briefly describe a few.

Coupling methods have been extensively used in the study of spatial epidemics. A simple (to describe!) spatial epidemic model is a contact distribution model (Mollison (1977)), in which individuals are located at the points of a two-dimensional square lattice and infectives make contacts at the points of a Poisson process with rate β during an infectious period distributed according to T_I. The locations (relative to the infective) of successive contacts are chosen independently from a specified contact distribution. The epidemic is started by introducing one infectious individual at the origin. Mollison (1977) coupled such an epidemic to two-dimensional bond percolation to prove that, provided the contact distribution attributes some weight to each of the four nearest neighbours, there is a threshold value β_0 such that if $\beta < \beta_0$ then the epidemic will almost surely ultimately infect only finitely many susceptibles, whilst if $\beta > \beta_0$ there is a non-zero probability of infinitely many susceptibles being infected. Kuulasmaa and Zachary (1984) compared the above epidemic with one in which $T_I = \tau$, where the constant τ is chosen so that infectives in the two epidemics have the same probability of infecting nobody. They showed that the number of contacts made by a typical infective in the epidemic with infectious period τ is stochastically larger than in the epidemic with infectious period T_I. Thus it is straightforward to couple the epidemics so that the τ epidemic spreads faster than the T_I epidemic. It follows that the τ epidemic will have a lower threshold value of β. Mollison (1972) considered the one-dimensional version of the above model with $T_I = \infty$, i.e. without removal of infectives. He used a coupling argument to sandwich the epidemic between one in which only the initial infectives are infectious (c.f. Weiss's (1965) carrier-borne epidemic) and one in which whenever a susceptible (at i say) is infected then all the susceptibles located at or to the left of i are simultaneously infected. He was then able to show that the front velocity is finite if and only if the contact distribution has finite variance. Another spatial epidemic which has seen considerable use of coupling techniques is the contact process, a stochastic spatial SIS epidemic, see e.g. Liggett (1985, Chapter 6).

Coupling can often be used profitably in simulation studies, particularily if we want our simulated realisations to reflect a property that we know theoretically to be true. For example, Ball (1985b) considered a model for fox rabies in which fox groups are located at the points of a two-dimensional square lattice and a rabid group infects each of its four nearest neighbouring groups independently with probability p. The model was used to evaluate the efficacy of control strategies that reduce the number of susceptible foxes, and hence p, in a region surrounding the initial case at the origin. Using a device of Hammersley and Handscomb (1964, Chapter 11), simulated realisations were obtained simultaneously for all values of p by assigning independent uniform $(0,1)$ random variables to all arcs connecting neighbouring groups, with the interpretation that for a particular value of p the infection will only spread between two groups if the associated uniform random variable is less than p. Note that the simulated realisations were necessarily increasing with p. The coupled simulations enabled success probabilities of the above control measures to be estimated simultaneously for all values of p.

Donnelly (1993) used coupling methods in a study of the correlation structure of a variety of epidemic models, in particular to answer questions such as: does knowledge that a certain group of individuals is infected make it more or less likely that other specified individals are infected? A key tool was a theorem of Harris (1977), which broadly states (in appropriately defined terms) that if a stochastic process is monotone and its initial distribution has positive correlations, then so does its distribution at time t, for any $t \geq 0$. Donnelly considered a very general SIS epidemic model and used a coupling argument to show that it is monotone in the initial set of infectives. In the presence of certain types of competition and interference between diseases he used coupling techniques to show, for example, with two diseases that increasing the initial number of infectives with one stochastically decreased the number of infectives with the other disease at later times. An unusual choice of partial order then allows Harris's result to prove (negative) correlation results "between" the diseases. He also used a graphical construction of a very general SIR model to prove correlation results in that context.

8.2   Generalisations of basic model

The basic model of Section 3 can be generalised in several ways to make it more realistic. We can introduce an infectivity profile $\xi(t)$, with the interpretation that $N\xi(t)$ is the rate that a typical infective makes contacts t units of time after its initial infection. Note that $\xi(t)$ may be both random and time-inhomogeneous. Also, both an infectious period, T_I, and a latent period, T_L, are implicitly incorporated, since $\xi(t) = 0$ unless $T_L \leq t < T_L + T_I$. Let $\xi_{-(a-1)}(t), \xi_{-(a-2)}(t), \ldots, \xi_N(t)$ be i.i.d. realisations of the infectivity profile $\xi(t)$. The Sellke construction can be modified by letting $\beta = 1$ and $A(t) = \sum_{i=-(a-1)}^{N(t)} \xi_i(t - \tau_i)$, where $\tau_i = 0$ $(i = -(a-1), -(a-2), \ldots, 0)$, $N(t)$ is the number of susceptibles that have been infected by time t and $\tau_1, \tau_2, \ldots, \tau_{N(t)}$ are the corresponding infection times. If we also let $R_i = \int_0^\infty \xi_i(t)\,dt\,(i = -(a-1), -(a-2), \ldots, N)$ and $\phi(\theta) = \mathrm{E}\left[\exp(-\theta \int_0^\infty \xi_i(t)\,dt)\right]$ then all the results of Sections 4, 5 and 7 go through with obvious modifications. The methods of Section 6 also apply to the present model but now the point process η is Poisson with intensity $\xi(t)$, see Ball and Donnelly (1992, 1995).

The assumption of homogeneous mixing can be relaxed. Specifically, our methods extend to the spread of an epidemic amongst a population split into groups labelled $1, 2, \ldots, m$, with infection rate β_{ij} between groups i and j $(i, j = 1, 2, \ldots, m)$. The final outcome results are given in Ball (1986) and the branching process approximation in Ball (1983). We can also allow the infectives to move amongst the groups (Ball and Clancy (1993)). Other treatments of multipopulation epidemics include Picard and Lefèvre (1990) (mainly exact results), and Scalia-Tomba (1986) and Andersson (1993) (mainly asymptotic results).

We can also allow the possibility that the infectious periods of the initial infectives follow a different distribution than those of the infected susceptibles. A case in point is the carrier-borne model of Downton (1968), in which a proportion $1 - \pi$ of infected susceptibles are removed immediately on infection and play no further part in the epidemic. Ball (1990) describes the extension of our arguments to such a situation.

References

Altmann, M. (1993) 'Limits of stochastic epidemics in large populations', *in preparation*.

Andersson, H. (1993) 'A threshold limit theorem for a multitype epidemic model', *Math. Biosci.* **117**, 3–18.

von Bahr, B., and Martin-Löf, A. (1980) 'Threshold limit theorems for some epidemic processes', *Adv. Appl. Prob.* **12**, 319–349.

Bailey, N.T.J. (1975) *The Mathematical Theory of Infectious Diseases and its Applications*, Griffin, London.

Ball, F.G. (1983) 'The threshold behaviour of epidemic models', *J. Appl. Prob.* **20**, 227–241.

Ball, F.G. (1986) 'A unified approach to the distribution of total size and total area under the trajectory of infectives in epidemic models', *Adv. Appl. Prob.* **18**, 289–310.

Ball, F.G. (1990) 'A new look at Downton's carrier-borne epidemic model'. In *Stochastic Processes in Epidemic Theory*, J-P. Gabriel, C. Lefèvre, and Ph. Picard, (eds.), *Lecture Notes in Biomathematics* **86**, 71–85.

Ball, F.G. (1985a) 'Deterministic and stochastic epidemics with several kinds of susceptibles', *Adv. Appl. Prob.* **17**, 1–22.

Ball, F.G. (1985b) 'Spatial models for the spread and control of rabies incorporating group size'. In *The Population Dynamics of Rabies in Wildlife*, P.J. Bacon (ed.), Academic Press, London, 197–222.

Ball, F.G. and Clancy, D. (1992) 'The final outcome of a generalised stochastic multitype epidemic model', Technical Report 92-4, Nottingham Statistics Group.

Ball, F.G. and Clancy, D. (1993) 'The final size and severity of a generalised stochastic multitype epidemic model', *Adv. Appl. Prob.* **25**, 721–736.

Ball, F.G. and Donnelly, P. (1992) 'Branching process approximation of epidemic models'. In *Proc. 2nd World Congress of the Bernoulli Society, Uppsala, 1990*, 144–147.

Ball, F.G. and Donnelly, P. (1995) 'Strong approximations for epidemic models' *Stoch. Proc. Appl.* (to appear).

Ball, F.G. and O'Neill, P.D. (1994) 'Strong convergence of general SIR stochastic epidemics', *Adv. Appl. Prob.* **26**, 629–655.

Barbour, A.D. (1974) 'On a functional central limit theorem for markov population processes', *Adv. Appl. Prob.* **6**, 21–39.

Barbour, A.D., Holst, L. and Janson, S (1992) *Poisson Approximation*, Clarendon Press, Oxford.

Barbour, A.D., Lindvall, T. and Rogers, L.C.G. (1991) 'Stochastic ordering of order statistics', *J. Appl. Prob.*, **28**, 278–286.

Bartlett, M.S. (1955) *An Introduction to Stochastic Processes*, Cambridge University Press, Cambridge.

Becker, N.G. (1973) 'Carrier-borne epidemics in a community consisting of different groups', *J. Appl. Prob.* **10**, 491–501

Becker, N.G. and Marschner, I.C. (1990) 'The effect of heterogeneity on the spread of disease'. In *Stochastic Processes in Epidemic Theory*, J.-P. Gabriel, C. Lefévre and P. Picard (eds.), Lecture Notes in Biomathematics **86**, Springer-Verlag, New York, 90–103.

Billard, L. (1973) 'Factorial moments and probabilities for the general stochastic epidemic', *J. Appl. Prob.* **10**, 277–288.

Donnelly, P.J. (1993) 'The correlation structure of epidemic models', *Math. Biosci.* **117**, 49–75.

Downton, F. (1968) 'The ultimate size of carrier-borne epidemics', *Biometrika* **55**, 277–289.

Downton, F. (1972) 'A correction to "The area under the infectives trajectory of the general stochastic epidemic" ', *J. Appl. Prob.* **9**, 873–876.

Grimmett, G.R. and Stirzaker, D.R. (1992) *Probability and Random Processes*, Clarendon Press, Oxford.

Hammersley, J.M. and Handscomb, D.C. (1964) *Monte Carlo Methods*, Methuen, London.

Harris, T. (1977) 'A correlation inequality for Markov processes in partially ordered state spaces', *Ann. Prob.* **5**, 451–454.

Jagers, P. (1975) *Branching Processes with Biological Applications*, Wiley, New York.

Karlin, S. and Taylor, H.M. (1975) *A First Course in Stochastic Processes* Academic Press, New York.

Kendall, D.G. (1956) 'Deterministic and stochastic epidemics in closed populations', in *Proc. 3rd Berkeley Symp. Math. Statist. Prob.* **4** 149–165.

Kendall, W.S. (1994) *In discussion of* Mollison *et al.*, *J. R. Statist. Soc. A* **157**, 143.

Kendall, W.S. and Saunders, I.W. (1983) 'Epidemics in competition II: the general epidemic', *J. R. Statist. Soc. B* **45** 238–244.

Kryscio, R.J. (1975) 'The transition probabilities of the general stochastic epidemic', *J. Appl. Prob.* **12**, 415–424.

Kurtz, T.G. (1970) 'Limit theorems for sequences of jump Markov processes approximating ordinary differential processes', *J. Appl. Prob.* **7**, 344–356.

Kurtz, T.G. (1981) *Approximation of Population Processes* SIAM, Philadelphia.

Kuulasmaa, K. and Zachary, S. (1984) 'On spatial general epidemics and bond percolation processes', *J. Appl. Prob.* **21**, 911–914.

Lefèvre, C. (1990) 'Stochastic epidemic models for S-I-R infectious diseases: a brief survey of the recent general theory', in *Stochastic Processes in Epidemic Theory*, Lecture Notes in Biomathematics **86** J.-P. Gabriel, C. Lefévre and P. Picard (eds.), Springer-Verlag, New York, pp. 1–12.

Lefèvre, C. (1995) 'Collective Reed-Frost epidemic processes', this volume.

Lefèvre, C. and Malice, M.-P. (1988) 'Comparisons for carrier-borne epidemics in heterogeneous and homogeneous populations', *J. Appl. Prob.* **25**, 663–674.

Liggett, T.M. (1985) *Interacting Particle Systems*, Springer-Verlag, New York.

Lindvall, T. (1992) *Lectures on the Coupling Method*, Wiley, New York.

Marschner, I.C. (1992) 'The effect of preferential mixing on the growth of an epidemic', *Math. Biosci.* **109**, 39–67.

Marshall, A.W. and Olkin, I. (1979) *Inequalities: Theory of Majorization and its Applications*, Academic Press, New York.

Martin-Löf, A. (1986) 'Symmetric sampling procedures, general epidemic processes and their threshold limit theorems', *J. Appl. Prob.* **23**, 265–282.

Metz, J.A.J. (1978) 'The epidemic in a closed population with all susceptibles equally vulnerable; some results for large susceptible populations and small initial infections', *Acta Biotheoretica* **27**, 75–123.

Mollison, D. (1972) 'The rate of spatial propogation of simple epidemics', in *Proc. 6th Berkeley Symp. Math. Statist. Prob.* **3**, 579–614.

Mollison, D. (1977) 'Spatial contact models for ecological and epidemic spread', (with discussion) *J. R. Statist. Soc. B* **39**, 283–326.

Nåsell, I. (1995) 'The threshold concept in stochastic epidemic and endemic models', this volume.

Picard, P. and Lefèvre, C. (1990) 'A unified analysis of the final size and severity distribution in collective Reed-Frost epidemic processes', *Adv. Appl. Prob.* **22**, 269–294.

Proschan, F. and Sethuraman, J. 'Stochastic comparisons of order statistics from heterogeneous populations, with applications in reliability', *J. Multivariate Anal.* **6**, 608–616.

Ross, S.M. (1983) *Stochastic Processes*, Wiley, New York.

Scalia-Tomba, G. (1985) 'Asymptotic final-size distribution for some chain-binomial processes', *Adv. Appl. Prob.* **17**, 477–495.

Scalia-Tomba, G. (1986) 'Asymptotic final-size distribution of the multitype Reed-Frost process', *J. Appl. Prob.* **23**, 565–584.

Sellke, T. (1983) 'On the asymptotic distribution of the size of a stochastic epidemic', *J. Appl. Prob.* **20**, 390–394.

Watson, R.K. (1980) 'On the size distribution for some epidemic models', *J. Appl. Prob.* **17**, 912–921.

Watson, R.K. (1981) 'An application of a martingale central limit theorem to the standard epidemic model', *Stoch. Proc. Applics.* **11**, 79–89.

Weiss, G.H. (1965) 'On the spread of epidemics by carriers', *Biometrics* **21**, 481–490.

Whittle, P. (1955) 'The outcome of a stochastic epidemic — a note on Bailey's paper', *Biometrika* **42**, 116–122.

Williams, T. (1971) 'An algebraic proof of the threshold theorem for the general stochastic epidemic' (abstract), *Adv. Appl. Prob.* **3**, 223.

Collective Epidemic Processes:
a general modelling approach to the final outcome of SIR infectious diseases

Claude Lefèvre

Philippe Picard

Summary

This paper presents a brief overview of the collective (Reed-Frost) epidemic process introduced by Picard and Lefèvre (1990). The model is shown to provide a unified and flexible approach to the study of the final outcome of SIR infectious diseases. Attention is paid to essential aspects first of the construction of the model and then of the distribution of the ultimate state.

1 Introduction

There is an important mathematical literature devoted to the analysis of the spread of an infectious disease of the SIR (Susceptible→ Infected→ Removed) type. The main characteristics of this epidemic process are roughly as follows. A closed population is subdivided into susceptibles, infectives and removed individuals. Each infective is infectious during a random period of time. While infected, it behaves independently of the others and is able to contact susceptibles, who will then become infectives. After that period, the individual is removed, by immunization or by death for example, and plays no further role in the propagation of the disease.

Until twenty years ago, most investigations in the field dealt with two special models, the general epidemic process and the Reed-Frost epidemic process (see e.g. Bailey 1975). Since then, increasing interest has been concentrated on the final outcome of the epidemic, when there are no more infectives present in the population. This led, in a natural way, to various generalizations of the two basic models. In particular, Picard and Lefèvre (1990) introduced recently a quite general process called the collective (Reed-Frost) epidemic model. The process was originally built from considerations of essentially analytical character. It appeared later on that its construction follows too from an appropriate probabilistic argument when describing the transmission of the infection.

The primary purpose of this work is to emphasize that the collective model provides a global and flexible modelling approach to the final outcome of SIR infectious diseases. This will be done by presenting a brief overview of current knowledge concerning first the building of the process, and then the distribution of the ultimate state. The matter thus is not new nor studied in depth. Real effort, however, has been made to obtain what we hope to be a clear and convincing presentation.

The paper is structured as follows. A crucial point here is that only the final outcome of the epidemic is concerned. Section 2 then explains how and why to represent the infection process through successive generations of infectives. In Section 3, we formulate the collective epidemic model and we point out that its construction is very simple, natural and general. Section 4 shows that most standard models for SIR infectious diseases can be obtained as special cases. We indicate in Section 5 how to adapt the model in order to account for variability in infectiousness. Section 6 provides a short summary of the results obtained so far for the exact and asymptotic distributions of the ultimate state and the total area under the trajectory of infectives. In Section 7, we tackle similar questions for those situations where the susceptible population is not uniform but subdivided into several groups homogeneous and different from each other.

Our list of references reflects only the topics we chose to discuss within the framework of SIR epidemic models. It is certainly not complete and may sometimes correspond to personal attraction rather than relative importance. A general survey of mathematical modelling work on SIR infectious diseases prior to 1990 is given in Lefèvre (1990).

2 Describing the infection process in terms of generations of infectives

As a first step in our model building, we are going to point out that

> when attention is focused on the final outcome of the epidemic, standard epidemic models for SIR infectious diseases can be treated in a unified way by describing the infection process through successive generations of infectives.

This observation is due to Ludwig (1975) and has been emphasized later by Von Bahr and Martin-Löf (1980). For clarity, it is reexplained below within the framework of the general epidemic model.

Specifically, under its usual formulation, the general epidemic is represented by the following continuous-time Markov process. At time τ, $\tau \in \mathcal{R}^+$, the population state is defined by the vector (X_τ, Y_τ), where X_τ denotes the number of susceptibles present and Y_τ the number of infectives. Initially, $(X_0, Y_0) = (n, m)$, and given (X_τ, Y_τ), two state changes can occur during the time increment $(\tau, \tau + d\tau)$:

the infection of a susceptible, with probability $\beta X_\tau Y_\tau d\tau + o(d\tau)$, (2.1)

the removal of an infective, with probability $\mu Y_\tau d\tau + o(d\tau)$, (2.2)

with β and $\mu > 0$. The epidemic terminates at the instant $\bar{T} = \inf\{\tau : Y_\tau = 0\}$ where there are no more infectives in the population. Then, $X_{\bar{T}}$ represents the ultimate number of susceptibles, which provides a main measure of the total damage caused by the disease. This is the statistic under investigation here.

An equivalent description of the model is as follows. An individual, if ever infected, is infectious during a random period of time with an exponential distribution of parameter μ. During that period, it is able to contact any susceptible according to a Poisson process of rate β. All the infectious periods and contact processes are independent of each other.

Now, in that model, let us forget the true time order of events and substitute for the original time-scale the following representation by artificial 'generations' of infectives. The initial infectives form generation 0. Generation 1 contains all those who have been contacted by the initial infectives, even after being infected by an infective of a later generation. Similarly, for $t \in \mathcal{N}$, those who have avoided contact with all infectives of generations less than t but have been contacted by an infective of generation t are assigned generation $t+1$. Consider the process $\{S_t, I_t; t \in \mathcal{N}\}$, where S_t is the number of individuals who have escaped contact with all the infectives of generations $0, \ldots, t-1$, and I_t the number of infectives of generation t. For each infective i of generation t, $t \in \mathcal{N}$, let $T_{t,i}$ denote the random length of the associated infectious period. During this period, the infective can contact any of the S_t individuals independently and at the points of a Poisson process of rate β; all the $T_{t,i}$'s are independent and identically distributed (i.i.d.) with an exponential distribution of parameter μ and are independent of the contact processes. Therefore, we see that $\{S_t, I_t; t \in \mathcal{N}\}$ is a discrete-time Markov chain characterized by the relation

$$S_t = S_{t+1} + I_{t+1}, \quad t \in \mathcal{N}, \tag{2.3}$$

and such that given (S_t, I_t), S_{t+1} has a mixed binomial distribution with exponent S_t and random parameter $\exp[-\beta(T_{t,1} + \ldots + T_{t,I_t})]$, written

$$S_{t+1}|(S_t, I_t) =_d MBin[S_t, \prod_{i=1}^{I_t} \exp(-\beta T_{t,i})], \quad t \in \mathcal{N}. \tag{2.4}$$

The process will continue until the instant $T = \inf\{t : I_t = 0\}$. Thus S_T is the number of individuals who have escaped all infectious contacts.

What information can this representation by generations of infectives provide with regard to the original model? We have indicated that the assignment of a generation to an infective may modify artificially the origin of his infection. However, this does not alter the status itself of the infective. Consequently, at the end of the infection both processes yield the same numbers of survivors, i.e., $X_{\hat{T}}$ and S_T are identically distributed.

We note that the argument is closely related to the one usually followed, in a similar context, to establish that the total number of individuals generated by a linear birth-and-death process corresponds to the total progeny of an appropriate branching process (see e.g. Galambos 1988).

What is the advantage of this alternative approach? We observe that in fact, (2.3) and (2.4) hold true whatever the distribution attributed to the infectious periods. Moreover, these relations can be easily adjusted to incorporate more complex infectiousness structures. This is shown in Section 5 for those situations where the infectives pass through successive stages of infection and/or there are several types of infectives with different infectious periods.

Why is it interesting to generalize further this model with the various extensions already mentioned? In fact, (2.4) relies, especially, on the hypothesis that contacts between any given infective and susceptible occur according to a Poisson process. This may be rather restrictive in practice. In particular, a broader and more natural assumption is that an infective contacts susceptibles by applying a sampling procedure within the population. We will see in Section 4 that the proposed extension does allow to cover such a situation, inter alia.

3   Construction of the collective epidemic model

Recently, Picard and Lefèvre (1990) introduced a new epidemic model, similar to that of Martin-Löf (1986), called the collective (Reed-Frost) epidemic process, which generalizes the infection model in terms of generations of infectives presented above. The process is based on two hypotheses. Firstly,

> (a) *the spread of the disease is described again through successive generations of infectives. Thus, at time t, $t \in \mathcal{N}$, the population state is defined, as before, by (S_t, I_t), and the damage relation (2.3) is still applicable.*

It remains to model the survival process during any generation. The previous Markovian formulation is retained, but it is now represented in a quite general way:

(b) $\{S_t, I_t; t \in \mathcal{N}\}$ *is a Markov chain whose transitions are governed by the following rule. Consider, among the n initial susceptibles, any possible subset of size k, $k \in [1, n]$. Then, all the infectives of every generation behave independently. Moreover, each of them fails to transmit infection within such a subset of susceptibles actually present, with the (known) probability $q(k; n)$ which depends only on the sizes k and n.*

We underline that in $q(k; n)$, $k \in \mathcal{N}$, no information is stipulated on the fate of the susceptibles present outside the subset.

This description has been studied in detail by Kissami, Lefèvre and Picard (1993). Let us summarize their analysis. Given the population state (S_t, I_t), the problem addressed is how to determine the number S_{t+1} of surviving susceptibles while being as little specific as possible on the infectious contact process. For that, we begin by associating with each susceptible l, $l = 1, \ldots, S_t$, the random event $A_l \equiv [l$ escapes contacts with the I_t infectives]. Obviously, S_{t+1} is just the exact number of these [non-infection] events that occur. We point out that the A_l's are correlated through the infectiousness exerted by the infectives. In fact, since the susceptibles have similar behaviours, the A_l's form exchangeable events (in de Finetti's sense, that is, the probability of occurrence of every subset of k events, $k = 1, \ldots, S_t$, depends only on the size k; see e.g. Galambos 1988).

Now, putting the epidemic context apart, the problem is in fact closely related to the realization of events among a fixed number, $\bar{n}$ say, of exchangeable events. This leads us back to a classical subject in the basic theory of probability, which has been widely discussed for $\bar{n}$ totally arbitrary events. In the exchangeable case, the approach followed relies on the use of the probabilities

$$P(A_1 \cap \ldots \cap A_k), \quad k = 1, \ldots, \bar{n}. \tag{3.1}$$

Observe that by symmetry (3.1) gives the probability of realization of any given set of k events, with no condition on the fate of the $\bar{n} - k$ others. Standard results then state how the distribution of the exact number of events that occur can be written, in an elegant way, in terms of the probabilities (3.1). These will directly yield the formulae (3.3) and (3.4) below.

Returning to the epidemic model, let us consider, for (S_t, I_t) fixed, the [non-infection] events A_l, $l = 1, \ldots, S_t$, with the survival process such as described in b). For that case, we see that (3.1) is given by

$$P(A_1 \cap \ldots \cap A_k) = [q(k; n)]^{I_t}, \quad k = 1, \ldots, S_t. \tag{3.2}$$

As announced, these probabilities constitute a collection of parameters that allow the conditional distribution of S_{t+1} to be determined. In particular, we obtain for the state probabilities

$$P(S_{t+1} = s | S_t, I_t) = \sum_{k=s}^{S_t} \binom{k}{s}(-1)^{k-s}\binom{S_t}{k}[q(k;n)]^{I_t}, \quad s = 0,\ldots,S_t, \quad (3.3)$$

where $q(0;n) \equiv 1$; and for the descending factorial moments

$$E(S_{t+1,[k]} | S_t, I_t) = S_{t,[k]}[q(k;n)]^{I_t}, \quad k = 1,\ldots,S_t, \quad (3.4)$$

where we put $u_{[k]} = u(u-1)\ldots(u-k+1)$, for $u, k \in [1,n]$.

Finally, we note that in order to implement the model, we have, of course, to be able to evaluate the probabilities $q(k;n)$. This raises the natural question: given a set of n arbitrary numbers $g(k;n)$, $k \in [1,n]$, what conditions should they satisfy to be viewed as a plausible set of $q(k;n)$'s, $k \in [1,n]$? It can be proved that a necessary and sufficient condition is

$$(-1)^{n-k}\Delta^{n-k}g(k;n) \geq 0, \quad k = 1,\ldots,n, \quad (3.5)$$

where $g(0;n) \equiv 1$, Δ denotes the forward difference operator with respect to k (*i.e.* $\Delta g(k;n) = g(k+1;n) - g(k;n)$) and Δ^{n-k} the $(n-k)$th iterate of Δ. To guarantee (3.5), a sufficient condition easy to handle is, for instance, that the $g(k;n)$'s can be expressed as

$$g(k;n) = \phi(1 - k/n), \quad k = 1,\ldots,n, \quad (3.6)$$

where $\phi(\cdot)$ represents an appropriate probability generating function. In practice, especially in epidemic theory, $q(k;n)$'s satisfying (3.5) can generally be readily deduced from the formulation of the model under study. This is illustrated in Sections 4 and 5 with the general epidemic and various extensions.

4 Standard epidemic models derived as special cases

Let us refer to the stochastic models usually proposed for SIR infectious diseases. We are going to show that

> as far as the final outcome of the epidemic is concerned, the collective epidemic process includes standard models for SIR infectious diseases.

The most famous model is the general epidemic process described in Section 2. Its success comes from its original formulation as a continuous-time Markovian process. Indeed, an advantage is that this allows us to obtain not only the final state distribution, but also, at least after some ingenious computations, the time-dependent probabilities of the (true) state (X_τ, Y_τ) (see the references given in Lefèvre 1990). Moreover, a deterministic version is easily associated in a natural way, and although such a construction is questionable, deterministic models are very popular in epidemic theory because of their tractability. The probabilistic approach, however, when it can be performed, is more realistic, powerful and flexible.

In recent years, much effort has been made to derive the final outcome of an epidemic model ruled by a more general (non-Markovian) infection process. A number of those extensions that can be covered by the collective model are presented below chronologically.

4.1 General infectious period distribution

A direct extension of the general epidemic (see e.g. Ludwig 1975) consists in supposing that while infected, each individual can again contact any susceptible according to a Poisson process of rate β, all these processes being independent; and that the corresponding infectious periods are still i.i.d. and independent of the contact processes, but this time with any specified distribution, that of the random variable D say. Obviously, this model is a collective process, and we see that

$$q(k;n) = E[\exp(-k\beta D)], \quad k = 1, \ldots, n. \tag{4.1}$$

For the general epidemic, (4.1) becomes

$$q(k;n) = \mu/(\mu + k\beta), \quad k = 1, \ldots, n. \tag{4.2}$$

Note that when D is equal to some constant d,

$$q(k;n) = [q(n)]^k, \quad k = 1, \ldots, n, \tag{4.3}$$

with $q(n) \equiv \exp(-\beta d)$: the model then can be viewed as equivalent to the standard Reed-Frost epidemic.

It is worth mentioning that $q(k;n)$ given in (4.1) generally depends on the initial susceptible size n through the contact rate β. In particular, for large values of n, it is usually recognized that the probability $1 - q(1;n)$ for any given susceptible to be infected (disregarding the fate of the others) is of order $0(1/n)$. This then means that β be approximately equal to $\hat{\beta}/n$ with $\hat{\beta}$ independent of n.

4.2 The randomized Reed-Frost epidemic

A further generalization is the so-called randomized Reed-Frost epidemic process introduced by Von Bahr and Martin-Löf (1980). This model does not

make any more the restricting assumption that infectives contact susceptibles according to Poisson processes. Instead, each infective i of generation t,
$t \in \mathcal{N}$, is now supposed to fail to infect any given susceptible with the random probability $Q_{t,i}$; all the random variables $Q_{t,i}$ are i.i.d., with any given
distribution, that of the random variable Q say. Thus, we have that

$$q(k;n) = E(Q^k), \quad k = 1,\ldots,n. \tag{4.4}$$

Comparing this with (4.1), we see that that model 4.1 corresponds to the
special case of (4.4) where $Q = \exp(-\beta D)$.

Observe from (4.4) that for Q fixed the fates of the susceptibles are independent. This means that as in (2.4), given (S_t, I_t), S_{t+1} has a mixed
binomial distribution:

$$S_{t+1}|(S_t, I_t) =_d MBin[S_t, \prod_{i=1}^{I_t} Q_{t,i}], \quad t \in \mathcal{N}. \tag{4.5}$$

4.3   Infection through sampling without replacement

Later, Martin-Löf (1986) developed a broader model by representing the infection process originated by any infective through a sampling procedure.
This time, each infective i of generation t, $t \in \mathcal{N}$, is supposed to contact
susceptibles by drawing a sample without replacement, of random size $R_{t,i}$,
from among the n initial susceptibles; all the random variabless $R_{t,i}$ are i.i.d.,
with any given distribution, that of the random variable R say. Therefore,

$$q(k;n) = E\left[\binom{n-k}{R} \middle/ \binom{n}{R}\right], \quad k = 1,\ldots,n. \tag{4.6}$$

From (4.6) and (4.3), it is directly verified that the model 4.2 corresponds to
the particular situation where $R =_d MBin\,(n, 1 - Q)$.

We see in (4.6) that the fates of the susceptibles are interdependent even
when R is fixed. This implies that in general, the conditional distribution of
S_{t+1} will not be of mixed binomial type. We recall that the distribution is
provided by (3.3).

4.4   Infection through sampling with replacement

A closely related process has been examined by Lefèvre and Picard (1989)
(see also Ball 1983). Here, each infective i of generation t, $t \in \mathcal{N}$, is still
supposed to make contacts by sampling a random number $R_{t,i}$ of individuals
among the n initial susceptibles, but now with replacement; all the $R_{t,i}$'s are
i.i.d. and distributed as the random variable R say. This yields

$$q(k;n) = E[(1 - k/n)^R], \quad k = 1,\ldots,n. \tag{4.7}$$

Note from (4.7) and (4.3) that the model 4.2 can be viewed as the special case where R has a mixed Poisson distribution with random parameter $-n ln(Q)$.

In that model too, the conditional distribution of S_{t+1} given by (3.3) does not reduce, generally, to a mixed binomial distribution.

We point out that (4.7) is precisely of the form (3.6) presented as admissible for the $q(k; n)$'s. This is also true for (4.1) in the usual situation where $\beta = \hat{\beta}/n$ with $\hat{\beta}$ independent of n. Equation (4.6), on the contrary, cannot be expressed as (3.6); it satisfies, of course, condition (3.5).

5 Accounting for different degrees in infectiousness

So far, it has been assumed that all the infectives display the same potential of infectiousness. In this section, we point out that

the collective epidemic model can be easily adapted to incorporate different degrees in infectiousness.

Coming back to the general epidemic process, two variants of the model have been mainly proposed to account for differences in the infection levels. They are reformulated below within the wider framework of the model 4.1. Their extensions to the general collective process are straightforward; they can be found in Picard and Lefèvre (1990).

5.1 Epidemic with multi-stage infectious period

A modified version of the model 4.1 supposes that once contacted, an individual passes through successive stages of infection, in number l say, with different levels of infectiousness, before being permanently removed. Numbering the stages of infection $l, l-1, \ldots, 1$, the diagram of the disease process is thus as follows:

susceptible $\rightarrow$ inf.(l) $\rightarrow$ inf.$(l$-$1)$ $\rightarrow \ldots \rightarrow$ inf.(1) $\rightarrow$ removed

where 'inf.(j)' is short for 'infected in stage j'. Initially, there are $m_l, m_{l-1}, \ldots, m_1$ infectives present in the successive stages. While in stage $j, j = l, \ldots, 1$, an infective can contact any susceptible at the points of a Poisson process of rate β_j; all these processes are independent. The infectious periods of all the infectives are independent of each other and of the contact processes. If ever contacted, an individual will sojourn in the l stages of infection for periods distributed as the random variables $(D_l, D_{l-1}, \ldots, D_1)$ say; these random variables may have any specified distribution and may be correlated. For infectives initially in stage $j, j = l, \ldots, 1$, the sojourn periods in the j remaining stages are distributed as $(D_j, \ldots, D_1)$.

Specific applications of this model are numerous. For example, Anderson and Watson (1980) considered the continuous-time Markovian version where the D_j's are independent and exponentially distributed of parameter μ_j, and they then subdivided the l stages into two subsets corresponding to l' periods of latency followed by $l - l'$ periods of infection – with $\beta_l = \ldots = \beta_{l-l'+1} = 0$, $\mu_l = \ldots = \mu_{l-l'+1}$ and $\beta_{l-l'} = \ldots = \beta_1$, $\mu_{l-l'} = \ldots = \mu_1$. In AIDS modelling, Anderson (1988), inter alia, developed a deterministic model with three stages to account for the tentative hypothesis that there are two phases of peak infectiousness during the long incubation period – β_3 and β_1 are thus taken much larger than β_2. Recently, Choi and Severo (1992) examined the Markovian process with two stages of infection, stage 2 being associated with mild symptoms and stage 1 with more serious symptoms – here, $\beta_2 < \beta_1$.

Now, arguing in tems of generations of infectives, we can construct again the Markovian chain $\{S_t, I_t; t \in \mathcal{N}\}$ with the interpretation given earlier. Clearly, the damage relation (2.3) holds true. For the conditional survival distribution of S_{t+1}, distinction has to be made between the cases $t \geq 1$ and $t = 0$. Note that any infective of generation t, $t \geq 1$, will pass necessarily through the l stages of infection. Thus, for $t \geq 1$, the conditional distribution of S_{t+1} is given by (3.3) with

$$q(k; n) = E\{\exp[-k(\beta_l D_l + \ldots + \beta_1 D_1)]\}, \quad k = 1, \ldots, n; \tag{5.1}$$

inserting (5.1) in (3.4) yields the associated factorial moments. For $t = 0$, the situation is not the same because the infectives of generation 0 differ in the number of stages of infection to pass through. In fact, from (3.2), we easily see that the conditional distribution of S_1 is still provided by (3.3) but with the substitution

$$[q(k; n)]^{I_0} \equiv \prod_{j=1}^{\ell} [q_j(k; n)]^{m_j}, \quad k = 1, \ldots, n, \tag{5.2}$$

where we put

$$q_j(k; n) = E\{\exp[-k(\beta_j D_j + \ldots + \beta_1 D_1)]\}, \quad j = 1, \ldots, l; \tag{5.3}$$

the same substitution is applied to (3.4) for the factorial moments.

5.2   Epidemic with several types of infectives

Another variant of the model 4.1 supposes that once contacted, an individual becomes infected of a certain type among several possible types, in number l say, characterized by different levels of infectiousness, before being removed. Here thus, the diagram of the disease process is as follows:

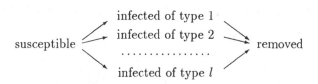

Initially, there are m_1 infectives of type $1, \ldots, m_l$ infectives of type l. While of type j, $j = 1, \ldots, l$, an infective can contact any susceptible at the points of a Poisson process of rate β_j; all these processes are independent. The infectious periods of all the infectives are independent of each other and of the contact processes; for type j, they are distributed as the random variable D_j say, with any specified distribution. If ever contacted, an individual will become of type j, $j = 1, \ldots, l$, with the given probability π_j; obviously, $\pi_1 + \ldots + \pi_l = 1$.

Situations with $l = 2$ types arise when modelling, in particular, infectious diseases spread by both clinically infected persons, called the infectives (type 1), and subclinically infected persons, called the carriers (type 2). Here, a classical epidemic model is the continuous-time Markovian process proposed by Pettigrew and Weiss (1967) where D_1 and D_2 are exponentially distributed with parameters μ_1 and μ_2, and $\beta_1 = \beta_2$. The associated deterministic version was considered by Isham (1988) to describe the initial stages of the spread of AIDS – infectives represent those infected persons who will ultimately develop AIDS, and carriers those seropositives who will not develop AIDS. The carrier-borne model discussed by Downton (1968) corresponds to the special situation where the infectives are immediately detected and removed ($\mu_1 = \infty$), so that infection is transmitted only by the carriers. In case of no carrier birth ($\pi_2 = 0$), the Downton process reduces to the model introduced by Weiss (1965); when infective birth is not allowed ($\pi_1 = 0$), it is equivalent to the general epidemic, with the carriers in the role of the infectives.

As above, we may associate with this model the process $\{S_t, I_t; t \in \mathcal{N}\}$ based on successive generations of infectives. The relation (2.3) remains valid. Now, let us derive the conditional survival distribution of S_{t+1}, by distinguishing again between the cases $t \geq 1$ and $t = 0$. An infected person of generation t, $t \geq 1$, can belong to any of the l types of infective. Thus, for $t \geq 1$, the conditional distribution of S_{t+1} is given by (3.3) with

$$q(k; n) = \sum_{j=1}^{l} \pi_j E[\exp(-k\beta_j D_j)], \quad k = 1, \ldots, n; \qquad (5.4)$$

combining (3.4) and (5.4) yields the factorial moments. The initial infectives being already of a specific type, the conditional distribution of S_1 is provided by (3.3) but now with the substitution (5.2) where we put

$$q_j(k; n) = E[\exp(-k\beta_j D_j)], \quad j = 1, \ldots, l; \qquad (5.5)$$

the same substitution is made in (3.4) for the factorial moments.

6   Distribution of the final outcome of the collective epidemic

We focus our attention on the distribution, exact and asymptotic, of the final number S_T of susceptibles surviving in the collective epidemic process of Section 3. We will close with some comments on another measure of the total damage caused by the disease.

6.1   Equations for the final state probabilities

The exact distribution of S_T has no simple explicit expression, even for the special cases mentioned earlier. A general and fundamental result, however, is that

> the ultimate state probabilities $P(S_T = s)$, $s = 1,\dots,n$, can be
> determined by solving a triangular system of n linear equations.

More precisely, it is easily proved that the n following identities relating to S_T hold true:

$$E\{S_{T,[k]}[q(k;n)]^{S_T}\} = n_{[k]}[q(k;n)]^{n+m}, \quad k = 1,\dots,n, \qquad (6.1)$$

i.e. equivalently,

$$\sum_{s=k}^{n} s_{[k]}[q(k;n)]^s P(S_T = s) = n_{[k]}[q(k;n)]^{n+m}, \quad k = 1,...,n. \qquad (6.2)$$

We emphasize that (6.2) constitutes a triangular system of n linear equations in the n unknown probabilities $P(S_T = s)$, $s = 1,\dots,n$. These can thus be computed recursively for $s = n,\ n-1,\dots,1$. The probability $P(S_T = 0)$ is then given by $1 - P(S_T = 1) - \dots - P(S_T = n)$.

This result was obtained by Picard and Lefèvre (1990); it had been derived previously for the standard models of Section 4. The method followed there is direct and global. It proceeds in two steps: first, a family of n martingales is identified from the relations (3.4); then, the optional stopping theorem is applied with respect to the stopping time T.

In the same work, Picard and Lefèvre (1990) exploited the system (6.1) to construct the probability generating function of S_T and to point out some properties of the distribution. To this end, a powerful key tool is a non-standard family of polynomials introduced by Gontcharoff (1937) and re-examined, in the epidemic context, by Lefèvre and Picard (1990). These developments are beyond the scope of this review.

We indicate that for the modified models (5.1) and (5.2), the system (6.1) has, of course, to be adapted. With the notations (5.1), (5.3) and (5.4), (5.5), this becomes

$$E\{S_{T,[k]}[q(k;n)]^{S_T}\} = n_{[k]}[q(k;n)]^n \prod_{j=1}^{\ell} [q_j(k;n)]^{m_j}, \quad k = 1, ..., n. \quad (6.3)$$

6.2   The asymptotic final state distribution

The asymptotic distribution of S_T *as the initial susceptible population becomes large has been investigated extensively for the special models of Section 4.* Some recent references are Von Bahr and Martin-Löf (1980), Ball (1983), Scalia-Tomba (1985) and Martin-Löf (1986). For the collective process, Kissami (1993) proved that these approximation results can be slightly generalized along similar lines. In particular, there exists a threshold theorem which states roughly that

a true epidemic infecting infinitely many susceptibles can occur with non-zero probability if and only if an appropriate measure of the infection process is above a critical level.

This analysis requires certain conditions on the parameters $q(k;n)$. For simplicity, we limit ourselves to the situation (3.6) where for all $n \in \mathcal{N}$, each $q(k;n)$ corresponds to the value of a probability generating function $\phi(\cdot)$ calculated at the point $1 - k/n$. In other words, there exists a random variable R say, such that all the $q(k;n)$'s can be expressed as in (4.7). The model is thus equivalent to the model 4.4 where an infective makes contacts by sampling R susceptibles with replacement among the n initial ones. It is assumed that the mean λ and the variance ν^2 of R are finite.

Let n tend to ∞. We note that, as announced after (4.3), the probability of infection per individual $1 - q(1;n)$ is then of order $O(1/n)$. Now, the asymptotic results for that case (3.6) are in fact identical with those derived by Martin-Löf (1986) for the model 4.3. This is not surprising since in 4.3 the infectives contact susceptibles by sampling similarly but without replacement, and for n large, that procedure is expected to be equivalent to the former with replacement. Specifically, the following threshold theorem holds.

(i)   Suppose that the initial number of infectives m is finite. Then a true epidemic can occur with non-zero probability if and only if $\lambda > 1$.

If $\lambda \leq 1$, $n - S_T$ is finite and has the same limit distribution as the total progeny of a branching process initiated by m ancestors and with $\phi(\cdot)$ as the offspring probability generating function. The corresponding p.g.f. is given by $[\psi(z)]^m$, $0 \leq z \leq 1$, where $\psi(z)$ is determined by the equation $\psi(z) = \phi[z\psi(z)]$.

If $\lambda > 1$, two opposite behaviours are possible. Let ρ be the root, less than 1, of the equation $z = \phi(z)$, $0 \leq z \leq 1$. With probability ρ^m, $n - S_T$ is finite and is asymptotically distributed as the total progeny in the above associated branching process, but conditional on extinction. With probability $1 - \rho^m$, a true epidemic occurs and $(S_T - n\eta)/\sqrt{n}$ has then a Gaussian limit distribution with mean 0 and variance θ^2. Here, η is the solution, less than 1, of the equation $z = \exp[-\lambda(1 - z)]$, $0 \leq z \leq 1$, and θ^2 denotes the quantity $\eta[1 - \eta + \eta(\nu^2 - \lambda)(1 - \eta)]/(1 - \lambda\eta)^2$.

(ii) Suppose that m is large with $m/n \to a$. Then, there is always a true epidemic and $(S_T - n\eta_a)/\sqrt{n}$ has a Gaussian limit distribution with mean 0 and variance θ_a^2. Here, η_a is the solution of the equation $z = \exp[-\lambda(1+a-z)]$, $0 \leq z \leq 1$, and θ_a^2 is given by $\eta_a[1 - \eta_a + \eta_a(\nu^2 - \lambda)(1 + a - \eta_a)]/(1 - \lambda\eta_a)^2$.

6.3   The final severity of the epidemic

To measure the damage caused by the disease, another statistic of interest introduced by Gani and Jerwood (1972) is *the final severity of the epidemic*, which is defined as the total area under the trajectory of the infectives. Denoted by A_T, it is usually interpreted as the total personal time units of infection during the course of the epidemic.

Clearly, A_T is equal to the sum of the lengths of the infectious periods of all the infectives. Its computation thus requires to make explicit the role of the infectious periods in the modelling. In analogy with the randomized model 4.3, Picard and Lefèvre (1990) adapted the general formulation of the collective process by supposing that each infective i of generation t, $t \in \mathcal{N}$, fails to transmit infection, during his survival time $T_{t,i}$, within any given subset of k susceptibles, $k \in [1, n]$, with the random probability $Q_{t,i}(k; n)$. All the random variables $T_{t,i}$ are i.i.d. and distributed as the random variable D say; all the random variables $Q_{t,i}$ are i.i.d. and distributed as the random variable $Q(k; n)$ say.

The exact joint distribution of (S_T, A_T) has been investigated by Picard and Lefèvre (1990) using the method mentioned in Section 6.1. They first identified a family of $n+1$ martingales involving S_T and A_T; a Wald's identity was deduced that yields, in particular, for the means

$$E(A_T) = [n - E(S_T) + m]\, E(D). \qquad (6.4)$$

They then exploited these martingales to express the joint p.g.f. and Laplace transform of (S_T, A_T) in terms again of the Gontcharoff polynomials.

The asymptotic distribution of A_T has been examined by Ball and Clancy (1993) for the special model 4.1. They proved that A_T can have different limit behaviours similar in form to those indicated in Section 6.2 for S_T. In fact, under the conditions on m and λ stated above, A_T either converges to the corresponding quantity in the associated branching process or it has a Gaussian limit distribution with appropriate parameters.

7 The multipopulation extension of the collective process

The assumption of a homogeneous susceptible population is unlikely to be realised with certain infectious diseases. In AIDS epidemics, for example, it is well recognized that prostitutes, drug users, homosexual, bisexual and heterosexual men and women do constitute groups of variable risks. In this section we are going to indicate, very succinctly, that

> *the collective modelling approach can be extended to the case of a multipopulation which is subdivided into several groups homogeneous and different from each other.*

7.1 Epidemic among a number of homogeneous groups

Following Picard and Lefèvre (1990), we consider a population split into J groups such that the behaviours of the individuals are identical within groups but vary between groups. In each group, susceptibles can be contacted by infectives of any group, and infectives remain active during a random period before being removed. Thus, the diagram of the disease process is of the form:

susceptible of group 1 $\rightarrow$ infected $\rightarrow$ removed
susceptible of group 2 $\rightarrow$ infected $\rightarrow$ removed
$$\vdots$$
susceptible of group J $\rightarrow$ infected $\rightarrow$ removed

Initially, there are $n_1, \ldots, n_J$ susceptibles and $m_1, \ldots, m_J$ infectives present in the J groups. The spread of the epidemic is then described according to the extended collective schema below.

(a) The infection process is represented through successive generations of infectives. At time t, $t \in \mathcal{N}$, the population state is given by $(S_t^{(j)}, I_t^{(j)}, j = 1, \ldots, J)$, where $S_t^{(j)}$ and $I_t^{(j)}$ denote the numbers of susceptibles and infectives (defined as before) in group j, respectively. The damage relation (2.3) is here valid within each group j.

(b) $\{(S_t^{(j)}, I_t^{(j)}, j = 1, \ldots, J); t \in \mathcal{N}\}$ is a Markov chain whose transitions are governed by the following rule. Consider any possible subsets in the J initial classes of susceptibles, of sizes $k_1 \in [0, n_1], \ldots, k_J \in [0, n_J]$, respectively, with $k_1 + \ldots + k_J \geq 1$. Then, all the infectives of every generation behave independently. Moreover, each of those in group j, $j = 1, \ldots, J$, fails to transmit infection within such J subsets of susceptibles actually present, with the (known) probability $q_j(k_1, \ldots, k_J; n_1, \ldots, n_J)$ which depends only on the current group j and on the sizes $k_1, \ldots, k_J$ and $n_1, \ldots, n_J$. Obviously, $k_j = 0$ for any given j means that no specification is made for the susceptible class j. We observe that the probabilities $q_j(\cdot)$ are evaluated independently of the fate of the susceptibles outside the subsets.

For a discussion of this modelling, the reader is referred to Kissami, Lefèvre and Picard (1993). It is shown there that the conditional survival distribution per generation can indeed be expressed in terms of the parameters $q_j(\cdot)$. We note that the fates of all the susceptibles are correlated and they form exchangeable events within every group.

The multipopulation versions of the special models of Section 4 are easily constructed. So, the extended model 4.1 supposes that while infected, an individual in group j, $j = 1, \ldots, J$, can contact any susceptible in each of the J classes at the points of independent Poisson processes, with rates $\beta_{j,1}, \ldots, \beta_{j,J}$ respectively. The infectious periods of all the infectives are independent of each other and of the contact processes; for group j, $j = 1, \ldots, J$, they are distributed as the random variable D_j say. Therefore, we obtain that for $j = 1, \ldots, J$,

$$q_j(k_1, \ldots, k_J; n_1, \ldots, n_J) = E\{\exp[(-k_1\beta_{j,1} - \ldots - k_J\beta_{j,J})D_j]\}, \qquad (7.1)$$
$$k_1 \in [0, n_1], \ldots, k_J \in [0, n_J], \quad k_1 + \ldots + k_J \geq 1$$

7.2   The final outcome of the multi-group epidemic

Now, let us examine the final outcome of the epidemic, at the time $T = \inf\{t : I_t^{(1)} = \ldots = I_t^{(J)} = 0\}$ where there are no more infectives present in the J groups. We denote by $S_T^{(j)}$, $j = 1, \ldots, J$, the ultimate number of susceptibles in group j. The exact distribution of $(S_T^{(1)}, \ldots, S_T^{(J)})$ has been derived and analyzed in Picard and Lefèvre (1990). In particular, they generalized the identities (6.1) by establishing that

$$E\{\prod_{j=1}^{J} S_{T,[k_j]}^{(j)} [q_j(k_1, \ldots, k_J; n_1, \ldots, n_J)]^{S_T^{(j)}}\}$$
$$= \prod_{j=1}^{J} n_{j,[k_j]} [q_j(k_1, \ldots, k_J; n_1, \ldots, n_J)]^{n_j + m_j},$$
$$k_1 \in [0, n_1], \ldots, k_J \in [0, n_J], \quad k_1 + \ldots + k_J \geq 1. \qquad (7.2)$$

The relations (7.2) constitute a system of $[(n_1 + 1)\ldots(n_J + 1) - 1]$ linear equations in the unknown state probabilities $P(S_T^{(1)} = s_1, \ldots, S_T^{(J)} = s_J)$, $s_1 \in [0, n_1], \ldots, s_J \in [0, n_J]$, $s_1 + \ldots + s_J \geq 1$. This can be solved recursively for $s_1 + \ldots + s_J$ equal to $n \equiv n_1 + \ldots + n_J$, then to $n - 1, \ldots, 1$; the probability $P(S_T^{(1)} = \ldots = S_T^{(J)} = 0)$ follows directly.

The limit distribution of $(S_T^{(1)}, \ldots, S_T^{(J)})$ has been investigated by Ball and Clancy (1993) for the above multitype model 4.1. They supposed that the initial size n_j of each susceptible class j is large, and each rate $\beta_{j,l}$ is normalized as $\hat{\beta}_{j,l}/(n_1 + \ldots + n_J)$ with $\hat{\beta}_{j,l}$ independent of $n_1, \ldots, n_J$. The main result stipulates that approximations similar to those obtained for a single population are applicable here too. We note that the particular case of the Reed-Frost process has been examined previously by Scalia-Tomba (1986) and Andersson (1993; contrary to what is claimed by Andersson, his study is not valid for the multitype model 4.3). We also mention that their study is made for a more general process that allows possible movements of infectives (but not of susceptibles) between groups.

To close, let us define the final severity $A_T^{(j)}$, $j = 1, \ldots, J$, as the total area under the trajectory of the infectives in group j. The exact joint distribution of $(S_T^{(1)}, \ldots, S_T^{(J)}; A_T^{(1)}, \ldots, A_T^{(J)})$ has been derived by Picard and Lefèvre (1990). Ball and Clancy (1993) have obtained the asymptotic distribution of $(A_T^{(1)}, \ldots, A_T^{(J)})$ for the previous extended process 4.1.

References

Anderson, D.A. and Watson, R.K. (1980) 'On the spread of a disease with gamma distributed latent and infectious periods', *Biometrika* **67**, 191–198.

Anderson, R.M. (1988) 'The epidemiology of HIV infection: variable incubation plus infectious periods and heterogeneity in sexual activity', *J. R. Statist. Soc. A* **151**, 66–93.

Andersson, H. (1993) 'A threshold limit theorem for a multitype epidemic model', *Math. Biosci.* **117**, 3–18.

Bailey, N.T.J. (1975) *The Mathematical Theory of Infectious Diseases and its Applications*, Griffin, London.

Ball, F.G. (1983) 'The threshold behaviour of epidemic models', *J. Appl. Prob.* **20**, 227–241.

Ball, F.G. and Clancy, D. (1994) 'The size and severity of a generalised stochastic multitype epidemic model', *Adv. Appl. Prob.* **25**, 721–736.

Choi, Y.J. and Severo, N.C. (1992) 'Transition probabilities for a modified general stochastic epidemic model', *Statist. Prob. Lett.* **13**, 401–404.

Downton, F. (1968) 'The ultimate size of carrier-borne epidemics', *Biometrika* **55**, 277–289.

Galambos, J. (1988) *Advanced Probability Theory*, Marcel Dekker, New York.

Gani, J., and Jerwood, D. (1972) 'The cost of a general stochastic epidemic', *J. Appl. Prob.* **9**, 257–269.

Gontcharoff, W. (1937) *Détermination des Fonctions Entières par Interpolation*, Hermann, Paris.

Isham, V. (1988) 'Mathematical modelling of the transmission dynamics of HIV infection and AIDS: a review', *J. R. Statist. Soc. A* **151**, 5–30.

Kissami, A. (1993) *Problèmes d'Urnes et Processus Epidémiques: Modélisation et Résultats Asymptotiques*, PhD Thesis, Université Libre de Bruxelles.

Kissami, A., Lefèvre, C. and Picard, P. (1993) 'A partially exchangeable model for the final outcome of an epidemic', *Working paper, Institute de Statistique, Université de Bruxelles*.

Lefèvre, C. (1990) 'Stochastic epidemic models for SIR infectious diseases: a brief survey of the recent general theory'. In *Stochastic Processes in Epidemic Theory*, J-P Gabriel, C Lefèvre and P Picard (eds.), *Lecture Notes in Biomath.* **86**, Springer, New York, 1–12.

Lefèvre, C. and Picard, P. (1989) 'On the formulation of discrete-time epidemic models', *Math. Biosci.* **95**, 27–35.

Lefèvre, C. and Picard, P. (1990) 'A non-standard family of polynomials and the final size distribution of Reed-Frost epidemic processes', *Adv. Appl. Prob.* **22**, 25–48.

Lefèvre, C., Kissami, A. and Picard, P. (1993) 'On the realization of n (partially) exchangeable events: a further look motivated by the modelling of epidemic processes', *submitted for publication*.

Ludwig, D. (1975) 'Final size distributions for epidemics', *Math. Biosci.* **23**, 33–46.

Martin-Löf, A. (1986) 'Symmetric sampling procedures, general epidemic processes and their threshold limit theorems', *J. Appl. Prob.* **23**, 265–282.

Pettigrew, H.M. and Weiss, G.H. (1967) 'Epidemics with carriers: the large population approximation', *J. Appl. Prob.* **4**, 257–263.

Picard, P. and Lefèvre, C. (1990) 'A unified analysis of the final size and severity distribution in collective Reed-Frost epidemic processes', *Adv. Appl. Prob.* **22**, 269–294.

Scalia-Tomba, G. (1985) 'Asymptotic final size distribution for some chain-binomial processes', *Adv. Appl. Prob.* **17**, 477–495.

Scalia-Tomba, G. (1986) 'Asymptotic final size distribution of the multitype Reed-Frost process', *J. Appl. Prob.* **23**, 563–584.

Von Bahr, B. and Martin-Löf, A. (1980) 'Threshold limit theorems for some epidemic processes', *Adv. Appl. Prob.* **12**, 319–349.

Weiss, G.H. (1965) 'On the spread of epidemics by carriers', *Biometrics* **21**, 481–491.

The Threshold Concept in Stochastic Epidemic and Endemic Models

Ingemar Nåsell

Summary

The threshold concept that has been used so far in mathematical epidemiology is based on the bifurcation caused by nonlinearities in the deterministic models. New definitions are given of thresholds for stochastic models. The threshold for epidemic models is based on the form of the distribution of the final size of the epidemic, and the threshold for endemic models is based on the expected time to extinction. The two types of model are shown to have thresholds that depend on the population size N in different ways. Thus, the threshold for the epidemic SIR model takes the form $R_0 \approx 1 + K_R/N^{1/3}$, where $K_R > 0$. For the endemic SIS model there are two types of threshold: an invasion threshold and a persistence threshold. The former one is higher than the latter one. Both of them behave like $R_0 \approx 1 + K_S/\sqrt{N}$ with $K_S > 0$.

1 Introduction

Mathematical epidemiology is a part of applied mathematics where one establishes and studies models for the spread of infection in a population of hosts. The mechanisms that cause an infection to spread are highly variable and difficult to measure and assess. This fact puts special demands on the mathematical models that are used. It is highly desirable that the model predictions are robust. This means that qualitative properties of the models are especially attractive, and is one of the reasons for the importance of threshold results in mathematical epidemiology.

The threshold concept is reviewed in some detail. Since we are dealing with a subject that belongs to applied mathematics, we shall emphasize the nonmathematical basis for the threshold concept in terms of epidemiological interpretations of the models' properties.

We begin by considering the relation between deterministic and stochastic models. It is true for most model structures that each deterministic model has a natural stochastic counterpart, and vice versa. We adopt the view that the stochastic model is the primary one and that the corresponding deterministic model is an approximation. This approximation of the stochastic model becomes valid only if the population size approaches infinity. Thus, the ability to make statements about a population of finite size is lost when one resorts to a deterministic model. One of the reasons for studying stochastic models is their ability to deal with finite population sizes.

It is well-known that stochastic epidemiological models are difficult to analyse mathematically, while the deterministic ones are more amenable to analysis. It is noteworthy that the stochastic model can often from a certain standpoint be interpreted as a linear one, while the deterministic model is non-linear. Specifically, the stochastic versions of many models are Markov chains for which the problem of determining the state probabilities is linear. Thus, contrary to what is rather common in applied mathematics, in mathematical epidemiology we approximate a difficult linear problem by a less difficult nonlinear one.

Both deterministic and stochastic models make use of a concept called the basic reproduction ratio R_0. In simple cases it can be defined as the number of secondary cases that are produced in a completely susceptible population by one infected individual. This definition is easy to understand heuristically. It implies that there is a threshold at $R_0 = 1$: large epidemics can occur, or endemic infection levels can be established or maintained, if $R_0 > 1$, but not otherwise. A detailed discussion of thresholds for a multitude of deterministic models is given by Diekmann *et al.* (1990). The present paper supplements that of Diekmann *et al.* in a certain sense, since it proposes a threshold concept for stochastic models that generalizes the well-known one in the deterministic setting.

Historically, the deterministic models have been introduced and studied before the stochastic ones, and the threshold behaviour has first been established for deterministic models. The thresholds of the deterministic models are caused by the nonlinearities in these models. Indeed, the threshold in the simplest deterministic models corresponds to a bifurcation set, which is a set of parameter values with the property that small changes in these parameter values may lead to qualitative changes in the corresponding phase portraits. The threshold concept for deterministic models is clear and well-established both mathematically and epidemiologically.

If we now turn to consider stochastic models in mathematical epidemiology we find a rather different situation. I claim that a convincing definition of threshold concepts for stochastic models with finite population size is missing. This claim may appear surprising in view of the fact that many papers have been published that deal with thresholds of stochastic models, see e.g. Whittle (1955), Williams (1971), Ball (1983). However, the threshold results of all these papers are based on letting the population size approach infinity. In this way they recapture the same threshold value for the basic reproduction ratio as the corresponding deterministic model, i.e. the value $R_0 = 1$. (I exclude spatial models in this discussion.) The result is interpreted as saying that the threshold value of R_0 is one if the population size is 'large enough'. There is a difficulty in applying this result to any given community and that is that the model itself gives no guidance for determining if the given finite population size is so large that this limiting result is an acceptable approximation.

The definition of thresholds for stochastic models is the main contribution of this paper. The definitions take different forms for epidemic and endemic infection. Epidemic models are dealt with in Section 2 and endemic ones in Section 3. The definitions for both types of model are based on first interpreting the threshold of the deterministic model in epidemiological terms and then translating these terms to the stochastic model.

An awareness of the need to redefine thresholds because of stochastic phenomena is shown by Anderson and May (1991). They discuss this need in relation to the phenomena of epidemic and endemic fade-out.

The threshold definitions in Sections 2 and 3 aim to simplify the understanding of the intricate properties of the stochastic models by describing them in terms that are similar to those that have been used with success for many years on deterministic models. They also form a challenge on the mathematical level, asking for the analysis to be directed toward an investigation of certain properties of the models that have not been studied previously.

2   Models for epidemic infections

A large number of models can be used to study epidemic infections. For concreteness, we study one of the simplest of such models that possesses a threshold, the so-called general epidemic. This is an example of a so-called SIR model. The letters SIR refer to the consecutive possible states of an individual who is assumed to pass from a susceptible via an infected to a removed state. The reasons for removal can be different, but they all have the consequence that the removed individual no longer takes part in the transmission of the infection. The threshold definition given below can, with minor modifications, be used on a number of other models for epidemic infections.

The model that we study is described in detail by Bailey (1975). Briefly, it is a bivariate Markov chain $\{S(t), I(t)\}$, $t \geq 0$, where $S(t)$ and $I(t)$ are interpreted as the number of susceptible and infected individuals, respectively, at time t. The initial number of susceptible individuals is denoted by $S(0) = N$, and the initial number of infected individuals by $I(0) = I_0$. Transition from the state (m, n) to $(m - 1, n + 1)$ corresponds to infection of one individual. The rate of such a transition is βmn. Transition from the state (m, n)

to $(m, n - 1)$ corresponds to recovery of one individual. The rate of such a transition is γn.

The deterministic version of this model has a threshold behaviour in the sense that the number of infected individuals increases initially if $R_0 > 1$, while it decreases monotonically if $R_0 \leq 1$, where $R_0 = N\beta/\gamma$. This threshold behaviour allows us to answer the following epidemiological question: will there be an epidemic outbreak if we introduce a small amount of infection into a community free of infection? The answer to this question is yes if the basic reproduction ratio R_0 is above its threshold value of one and otherwise it is no. Both question and answer serve to describe the model in qualitative terms.

The behaviour of this stochastic SIR model can be described in terms of the distribution of the total size of the epidemic, i.e. the distribution of the number of individuals that ultimately become infected before the epidemic ceases. We shall use numerical methods for illustrating the form of these distributions. There are several formulas available for numerically determining the distribution of the size of the epidemic. All of them can be used for small population sizes, but the numerical demands inrease as the population size grows. From a numerical standpoint, the formulas given by (6.49) in Bailey (1975) (first derived by Bailey in 1953) are superior to several alternatives.

Distributions of the epidemic size for three values of the basic reproduction ratio R_0 and two values of the initial number of infected individuals I_0 are shown in Figures 1-3. In all of these distributions, the initial number of susceptibles is kept constant at $N = 100$. The distributions have been determined numerically by programming the algorithm given by (6.49) in Bailey (1975) in MATLAB on a SUN workstation.

Kendall (1956) has classified the distributions of the epidemic size as having one of two shapes, called J-shape and U-shape. The term J-shape refers to a distribution that either is monotonically decreasing (so it has a mode at the origin), or has a mode at some small positive value of the argument. Thus all four distributions shown in Figures 1 and 2 are J-shaped. The distribution is said to have U-shape if it is bimodal, as shown by both the distributions in Figure 3.

It is natural to interpret a distribution that has J-shape as describing a small epidemic, and to interpret a distribution that has U-shape as associated with either a small or a large epidemic. This interpretation embodies a qualitative result. The epidemiological question posed above in conjunction with our discussion of the deterministic version of the SIR model can be answered with yes only if there is a possibility of a large epidemic, i.e. only if the distribution of the epidemic size is U-shaped. It is therefore natural to suggest the following definition of a threshold for the stochastic SIR model:

Definition: The stochastic SIR model has its *threshold* at that

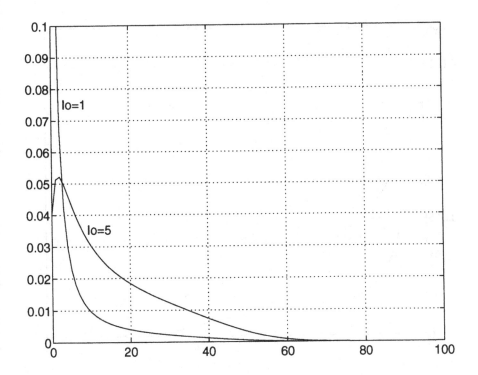

Figure 1.   Size distribution of the general epidemic ($N = 100$, $R_0 = 0.9$).

value of the basic reproduction ratio R_0 for which the distribution
of the total size of the epidemic makes a transition from J-shape
to U-shape.

Figure 2 illustrates the important fact that the transition from J-shape
to U-shape does not take place exactly at the deterministic threshold where
the basic reproduction ratio R_0 is equal to one. This fact was noted already
by Bailey (1975). On page 100 of his 1975 book he reports the result of a
calculation that shows that the distribution of the size of the epidemic is still
J-shaped when the population size is $N = 40$, the basic reproduction ratio is
$R_0 = 40/39$ and $I_0 = 1$. In view of our definition above, this result shows that
the threshold for the stochastc SIR model with a population size of $N = 40$
is larger than $40/39$.

I conjecture that the threshold for the SIR model, as defined above, varies

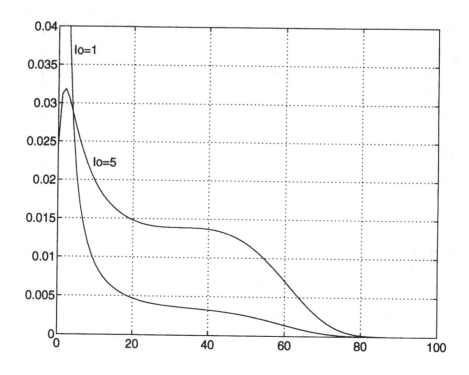

Figure 2.   Size distribution of the general epidemic ($N = 100$, $R_0 = 1.1$).

with the population size N according to the formula $R_0 \approx 1 + K_R/N^{1/3}$. The conjecture is based on numerical evaluations. Note that this conjectured result is consistent with the result that the threshold for the deterministic SIR model is at $R_0 = 1$, since the deterministic model becomes an acceptable approximation of the stochastic one when N approaches infinity. The deterministic threshold requires N to approach infinity, while the stochastic model threshold gives an approximation for finite value of N. The conjectured approximation of the threshold is supported by results by Ball and Nåsell (1994).

The first result showing a threshold that depends on the population size N for an epidemic model is reported by Andersson (1991). By using numerical methods he has found that the threshold (as defined above) of the Reed-Frost model is approximately equal to $R_0 \approx 1 + K/N^{1/3}$. The constant K will, as above, depend on the initial number of infected individuals. Its numerical

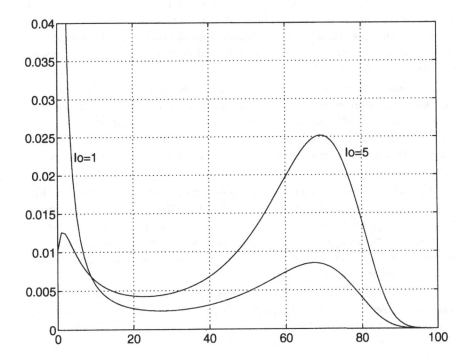

Figure 3. Size distribution of the general epidemic ($N = 100$, $R_0 = 1.5$).

value for the Reed-Frost model is different from that for the general epidemic.

3   Models for endemic infections

We proceed to consider endemic infections in the present section. As in the preceding section, the ideas will be advanced in a very concrete setting given by one of the simplest examples of endemic models, namely the so-called closed SIS model. The modifications necessary to deal with other stochastic endemic models should be obvious. In the SIS model, when an infected individual recovers he is transferred back to the susceptible state. This means that the infection does not lead to any immunity. The SIS model was first discussed by Weiss and Dishon (1971).

The model can be described as a univariate Markov chain $\{I(t)\}$, $t \geq 0$, where $I(t)$ can be interpreted as the number of infected individuals at time t. The state space is the set of all non-negative integers smaller than or equal to N, where N is the population size. Transition from the state n to the state $n + 1$ corresponds to infection of one individual and is hypothesized to take place with the rate $\beta n(N - n)$. Transition from the state n to the state $n - 1$ corresponds to recovery of one individual and is hypothesized in the model to take place with the rate γn.

The deterministic version of this model leads to a differential equation for the proportion of infected individuals $i = I/N$. By introducing the scaled time $\tau = \beta Nt$, we are led to the logistic differential equation $i' = ((R_0 - 1)/R_0 - i)i$ for the proportion i of infected individuals, where the basic reproduction ratio R_0 has the same formal definition as for the SIR model, namely $R_0 = N\beta/\gamma$.

There are two natural epidemiological questions that one can pose in this case. Both of them ask for the result of letting the processes of infection and recovery go on for a long time. In the first case we consider the invasion problem, when initially one (or a small number) of individuals is infected. In the second case we consider the persistence problem, when an endemic infection level is present at the outset.

The questions ask for qualitative answers; either the infection dies out or it establishes itself or persists. In addition, it is natural to ask for the threshold condition that separates these two possibilities from each other and to give the endemic level in case it is positive. We are going to pose these questions to both the deterministic and the stochastic versions of the model.

The simple nonlinear differential equation in the deterministic model has its bifurcation set at $R_0 = 1$, and we call this the threshold value for the model. The solution of the differential equation approaches the value 0 for all initial values if $R_0 \leq 1$, while the solution approaches the positive stationary solution $(R_0 - 1)/R_0$ if $R_0 > 1$, provided the initial value of i is positive. Thus, any amount of infection present initially will disappear with time if R_0 is less than or equal to its threshold value, while a positive endemic infection level will establish itself if R_0 is above its threshold value whenever the initial infection level is positive.

Therefore, the threshold in the deterministic model is the same for the invasion problem and the persistence problem. The two problems do however differ in the sense that the time required for getting close to the limiting value can be large in the invasion problem when the initial infection level is small, while the same time is equal to zero in the persistence problem.

If we now direct these two epidemiological questions to the stochastic model, we get different answers to both questions: the infection will ultimately die out, regardless of the value of the basic reproduction ratio R_0 and of the initial distribution. With this interpretation, the threshold found in the deterministic model is absent from the stochastic one. The reason is that the stochastic SIS model has an absorbing state at the origin. The probability of visiting the absorbing state is positive (although it can be small) for all initial states. Furthermore, if the process ever reaches the absorbing state, it will remain there for all future time.

If we are to understand what causes this difference between the deterministic and stochastic models, we need to analyze the latter model in more detail. One feature of the stochastic model that resembles the qualitative threshold behaviour of the deterministic model is the time to extinction. It has qualitatively different behaviours below and above the threshold for the deterministic model. Below the threshold it is small and practically independent of the population size N, while above the threshold it becomes large and grows exponentially with N. Indeed, it is easy to find examples where the expected time to extinction even for a rather small population exceeds the age of the universe. If the time to extinction is long, then the state of the process is for a long time well approximated by the so-called quasi-stationary distribution. This is the stationary solution of the set of equations that describe the time development of the process under condition of non-extinction. It is the natural counterpart in the stochastic model of the stationary solution for the deterministic model. Quasi-stationary distributions for continuous-time Markov chains with finite state space were first discussed by Darroch and Seneta (1967). Some results concerning both the quasi-stationary distribution and the times to extinction for the model discussed here are given by Kryscio and Lefèvre (1989). The times to extinction for a related SIS model with constant time of infection is studied by Longini (1980).

The properties of the stochastic model show that even though the infection will ultimately die out for all values of R_0, this fact is in itself of limited practical usefulness. Improved information requires us to quantify the term 'ultimately'. This can be done by pragmatically deciding when we regard the time to extinction as 'large' or 'small'. An endemic infection level will be established and maintained, respectively, if the expected time to extinction is 'large', and the infection will die out if the expected time to extinction is 'small'. Thus the two thresholds (for invasion and persistence, respectively) of the stochastic model appear where the expected time to extinction is at the boundary between 'large' and 'small'.

The need to decide when a waiting time is large or small is a new feature that has no counterpart in deterministic models. As a first step it is reasonable to require the waiting time to be related to the expected time for one infected individual to recover, $1/\gamma$, since this quantity is a natural time unit for the model. Second, one may want to allow for the waiting time to depend on the population size N. Thus we are led to propose that the boundary time is of the form $f(N)/\gamma$, where it remains to decide on the form of the function f.

We proceed to suggest the following definition of invasion and persistence thresholds for the stochastic SIS model:

> **Definition:** The stochastic SIS model has its *invasion* and *persistence thresholds* at those values of the basic reproduction ratio R_0 for which the expected time to extinction equals $f(N)/\gamma$ for some choice of nondecreasing function f. For the invasion threshold, time is measured from the moment when the initial number of infected individuals equals one, and for the persistence threshold time is measured from the moment when the initial distribution of infected individuals equals the quasi-stationary distribution.

Different choices of f are appropriate in different situations. One possibility is to let $f(N)$ be independent of N and equal to 10 or 100. This means that the boundary time is one or two orders of magnitude larger than the natural time unit $1/\gamma$. There is an apparent imprecision in this suggestion that may be surprising or even disturbing. It is clear that different choices of this boundary time will lead to different threshold values. However, most of them lie in an area where the expected time to extinction is making the transition from a small dependence on N to an exponential growth. Thus, the difference between two thresholds that are based on two waiting times that are an order of magnitude apart (i.e. differ by a factor of ten) can be expected to be small.

One can show that by choosing $f(N)$ to be constant in this way, we are led to a persistence threshold whose limiting value as $N \to \infty$ is less than one, and that the corresponding limiting value of the invasion threshold is equal to one. Since both of the threshold values are equal to one in the deterministic model, this choice of waiting time does not generalize the threshold concept of the deterministic model.

The two thresholds are illustrated in Figure 4 for the choice $f(N) = 2\sqrt{N}$. The figure indicates that each of the thresholds is asymptotically approximated by $R_0 \approx 1 + K_S/\sqrt{N}$ for some positive K_S value. One can show that $f(N)$ must asymptotically grow at least as $\sqrt{N}$ for large N if this asymptotic behaviour is to hold for both of the thresholds. Note that our choice of $f(N)$ for Figure 4 gives a boundary time that is described as small for the spatial epidemic model studied by Durrett (1995). Numerically we find that the invasion threshold is approximated by $R_0 \approx 1 + 3.4/\sqrt{N}$ and the persistence threshold by $R_0 \approx 1 + 1.1/\sqrt{N}$.

Jacquez and Simon (1993) define an invasion threshold for the stochastic SIS model in a different way. They consider the case where one individual is infected initially and show that the expected number of infected individuals then grows initially if $R_0 > N/(N-1)$ and that it decreases initially if

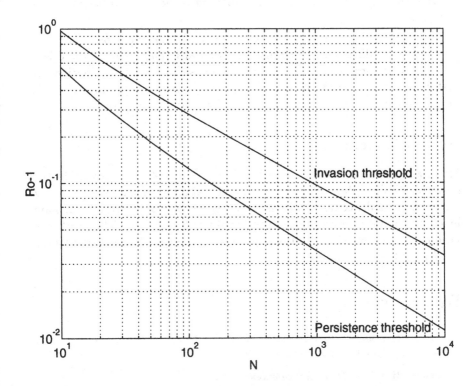

Figure 4. Threshold values for R_0 as a function of N.

$R_0 < N/(N-1)$. The behaviour of the stochastic SIS model is in this sense similar to that of the deterministic version of the SIR model. Based on this dichotomy in behaviour, Jacquez and Simon propose that the invasion threshold for the stochastic SIS model should be put at $R_0 = N/(N-1)$.

A detailed study of the quasi-stationary distribution and of the time to extinction for the stochastic SIS model is reported separately by Nåsell (1995). It is shown that the quasi-stationary distribution is approximated by a geometric distribution (discrete!) for $R_0 < 1$ and by a normal distribution (continuous!) for $R_0 > 1$. The approximation is uniform in R_0. By virtue of the uniformity we can study the transition between these two extreme distributions that takes place as R_0 passes the value one. These analytical results are derived by the use of asymptotic approximations that are uniform in R_0. The results are used to study the expected time to extinction from the quasi-stationary distribution needed for the persistence threshold. The expected time to extinction from the state one is also studied. It is needed for the invasion threshold. It does not require knowledge about the quasi-stationary distribution.

The fully stochastic version of the Ross malaria model can be interpreted as a bivariate SIS model. This model has an absorbing state at the origin and it is therefore of interest to study its quasi-stationary distribution. A first step in such a study is reported by Nåsell (1991). Our studies of this model have given insight into the phenomena studied in this section.

Acknowledgements

My ideas about a threshold concept for stochastic models were inspired by the results of Philippe Picard (1989); he showed that different ways of simplifying a stochastic model could lead to different expressions for the threshold. I am indebted to Håkan Andersson for stimulating discussions. This work has been partly supported by the Royal Swedish Academy of Sciences and by the Prudential Corporation plc.

References

Anderson, R.M. and May, R.M. (1991) *Infectious Diseases of Humans: Dynamics and Control*, Oxford Univ. Press, Oxford.

Andersson, H. (1991) *(Personal communication)*.

Bailey, N.T.J. (1975) *The Mathematical Theory of Infectious Diseases and its Applications*, Griffin, London.

Ball, F. (1983) 'The threshold behaviour of epidemic models', *J. Appl. Prob.* **20**, 227–241.

Ball, F. and Nåsell, I. (1994) 'The shape of the size distribution of an epidemic in a finite population', *Math. Biosci.*, to appear.

Darroch, J.N. and Seneta, E. (1967) 'On quasi-stationary distributions in absorbing continuous-time finite Markov chains', *J. Appl. Prob.* **4**, 192–196.

Diekmann, O., Heesterbeek, J.A.P. and Metz, J.A.J. (1990) 'On the definition and the computation of the basic reproduction ratio R_0 in models for infectious diseases in heterogeneous populations', *J. Math. Biol.* **28**, 365–382.

Durrett, R. (1995) 'Spatial epidemic models', this volume.

Jacquez, J.A. and Simon, C.P. (1993) 'The stochastic SI model with recruitment and deaths. I. Comparisons with the closed SIS model', *Math. Biosci.* **117**, 77–125.

Kendall, D.G. (1956) 'Deterministic and stochastic epidemics in closed populations', *Proc. Third Berkeley Symp. Math. Statist. and Prob.* **4**, 149–165.

Kryscio, R.J. and C. Lefèvre (1989) 'On the extinction of the S-I-S stochastic logistic epidemic', *J. Appl. Prob.* **27**, 685–694.

Longini, I.M. (1980) 'A chain binomial model of endemicity', *Math. Biosci.* **50**, 85–93.

Nåsell, I. (1991) 'On the quasi-stationary distribution of the Ross malaria model', *Math. Biosci.* **107**, 187–208.

Nåsell, I. (1995) 'The quasi-stationary distribution of the closed endemic SIS model', to appear.

Picard, P. (1989) 'Two variants of the first Nåsell-Hirsch model', *Math. Biosci.* **94**, 45–85.

Weiss, G.H. and M. Dishon (1971) 'On the asymptotic behavior of the stochastic and deterministic models of an epidemic', *Math. Biosci.* **11**, 261–265.

Whittle, P. (1955) 'The outcome of a stochastic epidemic – a note on Bailey's paper', *Biometrika* **42**, 211-222.

Williams, T. (1971) 'An algebraic proof of the threshold theorem for the general stochastic epidemic', *Adv. Appl. Prob.* **3**, 223.

How Does Transmission of Infection Depend on Population Size?

Mart C.M. de Jong

Odo Diekmann

Hans Heesterbeek

Summary

In this paper, the dependence of transmission on the total population size is studied, assuming that the relevant contacts between individuals occur by random encounters, i.e. by mass-action kinetics. We compare two different approaches for homogeneously mixing populations of constant density, which we shall distinguish as pseudo mass-action kinetics and true mass-action kinetics. In the first approach, pseudo mass-action, which is frequently used in the literature, the force-of-infection is described in terms of the population sizes of the susceptible and infectious subpopulations. Consequently, the transmission term used in pseudo mass-action models is βXY, where β is the transmission constant and X and Y are the sizes of the susceptible and infectious subpopulation respectively. In the second approach, called true mass-action, the transmission term is $\beta XY/N$, where N is the total population size. It is first shown that from a theoretical point of view the true mass-action approach is the correct one for modelling the transmission term. It is further shown that indeed some existing experimental and observational data are in agreement with the predictions made from true mass-action models. The aim of this paper, therefore, is to convince the user of homogeneous mixing models to use the true mass-action assumption, i.e. $\beta XY/N$.

1 Introduction

In mathematical models for the spread of infections, the force-of-infection, i.e. the probability per unit of time that a given susceptible individual becomes infected, is a crucial ingredient. Hence, the assumptions made regarding the force-of-infection deserve careful scrutiny (Mollison 1984, 1985). As a first step to examine the assumptions underlying the force-of-infection, it will be split in three factors. The first factor is the contact rate, i.e. the average number of relevant contacts with other individuals per unit of time.

The second is the probability that, if such a contact occurs, it is with an infectious individual. The third is the probability that such a contact with an infectious individual results in transmission of the infection. In this paper we are concerned with possible effects of population size on the contact rate and on the probability that such contacts are with infectious individuals. We assume that the probability that a susceptible individual gets infected, given that a contact occurs between that susceptible individual and an infectious one, is constant.

It has long been a standard approach in mathematical epidemiology to model the spatial density of contacts per unit of time between susceptible individuals and infectious individuals by analogy to chemical reaction kinetics (Hamer 1906, Kermack and McKendrick 1927, De Palma and Lefevre 1988). In that approach, the transmission term, i.e. the force-of-infection times the density of susceptible individuals, is derived from the mass-action assumption, which is the assumption that the density of relevant contacts per unit of time, i.e. the number of contacts occurring between a susceptible individual and an infectious individual per unit time per unit area, is proportional both to the density of susceptible individuals and to the density of infectious individuals. This particular formulation of the transmission term, where the force-of-infection is proportional to the density of infectious individuals, will be called the true mass-action assumption. The true mass-action assumption is valid whenever individuals move randomly within the space in which the population lives with 'contacts' corresponding to 'collisions'.

True mass-action implies that the contact rate increases linearly with population density, but is independent of the total area and, hence, of the total population size. It is likely that true mass-action is not an accurate description of the contact rate for high densities of individuals (Mollison 1985). Saturation of the contact rates will occur, because of time limitation or because of satiation effects in case of e.g. sexual contacts. It is possible to derive, from a mechanistic model which takes the duration of contacts into account, an expression for the contact rate, where the contact rate increases proportional to the density at low densities and is constant at high densities, see Heesterbeek and Metz (1993). However, in what is to follow we will only discuss populations with constant density, but different size, and thus saturation of contact rates with density is of no concern.

Anderson and May (1979) formulate transmission in terms of numbers of individuals instead of densities: they assume that the number of new infections per unit of time is proportional to the product of the number of susceptible individuals and the number of infectious individuals. This variant will be labelled the pseudo mass-action assumption. There the force-of-infection is proportional to the population size of the infectious subpopulation. It is not clear what mechanism could lead to a linear increase of contact rate with total population size as implied by pseudo mass-action. One way to arrive at such a linear increase with population size is to reason that the area considered is constant and hence any increase in numbers is an increase in density. This is the explanation given by Kermack and McKendrick (1927) and May and Anderson (1985). One should realise, however, that mass-action is concerned with local densities, e.g. the average distance to nearest neighbours, and not with 'formal' densities, obtained by including area not occupied by the population. There are mechanisms that could cause contact rates to increase with population size (although it's unlikely to be exactly linear) at least for small population sizes. For example: loss of infectious material over the borders of the area in which the population lives, and active search for contacts with individuals not encountered before.

For pseudo mass-action models, Dietz (1982) and Schenzle and Dietz (1987), have pointed out that one should at high numbers take saturation in contact rate into account. They argue correctly that it is unlikely that in a population of 1,000,000 each individual has ten times as many contacts as in a population of 100,000. Note, however, that an alternative argument is that the larger population probably occupies an area 10 times as large as the smaller population. Hence, densities are the same and therefore, assuming true mass-action, each individual has the same number of contacts.

Although we consider true mass-action to be more plausible than the pseudo mass-action this does of course not guarantee that real micro-organisms in real host populations behave accordingly. For example, Anderson and May (1979) obtained a good fit of both the qualitative and quantitative predictions of the pseudo mass-action model to experimental data, in spite of the fact that these data originated from an experiment where only the total population size was changing, and the density remained constant (see below). However, also Kermack and McKendrick (1939) obtained a very good fit using a true mass-action model on a similar data-set but for a different micro-organism. Kermack and McKendrick (1939) did not analyse the dynamics of their model when total population sizes change but densities are constant. Here, we will analyse the dynamics of both the true and pseudo mass-action models (Section 2, see also Thieme (1992)), and compare the predictions from these models to the experiments by Greenwood *et al.* (1936) that were used by Anderson and May (1979) (Section 3).

2   Theory

2.1   Pseudo mass-action

The consequences of using either true mass-action or pseudo mass-action are studied by formulating and analysing two models based upon these two assumptions, but which have otherwise the same ingredients. In these models population size changes but population density is constant. The first model to be described, is based upon the pseudo mass-action assumption and it was formulated by Anderson and May (1979). Let X, Y and Z be the numbers of susceptible, infectious and immune individuals respectively. The model is given by the following set of ordinary differential equations:

$$\frac{dX}{dt} = A - bX - \beta XY + \gamma Z$$
$$\frac{dY}{dt} = \beta XY - (b + \alpha + \nu)Y \qquad [\text{P}]$$
$$\frac{dZ}{dt} = \nu Y - (b + \gamma)Z$$

where A is the number of individuals added per unit of time, b is the probability per unit of time to die from causes unrelated to the infection, β is the transmission constant, γ is the probability per unit of time of losing immunity, α is the additional mortality due to the infection, and ν is the probability per unit of time that the individual recovers.

The model [P] has two steady states (Anderson and May 1979): (1) absence of infection, when $Y^* = Z^* = 0$ and the total population size $N^* = X^* = A/b$, and (2) presence of infection, when

$$N^* = \frac{A + DX^*}{b + D}$$

where $X^* = (\alpha + b + \nu)/\beta$ and $D = \alpha/(1 + \frac{\nu}{b+\gamma})$.

Note that the total population size in the steady state is a linear function of A, with positive intercept. The first stationary state, absence of infection, is a locally asymptotically stable steady state whenever $R_{0,P} < 1$, where

$$R_{0,P} = \frac{N^*\beta}{\alpha + b + \nu},$$

and the endemic steady state is locally asymptotically stable when $R_{0,P} > 1$. Note that $R_{0,P}$, the basic reproduction ratio for the pseudo mass-action model, depends on the total population size N. Hence, there is a critical population size above which the infection spreads and consequently a bifurcation occurs when the parameter A reaches a critical value (Figure 1).

2.2 True mass-action model

Next, this pseudo mass-action model [P] of Anderson and May will be compared to the corresponding true mass-action model. The only difference between true and pseudo mass-action model is in the formulation of the transmission term: for true mass-action the transmission 'constant' depends on N

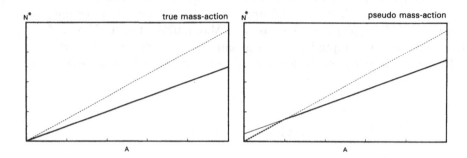

Figure 1. Steady state population size (N^*) as a function of the number of mice added per day (A) separated for the two models ([T] or [P]) having either variant of the transmission term. In each graph there is one (dashed) line for the relationship in the absence of the infection ($N^* = A/b$), and one (continuous) line for the presence of the infection. In the pseudo mass-action model the two lines intersect and there exists a critical rate of adding mice below which the infection cannot spread. In the true mass-action model the line for the presence of the infection lies either entirely below the line of absence of infection ($R_{0,T} > 1$), or it lies entirely above the line of absence of infection ($R_{0,T} < 1$). In both graphs the stable steady states are indicated by thick lines and the unstable by thin lines.

and for pseudo mass-action it is really a constant. The dependence of the transmission constant on N reflects the fact that, whereas for constant density and increasing population size the number of individuals encountered per individual does not change, the probability of encountering any particular individual decreases. The transmission term in the true mass-action model [T] can be 'derived' using a direct argument in terms of numbers: as a fraction Y/N of all encounters is with infectious individuals, and there is a constant number of effective encounters per unit of time (β), the total number of infections per unit of time for X susceptible individuals is ($\beta XY)/N$. The set of ordinary differential equations we will call the true mass-action model is:

$$\frac{dX}{dt} = A - bX - \beta\frac{XY}{N} + \gamma Z$$

$$\frac{dY}{dt} = \beta\frac{XY}{N} - (b + \alpha + \nu)Y \qquad\qquad [\text{T}]$$

$$\frac{dZ}{dt} = \nu Y - (b + \gamma)Z$$

The model [T] has two stationary states: (1) absence of the infection, when $Y^* = Z^* = 0$ and $X^* = N^* = A/b$, and (2) presence of the infection, when:

$$N^* = \frac{A}{b + D(1 - \frac{1}{R_{0,T}})}$$

with D as given above and $R_{0,T} = \beta/(\alpha+b+\beta)$. Note that N^* is again a linear function of A, but now the intercept is always equal to zero. The first stationary state, absence of disease, is locally asymptotically stable when $R_{0,T} < 1$. Note that $R_{0,T}$, the basic reproduction ratio for the true mass-action model, is independent of the total population size. The endemic stationary state is locally asymptotically stable when $R_{0,T} > 1$ (Figure 1). The stability results for both models have been obtained earlier by Mena-Lorca and Hethcote (1992). These authors also compare the predictions of the two models to the experimental data as presented in Anderson and May (1979). However, their observation that these data show that the pseudo mass-action assumption leads to a better fit than the true mass- action assumption is unwarranted, because in this particular case, as we will show in Section 3.2 there is no significant difference between the two predictions.

2.3   Theoretical justification

In this section we derive the analogue of models [T] and [P] formulated in terms of densities of susceptible and infectious individuals. This formulation is based on the original meaning of mass-action, i.e. that the transmission term is expressed in densities. We show that from this model, one obtains model [T] as the correct counterpart formulated in terms of numbers instead of densities. We follow as closely as possible the assumptions underlying the model [P], the model that Anderson and May (1979) used to describe the Greenwood *et al.* (1936) experiment where *Pasteurella muris* was studied in a mouse population that was artificially kept at a constant density. Let x denote the density of susceptible individuals, y the density of infectious individuals and z the density of immune individuals. The following equations provide a true mass-action model similar to Anderson and May's model:

$$\begin{aligned}
\frac{dx}{dt} &= \frac{A}{N} - \beta xy + \gamma z + \alpha yx \\
\frac{dy}{dt} &= \beta xy - (\alpha + \nu)y - \frac{A}{N}y + \alpha y^2 \qquad [d] \\
\frac{dz}{dt} &= \nu y - \gamma z - \frac{A}{N}z + \alpha yz
\end{aligned}$$

where we normalise $x + y + z = 1$ because the overall population density n $(= x + y + z)$ is assumed to be constant. Because we take as one unit of area the area available to one mouse (i.e. we assumed $n = 1$), it follows that the area available to N mice is N units Hence, adding A susceptible individuals increases the density of the susceptible individuals (x) by A/N. However, as the overall density is kept constant, all three densities (x, y and z) will decrease proportionally. Thus, due to our scaling for the area, the amounts Ax/N, Ay/N and Az/N have to be discounted for when A susceptible individuals are added. The same occurs with the per capita death rate due to the infection: the density of the infectious subpopulation decreases with αy and all densities have to be increased proportionally (αyx, αy^2 and αyz). The disease-unrelated death rate does not appear in the equations based on the densities as this death rate affected all individuals equally and therefore it does not change the densities. Now, note that $x = X/N$, $y = Y/N$, $z = Z/N$, and assume that the total number of individuals (and hence also the total area used by the population) changes as:

$$\frac{dN}{dt} = A - bN - \alpha Y.$$

Then if one rewrites Equations [d] using the above substitutions one obtains the true mass-action model [T].

3   Experimental and observational evidence for true mass-action

3.1   Evidence from published analyses

From the above it emerges that the predictions of simple epidemic models concerning the question how transmission of infections changes with population size, depend strongly on which mass-action assumption is used. Models with the true mass-action assumption have a transmission parameter that is inversely proportional to the population size, and a R_0 that is independent of population size. In contrast, models based on the pseudo mass-action assumption have a transmission parameter that is independent of population size, but an R_0 that is proportional to population size.

The next thing to do is compare these predictions with data. As far as we know there have been few attempts to confront predictions of simple epidemic models with data-sets. We know of two comparisons with observations and two comparisons with experimental data. None of these comparisons falsify the predictions of models based upon the true mass-action assumption, and three out of four data-sets falsify predictions of the models based upon the pseudo mass-action assumption.

Anderson and May (1979) fitted model [P] based on pseudo mass-action to the data-set of Greenwood *et al.* (1936) on *P. muris* in mice. As they obtained a good fit it seemed that this would refute the true mass-action assumption. However, as we show in Section 3.2, an equally good fit is obtained with model [T] based on the true mass-action assumption.

Becker and Angulo (1981) estimated the transmission parameter for small-pox from data on this infection in Brazil. Their estimate for the transmission parameter based on household data was 100,000 times as high as their estimate based on community data. This is not in agreement with the pseudo mass-action assumption: for the pseudo mass-action assumption to be true the transmission parameters had to be constant. The result is, however, in agreement with the true mass-action assumption, for which the transmission parameter should change in inverse proportion to population size. This was the case, as the population sizes were 5 for households and 500,000 for the community.

The next comparison of model prediction to observational data is by Anderson (1982): population sizes were plotted against R_0 for data-sets regarding measles, pertussis, diphtheria, and scarlet fever. Instead of showing a linear increase of R_0 with population size, as predicted by pseudo mass-action models, R_0 showed a weak non-linear increase with population size, $R_0 = \beta N^v$, with estimates of v for the different infections varying between 0.03 and 0.07. Significance testing against the hypothesis that in fact $v = 0$, or alternatively that $v = 1$, was not done, but from the estimations the conclusion that $v = 0$, which is compatible with the true mass-action assumption, seems more plausible.

A good method to compare the predictions of the two mass-action assumptions would be to compare the transmission parameter or R_0 in experimental populations that do not change in size during the experiment, but that differ in their preset sizes. Moreover, because experimental populations are usually small, stochastic models should be used to calculate exactly the probability of the outcomes under both variants. Bouma *et al.* did exactly this for Aujeszky's disease virus (ADV) in vaccinated populations of pigs. They showed that the R_0 in a population of 40 pigs was not significantly different from the R_0 in populations of 10 pigs. Moreover, the R_0 for 40 pigs was significantly smaller than the R_0 predicted from the pseudo mass-action model. Thus they falsified the pseudo mass-action assumption used for ADV infections in pigs by Smith and Grenfell (1990).

3.2   The Greenwood data-set

Because Anderson and May's comparison of a pseudo mass-action model with the data of Greenwood *et al.* (1936) on *P. muris* in mice suggested that the pseudo mass-action assumption was valid whereas all other data suggested that the pseudo mass-action assumption was not valid, a comparison of these

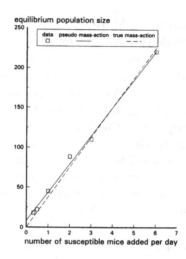

Figure 2. The observed steady state population sizes (X) for experimental mice populations infected with *P. muris* and where daily A mice were added (Greenwood *et al.* 1936). The thin line is the relationship predicted by the pseudo mass-action model as first analysed by Anderson and May (1979). The thick line is the true mass-action model, analysis of which is given in the text. Either predicted relationship gives a good fit to the data.

data with the true mass-action model was necessary. The relationship (Figure 2) between equilibrium population size (N^*) and the number of mice added per day (A) was used for the comparison. Both models lead to the prediction that the relationship between A and N^* is linear. The difference lies in the value at $A = 0$. The estimated relationship (Figure 2) for true mass-action is $N^* = 37.5A$ $(r^2 = 0.989)$ and for pseudo mass-action is $N^* = 35.4A + 8.15$ $(r^2 = 0.995)$. The ratio of the residuals of the two models is 5.55, a test statistic which is approximately distributed as an F-statistic with 1 and 4 degrees of freedom. Hence, the difference between the two models is not significant: both models fit the Greenwood data equally well.

4 Discussion

Both for small groups of individuals in experiments (the *P. muris* experiment as analysed above; Bouma *et al.*) and for more complex observational situations (Becker and Angulo 1981, Anderson 1982) the assumption of random encounters, i.e. true mass-action, was a good approximation. This contrasts with the pseudo mass-action assumption, which was falsified by one of the experiments (Bouma *et al.*) and both sets of observations (Becker and Angulo 1981, Anderson 1982). Because, moreover, true mass-action follows from the simple mechanistic notion of random encounters, true mass-action is the bench mark to which to compare observations.

Of course the simple model [T] is not realistic for several of the complex situations in which we want answers from modelling. The simple model [T] has to be extended to incorporate the details of a given problem. For example, this could mean using other scenarios for encounters between individuals, taking heterogeneity in the population into account, or allowing the density to change (for example as a function of population size). An extended scenario for encounters could include multiple groups with movements of individuals between groups or different individual behaviour, for instance when individuals are time limited with respect to the number of contacts (Heesterbeek and Metz 1993). A description of the change in density for a growing population could be that at first density does not change because the population expands the area on which it lives and later density does increase when all the available area is taken. For populations of approximately constant size it is plausible that density does not vary all that much, because the hosts regulate their local densities. However, different individuals in the population of hosts (e.g. males versus young animals) may experience different densities and in addition densities may vary with the seasons. Notwithstanding all these possible complications, we put confidence in the principle of true mass-action as a building block for epidemic models.

Acknowledgements

This paper was written when two of us (MdJ and HH) were working at the Isaac Newton Institute for Mathematical Sciences. HH was financially supported by the Netherlands Organisation for Scientific Research (NWO) and the Royal Society.

References

Anderson, R.M. (1982) 'Transmission dynamics and control of infectious disease agents'. In *Population Biology of Infectious Diseases*, R.M. Anderson and R.M. May (eds.), Springer-Verlag, Berlin, 149–176.

Anderson, R.M. and May, R.M. (1979) 'Population biology of infectious diseases: Part I', *Nature* **280**, 361–367.

Becker, N. and Angulo, J. (1981) 'On estimating the contagiousness of the disease transmitted from person to person', *Math. Biosci.* **54**, 137–154.

Bouma, A., De Jong, M.C.M., and Kimman, T.G. 'Transmission of pseudorabies virus in pig populations is independent of the size of the population', *Prev. Vet. Med.*, in press.

De Palma, A. and Lefevre C. (1988) 'Population systems with (non)-extensive interaction rates', *Math. Comput. Modelling* **10**, 359–365.

Dietz, K. (1982) 'Overall population patterns in the transmission cycle of infectious agents'. In *Population Biology of Infectious Diseases*, R.M. Anderson and R.M. May (eds.), Springer-Verlag, Berlin, 87–102.

Greenwood, M., Bradford Hill, A.T., Topley, W.W.C., and Wilson, J. (1936) *Experimental epidemiology*, MRC Special Report Series **209**.

Hamer, W. H. (1906) 'Epidemic disease in England – evidence of variability and of persistence of type', *The Lancet* **i**, 733–739.

Heesterbeek, J.A.P. and Metz, J.A.J. (1993) 'The saturating contact rate in marriage and epidemic models', *J. Math. Biol.* **31**, 529–539.

Kermack, W.O. and McKendrick, A.G. (1927) 'A contribution to the mathematical theory of epidemics', *Proc. R. Soc. Lond.* A **115**, 700–721.

Kermack, W.O. and McKendrick, A.G. (1939) 'Contributions to the mathematical theory of epidemics. V – Analysis of experimental epidemics of mouse typhoid: a bacterial disease conferring incomplete immunity', *J. Hyg. (Camb.)* **39**, 271–288.

May, R.M. and Anderson, R.M. (1985) 'Endemic infections in growing populations', *Math. Biosci.* **77**, 141–156.

Mena-Lorca, J. and Hethcote, H.W. (1992) 'Dynamic models of infectious diseases as regulators of population sizes', *J. Math. Biol.* **30**, 693–716.

Mollison, D. (1984) 'Simplifying simple epidemic models', *Nature* **310**, 224–225.

Mollison, D. (1985) 'Sensitivity analysis of simple endemic models'. In *Population Dynamics of Rabies in Wildlife*, P.J. Bacon (ed.), Academic Press, London, 223–234.

Schenzle, D., and Dietz, K. (1987) 'Critical population sizes for endemic virus transmission'. In *Raumliche Persistenz und Diffusion von Krankheiten* W. Fricke and E. Hinz (eds.), *Heidelberger geographische Arbeiten* **83**, 31–42.

Smith, G. and Grenfell, B.T. (1990) 'Population biology of pseudorabies in swine', *Am. J. Vet. Res.* **51**, 148–155.

Thieme, H.R. 'Epidemic and demographic interaction in the spread of potentially fatal disease in growing populations', *Math. Biosci.* **111**, 99–130.

The Legacy of Kermack and McKendrick

Odo Diekmann

Hans Heesterbeek

Hans Metz

Summary

Starting from the pioneering work by Kermack and McKendrick of 1927, we review some issues of recent interest in deterministic epidemic modelling such as: classification of dynamics, the influence of heterogeneity and submodels for the contact process.

1 Introduction

In 1927, Kermack and McKendrick published a contribution to the mathematical theory of epidemics in which they considered the following situation:

1. a single infection triggers an autonomous process within the host (i.e., they look at 'microparasites' and not at 'macroparasites');

2. the disease results in either complete immunity or death;

3. contacts are according to the law of mass-action;

4. all individuals are equally susceptible;

5. the population is *closed*, i.e. at the time-scale of disease transmission the inflow of new susceptibles into the population is negligible;

6. the population size is large enough to warrant a deterministic description.

The aim of this paper is first to review very briefly the results of Kermack and McKendrick and then to give an overview of some new issues which have received a lot of attention more recently, to wit

– more complicated dynamics (relaxing 5)

– heterogeneity (relaxing 4)

– submodels, in particular for the contact process (relaxing 3)

while staying within the deterministic setting (i.e. retaining 6, although we will make one or two remarks on the difficulty of defining the 'border' between those situations where a deterministic model makes sense and those where it does not). We will not consider partial and/or temporary immunity (Anderson and May 1991), nor say anything about models for macroparasites (see Adler and Kretzschmar (1992), Kretzschmar and Adler (1993) for a comparison of different approaches and Roberts, Smith and Grenfell (1994) for a recent review). For a general introduction to modelling infectious diseases, especially those incorporating vertical transmission, consult Busenberg and Cooke (1993).

Admittedly, the overview will be strongly biassed by personal interest and knowledge. At the positive side of this we want to acknowledge the pleasant cooperation over several years with M.C.M. de Jong and M. Kretzschmar which has contributed a lot to any insight we might have.

2   Invasion, time course and final size according to Kermack and McKendrick

The assumptions listed in section 1 directly lead to the integral equation

$$\dot{S}(t) = S(t) \int_0^\infty \bar{A}(\tau)\dot{S}(t - \tau)d\tau, \qquad (2.1)$$

where $S(t)$ denotes the (spatial) density of susceptibles (i.e., number of individuals per unit area) at time t and where, by definition,

$$\bar{A}(\tau) = \quad \text{expected infectivity of an individual that}$$
$$\text{became infected } \tau \text{ units of time ago.} \qquad (2.2)$$

In order to understand equation (2.1) one has just to realise that, by the closedness of the population, $-\dot{S}(t)$ is precisely the incidence at time t, so $-\dot{S}(t - \tau)$ is the number of individuals arising per unit of time who at time t have been infected for τ time-units.

At this point we make a short digression. Even though it has been emphasised repeatedly that Kermack and McKendrick deal with the case of a general time-kernel $\bar{A}(\tau)$ for infectivity, most people keep referring to the system of ordinary differential equations

$$\dot{S}(t) = -\beta S(t)I(t)$$
$$\dot{I}(t) = \beta S(t)I(t) - \gamma I(t) \qquad (2.3)$$

as *the* Kermack and McKendrick model. This should stop! [The often heard excuse for only citing but not reading the Kermack and McKendrick papers, namely that it is difficult to obtain them, can no longer be upheld, thanks to their recent reprinting (Kermack and McKendrick 1991a,b,c).] Note that (2.3) is derived from the special case

$$\bar{A}(\tau) = \beta e^{-\gamma \tau} \tag{2.4}$$

by defining $I(t) := -\frac{1}{\beta} \int_0^\infty \bar{A}(\tau) \dot{S}(t - \tau) d\tau = -\frac{1}{\beta} \int_{-\infty}^t \bar{A}(t - \tau) \dot{S}(\tau) d\tau$ and differentiating. In conclusion of our digression, we pass on the observation of Klaus Dietz that already in 1917, in a neglected paper, Ross and Hudson (1917) discussed a model where infectivity can be a general function of the time elapsed since infection took place (and, incidentally, also discuss (2.3) with differential mortality). Although Kermack and McKendrick were the first to give a detailed analysis of such a model, they were clearly influenced by Ross and Hudson (see Aitchison and Watson 1988). The spirit of the Kermack and McKendrick and Ross-Hudson papers is very much one of generality. Their aim is to analyse large classes of models in one go. In recent years, a trend in the opposite direction can be discerned, leading to page after page on the analysis of the umpteenth variant of model $4A\beta*$, without any more extensive insights or methods coming to the fore (see Hethcote (1993) for a critique of this phenomenon).

The definition of $\bar{A}(\tau)$ as an *expected* infectivity emphasises that some heterogeneity, viz. variability in infectivity, is already incorporated. Indeed, one should always realise that even deterministic models are built from stochastic considerations at the individual level. Sometimes it is clear how to take averages and sometimes, as we will see below, it is less clear or even not clear at all.

To illustrate this remark we recall the usual interpretation of (2.3): individuals are infected for an exponentially distributed period of time (with exponent γ) and have a constant infectivity β. Hence

$$\bar{A}(\tau) = \int_0^\infty A(\tau, \xi) f(\xi) d\xi, \tag{2.5}$$

where $f(\xi) = \gamma e^{-\gamma \xi}$ and $A(\tau, \xi) = \beta$ when $\tau \leq \xi$ and $A(\tau, \xi) = 0$ when $\tau > \xi$. So here the 'type' ξ of individuals refers to the length of their period of infectivity. In this manner any compartmental model (indicated as some finite sequence of characters from $\{S, E, I, R\}$) for a closed population may be reduced to (2.1) with an appropriate kernel $\bar{A}$, (see Metz 1978).

Kermack and McKendrick derive an invasion criterion and the equation for the final size of the epidemic in the general setting of (2.1) and they obtain more detailed information about the time course of the epidemic for the special case described by (2.3).

The *invasion* criterion is based on the linearisation in which at the right hand side of (2.1), $S(t)$ is replaced by S_0, the density of the population at the start of the epidemic with everyone susceptible. The linearised equation has a solution $\dot{S}(t) = ce^{rt}$ with $r > 0$ if and only if $R_0 > 1$ where, by definition,

$$R_0 = S_0 \int_0^\infty \bar{A}(\tau)d\tau. \tag{2.6}$$

Hence, R_0 can be interpreted as the expected number of secondary cases produced by one typical primary case and it describes the growth of the epidemic in the initial phase on a generation basis. In the same vein r, the real root of the characteristic equation

$$1 = S_0 \int_0^\infty \bar{A}(\tau)e^{-r\tau}d\tau \tag{2.7}$$

describes the 'real-time' growth in the initial phase. The positivity of $\bar{A}$ guarantees the equivalence

$$R_0 > 1 \Leftrightarrow r > 0 \tag{2.8}$$

but one should note that, if one compares different kernels, the ordering of the R_0-values does not necessarily correspond to the ordering of the r-values (early or late 'reproduction' does not matter for R_0 but it does matter for r). Anyhow, the invasion criterion clearly is $R_0 > 1$.

The invasion criterion is actually very often used negatively, viz. as an eradication/elimination criterion: whether or not a certain control measure (e.g. a vaccination programme) is strong enough to eradicate/eliminate the disease is determined by whether or not it is capable of reducing the value of the net reproduction ratio R to below 1. [One can argue whether or not a new symbol should be introduced in the case of a population that is not wholly susceptible because some control measures have been applied. One could denote the corresponding net reproduction ratio by R. However, from a mathematical point of view, R_0 and R are reproduction ratios calculated in precisely the same manner, the only difference being that the virgin and the controlled populations differ in density of susceptibles at the moment of invasion. Under the assumptions in this section $R = \frac{S}{S_0}R_0$, where S/S_0 is the fraction of the population that is actually susceptible.]

Incidentally, we remark that explicit expressions for R may be helpful in suggesting which component(s) of the transmission cycle are most sensitive to control measures. See Dietz (1993) for a more elaborate discussion.

Dividing (2.1) by $S(t)$ and integrating we obtain

$$\ln \frac{S(t)}{S_0} = \int_0^\infty \bar{A}(\tau)\{S(t-\tau) - S_0\}d\tau \tag{2.9}$$

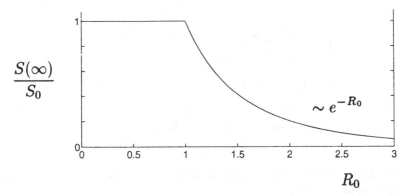

Figure 1.   Final size as a function of R_0.

and subsequently a limit argument yields the *final size* equation

$$\ln \frac{S(\infty)}{S_0} = R_0 \left(\frac{S(\infty)}{S_0} - 1 \right) \qquad (2.10)$$

which can easily be analysed graphically (here we are concentrating on a negligibly small inoculum; a more elaborate presentation of the arguments involved can be found in Metz and Diekmann (1986), section IV.4.1). The outcome is most conveniently presented pictorially as in Figure 1.

Concerning the *time course* of the epidemic when (2.3) is used, the density of infecteds reaches its peak value when $S = \frac{\gamma}{\beta}$. This can be seen directly from the second equation of (2.3).

3   The problem of endemicity

In 1932 and 1933, Kermack and McKendrick (1932,1933) addressed the problems that arise when one relaxes assumption 5 that the population is closed, and assumption 2 of permanent immunity. Here, possibly by the nature of the problem and by the lack of computers, they did not arive at such clear conclusions.

What type of model is appropriate depends on the *time-scale*

1. of disease transmission;

2. of population turnover (demography);

3. which interests us.

First of all one has to decide whether one takes the rate at which newborns are added to the population

a. constant

or

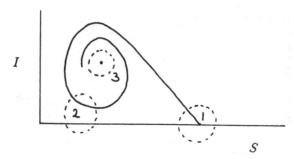

Figure 2.   Stages when stochastic aspects are important (see text for explanation of '1, 2, 3').

b. (linearly) related to population size.

In case *a*, demography influences the disease dynamics but not really vice versa, whereas in case *b* one can study the regulation problem: can an infectious agent control the size of its host population? Anderson and May called attention to this regulation problem in influential papers in 1978 and 1979.

Before briefly listing the typical results for cases *a* and *b*, we want to emphasise a problem which is, in our opinion, not understood at all: when can we expect *repeated outbreaks* (i.e. epidemics separated by disease free periods, e.g. measles in Iceland) and when an endemic situation? Here we touch upon the difficulty that deterministic dynamics may lead to a situation where the deterministic approximation ceases to be meaningful (the 'atto-fox' of D. Mollison 1991). If we draw the somewhat symbolic Figure 2, we can distinguish three types of stochastic aspects:

1. At the introduction of the infectious agent the possibility of a minor outbreak exists, but *if* a major outbreak starts off then the deterministic description applies.

2. If population turnover is slow relative to disease transmission, we reach almost the final size situation of the closed epidemic before the gradual inflow of new susceptibles has any effect. In this situation, there are very few infecteds and the density of susceptibles is of the order of $S_0 e^{-R_0}$, which is far below threshold. It will take a long time before the density is above threshold again, and during this period demographic stochasticity may easily lead to the extinction of the infectious agent. But when and how to switch to a stochastic model?

3. Even if the infective agent escapes extinction after the first outbreak and becomes established, there is still the possibility of extinction as a result of chance fluctuations. Relevant questions are: what is the expected time until extinction if we are currently in the 'endemic' regime? (see

Nåsell 1995); what is the expected total number of cases during that time?

A general feeling is that the possibility of extinction due to demographic stochasticity is strongly enhanced if the deterministic dynamics is characterised by oscillations, rather than by a stable endemic steady state.

Bartlett (1960), Dietz and Schenzle (1985) and others mainly concentrate on 3. The distinction between 2 and 3 is also mentioned in passing as epidemic fade-out versus endemic fade-out in the book by Anderson and May (1991, p. 20). The notion of a *critical community* size (Bartlett 1960, Dietz 1982, Schenzle and Dietz 1987) seems to come in for two reasons. The first is that Ne^{-R_0} may still be reasonably large if the total population size N is large (a low density over a large domain may yield an appreciable number). The second is that the geographical distribution by itself may necessitate a reconsideration of the process of disease transmission. If local epidemics are out of phase, then the proneness to extinction may be much smaller (cf. metapopulation models in ecology, Gilpin and Hanski 1991). See Grenfell (1992) for this aspect and others, related to age structure, of the fade-out phenomenon in the context of measles. Concerning 2, see Rand and Wilson (1991) for other aspects.

Let us now consider case a where the birthrate is assumed to be a constant. Basic issues are the existence, uniqueness, representation and stability of endemic *steady states*. The representation is important when one wants to use estimates of endemic levels for parameter estimation (cf. Hasibeder, personal communication). Stability has both a local aspect (where do the roots of the characteristic equation lie?) and a global aspect (e.g. can we find a Lyapunov function?). See e.g. Capasso (1993), Hethcote (1976), Bailey (1975). The generic picture that emerges is that there exists a (unique) steady state if and only if $R_0 > 1$ (but see section 5 below). Recent issues are: if the steady state is unstable, what sort of dynamics can we expect? Periodic oscillations or chaos? If contact rates are periodic (seasons, school system) then how are the periods of the solutions related to the driving period? For results in this line we refer to Smith (1983), Aron and Schwarz (1984), Dietz (1976), Kuznetsov and Piccardi (1992), Schenzle (1984), Schwarz (1985, 1988), Schaffer (1985), Hethcote and Levin (1989) and Grenfell (1992).

The regulation case b is characterised by the existence of multiple thresholds if there is differential mortality. Typically we find four regimes for a contact rate parameter according to the following types of dynamic behaviour:

- the infectious agent dies out;

- the infectious agent grows exponentially, but at a slower rate than the host population (the dilution effect is that the *proportion* of infecteds in the population goes to zero);

- host and infectious agent grow at the same rate, which is reduced relative to the host growth rate in the disease free situation;

- either the common growth rate is negative or a steady state obtains, depending on how exactly one models the contact rate (strictly homogeneous or only asymptotically homogeneous).

For this type of result see Anderson (1979), Diekmann and Kretzschmar (1991), Busenberg and Van den Driessche (1990), Busenberg and Hadeler (1990), Anderson and May (1991), Thieme (1992) and Mena-Lorca and Hethcote (1992).

Results become more subtle when one allows for the interaction of disease effects with other density dependent effects. This area currently receives much attention, see, e.g., Brauer (1990), Pugliese (1990), Greenhalgh (1992a,b), Greenhalgh and Das (1992) and Gao and Hethcote (1992), but we feel that time-scale aspects deserve more prominence (see Andreasen 1989, 1992a,b). For a recent general approach to SIS density-dependent models, see Zhou and Hethcote (1993).

The following table summarises our classification of aspects of infectious-disease dynamics.

closed population	$\left\{\begin{array}{l}\text{invasion/elimination} \\ \text{time course} \\ \text{final size}\end{array}\right.$
repeated outbreaks	
endemic situation	$\left\{\begin{array}{l}\text{steady state} \\ \text{periodic oscillations} \\ \text{chaos}\end{array}\right.$
feedback to demography	$\left\{\begin{array}{l}\text{independent growth} \\ \text{partial regulation: reduced growth of host} \\ \text{regulation}\end{array}\right.$

4   Heterogeneity

Suppose that not all individuals are equally susceptible, but that certain traits (e.g. age, gender or whether or not one suffers from a sexually transmitted disease causing ulcers, when we consider HIV transmission) have a marked influence. Of course one then has to specify these traits, their dynamics and their frequency in the susceptible population. Having done that, one question is: can we average and if so, how to do it?

In order to have a common formulation for both static and dynamic traits it is most convenient to parametrise by the trait an individual has at the moment it becomes infected (we will also write 'at birth'). Let now A be a function of three variables defined by

$$A(\tau,\xi,\eta) = \text{the expected infectivity of an individual that was}$$
$$\text{infected } \tau \text{ units of time ago while having trait}$$
$$\text{value } \eta \text{ towards a susceptible with trait value } \xi. \quad (4.1)$$

Then exactly the same reasoning which led to (2.1) yields, in the case of a closed population,

$$\frac{\partial S}{\partial t}(t,\xi) = S(t,\xi) \int_\Omega \int_0^\infty A(\tau,\xi,\eta) \frac{\partial S}{\partial t}(t-\tau,\eta) d\tau d\eta \quad (4.2)$$

where Ω denotes the set of trait values. So the structure remains essentially the same as in (2.1), but the way to proceed is slightly more involved. We have to deal with distributed quantities and replace straightforward multiplication by an operator mapping a function onto a new function. The linearised version of (4.2) has a solution of the form $\frac{\partial S}{\partial t}(t,\xi) = \Psi(\xi)e^{\lambda t}$ if and only if $\Psi(\cdot)$ is an eigenvector, corresponding to eigenvalue one, of the operator K_λ defined by

$$(K_\lambda \phi)(\xi) = S_0(\xi) \int_\Omega \int_0^\infty A(\tau,\xi,\eta) e^{-\lambda\tau} d\tau \phi(\eta) d\eta \quad (4.3)$$

(here $S_0(\cdot)$ is the demographic steady state at the start of the epidemic). Note that K_0 is the *next-generation operator* corresponding to the linearisation. This means that, given a generation of infecteds distributed as ϕ with respect to trait value at birth and of size $\int_\Omega \phi(\eta) d\eta$, the function $K_0\phi$ describes both the size and the distribution of the next generation. The positivity of A guarantees that K_0 is a positive operator on $L_1(\Omega)$, the space of integrable functions, and under appropriate minor extra conditions (minor in the sense that they will generally be fulfilled in practical situations) one can conclude that K_0 has a *strictly* dominant eigenvalue R_0. We can rightfully identify this eigenvalue with R_0 since, under those minor extra conditions, we have the asymptotic relation

$$K_0^n \phi \sim R_0^n c(\phi)\phi_d, \qquad n \to \infty, \quad (4.4)$$

where $c(\phi)$ is a scalar depending on the initial generation, and ϕ_d the eigenvector corresponding to R_0. So, if we iterate the next-generation operator, the distribution of infected individuals over all trait values stabilises to the form described by ϕ_d, while numbers are multiplied by R_0 from generation to generation. In other words, ϕ_d describes the distribution of the 'typical' infected individual and R_0 is the number of secondary cases. With the normalisation $\int_\Omega \phi_d(\eta) d\eta = 1$, the eigenvector has the interpretation of a probability distribution for the trait value at the moment of infection.

We remark that in the host-vector case the population can be divided into two subpopulations which do not communicate internally and hence transmission has a well-defined cycle (of length two). The next-generation matrix then has the anti-diagonal structure

$$K_0 = \begin{pmatrix} 0 & K_{hv} \\ K_{vh} & 0 \end{pmatrix}$$

and $R_0 = \sqrt{\lambda_d(K_{hv}K_{vh})} = \sqrt{\lambda_d(K_{vh}K_{hv})}$, where $\lambda_d(M)$ denotes the dominant eigenvalue of the (positive) matrix M. In this case it is, in the biological literature, more usual to choose R_0^2 for the quantity one calls R_0, in particular since R_0^2 admits a more direct interpretation, as the host-to-host (and vector-to-vector) multiplication factor. Useful as this may seem, one should realise that such a choice can lead to a proliferation of R_0's (think for example of two loosely coupled groups, where one can define R_0^{rig} ('return-in-group') as the number of first offspring in ones own group, i.e. the sum of the cases in ones own group produced either directly or indirectly via an arbitrarily long transmission chain in the other group). We therefore sympathise with Hasibeder's suggestion (Hasibeder, personal communication) to use the notation R_0^c for the dominant eigenvalue of the iterated next-generation matrix in the case of a well-defined transmission cycle.

In the heterogeneous case we have, as before, the equivalence

$$R_0 > 1 \Leftrightarrow r > 0 \tag{4.5}$$

where now r is defined as the (real) value of λ for which K_λ has dominant eigenvalue one, i.e. r is the 'real-time' growth rate (in contrast to the homogeneous case, the proof of the equivalence requires some work, see Heesterbeek (1992) for one possible proof).

Here a cautionary remark is in order. We have to worry about how irreducible the kernel A and how dominant r really is before we can rightfully conclude that the epidemic grows as e^{rt} in real time. For instance, when we consider a very large spatial domain, then the speed of the epidemic is not described by r but rather by the asymptotic speed of propagation c_0 (see Metz and van den Bosch, this volume). In this connection we also mention that the Perron root of K_0 – which is in a certain way a measure of *local* changes; see Jagers (1992), Shurenkov (1992) – and the spectral radius R_0 (which is more concerned with total growth) may differ when the epidemic drifts off towards infinity while growing (e.g. think of a focus of a fungal plant disease in a field of wheat where the spread of the epidemic can be heavily influenced by a strong prevailing wind direction). In the theory of branching processes r, there usually referred to as the Malthusian parameter, recently has become associated with the Perron root rather than the spectral radius, see Jagers (1992), Shurenkov (1992), Taib (1992). However, the two notions can only lead to different results for non-compact trait spaces (Shurenkov 1992). As another example, consider two very loosely coupled subpopulations, one small but highly active and one big with low activity. Then it may very well be that the nonlinearity comes into play in the small group before enough time has elapsed for the stable invasion distribution to be attained.

Anyhow, concerning the invasion/elimination criterion we can conclude that there is a systematic way of performing the right averaging: compute the dominant eigenvalue R_0 (R) of the next-generation operator and compare it with 1. This still leaves us with important basic problems:

- how to express the kernel A in terms of ingredients of submodels for the contact- and transmission process?

- how actually to compute R_0 (R) for a given kernel A?

We refer to Heesterbeek (1992), Diekmann, Heesterbeek and Metz (1990) and Diekmann (1991, 1993) and the references therein for various results in this direction. In de Jong, Diekmann and Heesterbeek (1994) an algorithm is given to compute the elements of the next-generation matrix for discrete-time multigroup models where the individuals are allowed to change their 'type'. Dietz (1993) gives a survey of various methods to estimate reproduction ratios.

The final size equation for the closed population takes the form

$$\ln \frac{S(\infty, \xi)}{S_0(\xi)} = \int_\Omega \int_0^\infty A(\tau, \xi, \eta) d\tau (S(\infty, \eta) - S_0(\eta)) d\eta \qquad (4.6)$$

and has, in particular when ξ is a discrete variable, been studied by Radcliffe and Rass (1984) – see also Diekmann (1978), Thieme (1977a). One can easily show that a nontrivial positive solution exists if and only if $R_0 > 1$, but apart from that very little can be said in any generality. The nonlinearity is an obstruction for a further simplification of (4.6), the problem remains higher-, usually even infinite-, dimensional and cannot be summarised in terms of one or two numbers as in the case of the invasion problem.

In heterogeneous populations, the invasion/elimination problem is the only part of the classification table in section 3 that has been addressed in some generality. As far as the other aspects listed in that table are concerned, results are only available for special kinds of structure. There are many results on age-structured models, on spatial structure and on models incorporating a finite number of groups. While not at all claiming to list all important contributions, we mention a few papers that tackle aspects of table 3 in heterogeneous populations. For a recent review of models for periodic outbreaks see Hethcote and Levin (1989) and Liu (1992). For the endemic equilibrium see for example Capasso (1993), Hethcote and Yorke (1984), Lajmanovich and Yorke (1976), Lin and So (1990), Busenberg and Van den Driessche (1992), Hethcote and Thieme (1985) and Beretta and Capasso (1986) in the case of a finite number of individual types, and Busenberg, Iannelli and Thieme (1991), Greenhalgh (1988) and Inaba (1990) in the case of age structure. For the interaction with demography see for example Busenberg, Cooke and Thieme (1991) for multigroup models, and May, Anderson and McLean (1988a,b), Tuljapurkar and John (1990) for age structured models.

5   Submodels for the contact process

What exactly constitutes a 'contact' depends on the disease being modelled. For example, for sexually transmitted diseases contacts take place at two levels (partners and sexual contacts within partnerships), and for some host-vector diseases a different type of contact is involved for the two transmission steps. Even if contacts are symmetric, the transmission probability, given contact, need not be so.

Disregarding heterogeneity for a moment, a first question is how many contacts an individual makes as a function of population size. (Here we have to carefully distinguish between the cases where our variables describe numbers and where they describe (spatial) densities (see de Jong, Diekmann and Heesterbeek (1995) for a discussion of both theoretical arguments and experimental results concerning this point); in this paper we consistently work with densities.) This is the functional response question from predator-prey ecology, but now in an epidemic context. The following approaches have been taken:

a. mass-action: the per capita number of contacts per unit of time is a linear function of density;

b. saturation: the linear function is replaced by $aN/(1 + bN)$ as a convenient phenomenological description without mechanistic underpinning (see Dietz 1982);

c. extreme saturation: the linear function is replaced by a constant. Even though this does not make sense at extremely low densities, it seems a reasonable assumption for, e.g., sexual contacts or blood meals taken by mosquitoes;

d. Holling squared: In Heesterbeek and Metz (1993) a submodel for the contact process is considered for pair formation at a short time-scale, together with a quasi-steady-state assumption to derive the functional response in much the same way as one derives the famous Holling disc

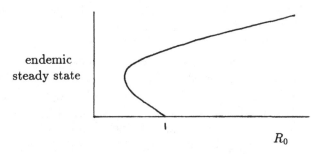

Figure 3. Possible bifurcation diagram for endemic steady states (see text).

expression of (b) above from a submodel of prey search and handling by a predator. In the simplest situation the argument works as follows. Let x denote the (local spatial) density of 'free' individuals and let c denote the density of pairs of individuals involved in a contact. One assumes that there are constants ρ and σ, respectively the contact rate parameter and the inverse of the average duration of contacts, such that

$$\frac{dx}{dt} = -\rho x^2 + 2\sigma c$$
$$\frac{dc}{dt} = \frac{1}{2}\rho x^2 - \sigma c. \tag{5.1}$$

Solving the steady state equations of (5.1) under the constraint that $x + 2c = n$, one obtains for the number of contacts per individual per unit of time $\frac{\rho x^2}{n}$, the expression

$$\frac{2\rho n}{1 + 2\rho n/\sigma + \sqrt{1 + 4\rho n/\sigma}} \tag{5.2}$$

which behaves like $2\rho n$ for small densities n, while approaching the limit σ for $n \to \infty$.

If we add heterogeneity again, matters quickly get complicated. The approach (d) still works but usually no longer leads to explicit expressions (for several possible 'next steps', e.g. numerical integration, this need not trouble us too much).

When one has a constant functional response, as in (c), strange things may happen since the reduction of the size of some groups may *increase* the infective 'pressure' on an other group. Indeed, Huang, Cooke, Castillo-Chavez (1992) showed by way of example that one may have a bifurcation diagram of the form shown in Figure 3, where there is bistability for $R_0 < 1$ (see Jacquez, Simon and Koopman (1995) for a related phenomenon: R_0

of the whole population may increase when some subpopulation reduces its contact intensity with another group, if one works with a constant functional response).

In addition, we have to face the consistency problem: the total number of contacts (per unit of time) of all individuals of type ξ with all individuals of type η has to be equal to the same quantity with ξ and η interchanged. This is automatically satisfied for the extended version of (5.1) and for the mass-action type selective mixing of Morris (1995) but has to be achieved by a suitable choice of mixing pattern in the case (c) of a constant functional response. In Busenberg and Castillo-Chavez (1991) all possibilities have been classified. In this purely descriptive approach, the free parameters have no clear interpretation. Other authors like Sattenspiel (1987), Sattenspiel and Castillo-Chavez (1990), and Jacquez *et al.* (1988) have introduced submodels which allow somewhat more of a mechanistic interpretation. However, the matching of supply and demand by a market mechanism incorporating preferences remains a difficult problem in combinatorial sociology. Of course, the acquisition and analysis of actual data adds another difficult component to this problem (see Morris 1995).

Another special case is when an individual is either single or paired to one other individual, where pairs remain together for a substantial period of time (as opposed to the short time-scale pairing of (d) above) which however may not cover the entire period of infectiousness (as opposed to the long time-scale bonds described in the previous paragraph), and where partnerships are formed at random. One can again derive a next-generation operator which has a dominant eigenvalue deserving the name R_0. This is explained in detail in Diekmann, Dietz and Heesterbeek (1991) and used in Dietz, Heesterbeek and Tudor (1993) to analyse, among other things, the effect that 'wasted' contacts (i.e. contacts between two infected partners) have on the value of R_0. An annoying feature of the comparison of various members of a family of models with each other, that arises here (and elsewhere), is that it is not directly obvious how to gauge the models in order to make them comparable in the first place.

A final question concerning the contact process is the following: is the deterministic limit meaningful? Clearly when individuals interact only with their nearest neighbours on a spatial lattice, the answer is no and one has to turn to cellular automata (or interacting particle systems, in another jargon; see Durrett and Levin (1992) for a nice overview; also see Mollison (1995), and Durrett (1995). If the neighbourhood structure has no regularity, but still individuals interact only with a fixed group of others, at least for some period of time, one is considering an epidemic on a random graph, see Blanchard, Bolz and Krüger (1990). However, very little headway with such models has been made on a general level.

6 Final remarks

Differences in behaviour necessitate subtle ways of averaging. In the linearisation appropriate for the initial phase of an epidemic one can do this in quite some generality and arrive at one or two numbers (R_0 and r or c_0 (the asymptotic speed of spatial propagation, see Metz and van den Bosch (1995)) to describe the dynamics. Things are far less clear for other aspects of the dynamics, such as the final size of an epidemic, the 'size' and stability of an endemic steady state, the growth rate reduction in the 'regulation' setting. Here we need clever case studies, where 'clever' means that one has to consider simplifications which are not too unrealistic while making the problem tractable.

In addition there is a need for quasi-mechanistic submodels especially for the contact process, dealing with such issues as handling time, satiation, virus transport by aerosols, modes of spore dispersal, lining up of seals on a sandbank, etc. (The last example illustrates a further difficulty in the modelling of contact rates: when numbers go down, the *effective* density may stay constant since the nearest neighbour distances remain roughly the same.)

We have to contemplate what is the time-scale of the various processes that we are combining into one model, in order to decide what should be considered as constant and what as variable on the time-scale that we focus on (see Andreasen (1992a,b) for a nice example of the power that the exploitation of differences in time-scale may have).

We reiterate that the border between stochastic and deterministic phases of the dynamics of disease is hard to define or to determine, yet is very relevant to our overall understanding.

In modelling one can either use a top-down approach, where one starts to build a general abstract framework and then gradually gives a more concrete specification of various ingredients, or a bottom-up approach, where one first concentrates on the data concerning a specific disease in a given population and then gradually tries to describe and analyse the essential mechanisms and phenomena. R_0 and c_0 are among the success-stories of the top-down approach, the current understanding of measles dynamics illustrates the potential power of the bottom-up approach. Although we classify ourselves as 'top-down' people, and have written this paper in a top-down spirit, we think that both approaches should be followed. A chain of people with partially overlapping interests and knowledge should bridge the gap between the two starting points by striving for unity in the formulation of mathematical models and the type of data that are collected. The Cambridge workshop was an excellent catalyst for the formation of such chains.

After these somewhat pedantic remarks we like to close with paraphrasing Simon Levin's observation during the conference dinner:

'to are or to R_0, that was the question.'

Acknowledgement

This paper was written during a stay at the Isaac Newton Institute for Mathematical Sciences; we thank the Newton Institute for its hospitality. The second author would like to thank the Netherlands Organisation for Scientific Research NWO and the Royal Society for financial support during the writing of this paper.

References

Adler, F.R. and Kretzschmar, M. (1992) 'Aggregation and stability in parasite-host models', *Parasitology* **104**, 199–205.

Aitchison, J. and Watson, G.S. (1988) 'A not-so-plain tale from the Raj'. In *The Influence of Scottish Medicine*, D. Dows (ed.), Parthenon, Park Ridge, New Jersey, 113–128.

Anderson, R.M. (1979) 'The persistence of direct life cycle infectious diseases within populations of hosts', *Lect. on Math. in Life Sciences* **12**, 1–67.

Anderson, R.M. and May, R.M. (1978) 'Regulation and stability of host-parasite population interactions. I. Regulatory processes', *J. Anim. Ecol.* **47**, 219–247.

Anderson, R.M. and May, R.M. (1979) 'Population biology of infectious diseases, part 1', *Nature* **280**, 361–367.

Anderson, R.M., and May, R.M. (1991) *Infectious Diseases of Humans, Dynamics and Control.* Oxford University Press, Oxford.

Andreasen, V. (1989) 'Disease regulation of age-structured host populations', *Theor. Pop. Biol.* **36**, 214–239.

Andreasen, V. (1992a) 'The effect of age-dependent host mortality on the dynamics of an endemic disease'. Preprint.

Andreasen, V. (1992b) 'Instability in an SIR-model with age-dependent susceptibility'. Preprint.

Aron, J.L. and Schwarz, I.B. (1984) 'Seasonality and period-doubling bifurcations in an epidemic model', *J. Theor. Biol.* **110**, 665–679.

Bailey, N.T.J. (1975) *The Mathematical Theory of Infectious Diseases and Its Applications*, Griffin, London.

Bartlett, M.S. (1960) *Stochastic Population Models in Ecology and Epidemiology*, Methuen, London.

Beretta, E. and Capasso, V. (1986) 'On the general structure of epidemic systems. Global asymptotic stability', *Comp. and Maths. with Appls.* **12A**, 677–694.

Blanchard Ph., Bolz, G.F. and Krüger, T. (1990) 'Modelling AIDS-Epidemics or any venereal disease on random graphs'. In *Stochastic Processes in Epidemic Theory*, J.-P. Gabriel, C. Lefèvre and P. Picard (eds.), Lecture Notes in Biomathematics **86**, 104–117.

Brauer, F. (1990) 'Models for the spread of universally fatal diseases', *J. Math. Biol.* **28**, 451–462.

Busenberg, S.N. and Castillo-Chavez, C. (1991) 'A general solution of the problem of mixing of subpopulations and its application to risk- and age-structured epidemic models for the spread of AIDS', *IMA J. Math. Appl. Med. Biol.* **8**, 1–29.

Busenberg, S.N. and Cooke, K. (1993) *Vertically Transmitted Diseases, Models and Dynamics*, Biomathematics vol. 23, Springer-Verlag, Berlin.

Busenberg, S.N., Cooke, K. and Thieme, H.R. (1991) 'Demographic change and persistence of HIV/AIDS in a heterogeneous population', *SIAM J. Appl. Math.* **51**, 1030–1052.

Busenberg, S.N. and Hadeler, K.P. (1990) 'Demography and epidemics', *Math. Biosci.* **101**, 63–74.

Busenberg, S.N., Iannelli, M. and Thieme, H.R. (1991) 'Global behavior of an age-structured SIS epidemic model', *SIAM J. Math. Anal.* **22**, 1065–1080.

Busenberg, S.N. and van den Driessche, P. (1990) 'Analysis of a disease transmission model in a population with varying size', *J. Math. Biol.* **28**, 257–270.

Busenberg, S.N. and van den Driessche, P. (1992) 'Disease transmission in multigroup populations of variable size'. To appear in *Proceedings 3rd International Conference on Mathematical Population Dynamics*, Pau, 1992.

Capasso, V. (1993) *Mathematical Structures of Epidemic Systems*, Lecture Notes in Biomathematics 97, Springer-Verlag, Berlin.

De Jong, M.C.M., Diekmann, O. and Heesterbeek, J.A.P. (1994) 'The computation of R_0 for discrete-time epidemic models with dynamic heterogeneity', *Math. Biosci.* **119**, 94–114.

De Jong, M.C.M., Diekmann, O. and Heesterbeek, J.A.P. (1995) 'How does infection-transmission depend on population size?', this volume.

Diekmann, O. (1978) 'Thresholds and travelling waves for the geographical spread of infection', *J. Math. Biol.* **6**, 109–130.

Diekmann, O. (1991) 'Modelling infectious diseases in structured populations'. In *Ordinary and Partial Differential Equations, vol. III*, B.D. Sleeman and R.J. Jarvis (eds.) Pitman RNiMS 254, Longman, Harlow, 67–79.

Diekmann, O. (1993) 'An invitation to structured (meta)population models'. In *Patch Dynamics*, S.A. Levin, T.M. Powell and J.H. Steele (eds.), Lecture Notes in Biomathematics 96, Springer-Verlag, Berlin, 162–175.

Diekmann, O., Dietz, K. and Heesterbeek, J.A.P. (1991) 'The basic reproduction ratio for sexually transmitted diseases, part 1: theoretical considerations', *Math. Biosci.* **107**, 325–339.

Diekmann, O., Heesterbeek, J.A.P. and Metz, J.A.J. (1990) 'On the definition and the computation of the basic reproduction ratio R_0 in models for infectious diseases in heterogeneous populations', *J. Math. Biol.* **28**, 365–382.

Diekmann, O. and M. Kretzschmar, M. (1991) 'Patterns in the effects of infectious diseases on population growth', *J. Math. Biol.* **29**, 539–570.

Dietz, K. (1976) 'The incidence of infectious diseases under the influence of seasonal fluctuations', Lecture Notes in Biomathematics, 11, Springer-Verlag, Berlin, 1–15.

Dietz, K (1982) 'Overall population patterns in the transmission cycle of infectious disease agents'. In *Population Biology of Infectious Diseases*, R.M. Anderson and R.M. May (eds.), Springer-Verlag, Berlin, 87–102.

Dietz, K. (1993) 'The estimation of the basic reproduction number for infectious diseases', *Stat. Meth. Med. Research* 2, 23–41.

Dietz, K., Heesterbeek, J.A.P. and Tudor, D.W. (1993) 'The basic reproduction ratio for sexually transmitted diseases, part 2: The influence of variable HIV-infectivity', *Math. Biosci.* **117**, 35-47.

Dietz, K. and Schenzle, D. (1985) 'Mathematical models for infectious disease statistics'. In *A Celebration of Statistics*, A.C. Atkinson and S.E. Feinberg (eds.), Springer, Berlin.

Durrett, R. (1995) 'Spatial epidemic models', this volume.

Durrett, R. and Levin, S.A. (1994) 'Stochastic spatial models: a user's guide to ecological applications', *Phil. Trans. R. Soc. London, B,* **343**, 329–350.

Gao, L.Q. and Hethcote, H.W. (1992) 'Disease transmission models with density-dependent demographics', *J. Math. Biol.* **30**, 717-731.

Gilpin, M.E. and Hanski, I. (1991) *Metapopulation Dynamics: Empirical and Theoretical Investigations*, Academic Press.

Greenhalgh, D. (1988) 'Threshold and stability results for an epidemic model with an age-structured meeting rate', *IMA J. Math. Appl. Med. Biol.* **5**, 81–100.

Greenhalgh, D. (1992a) 'Vaccination in density-dependent epidemic models', *Bull. Math. Biol.* **54**, 733–758.

Greenhalgh, D. (1992b) 'Some threshold and stability results for epidemic models with a density dependent death rate', *Theor. Pop. Biol.* **42**, 130–151.

Greenhalgh, D. and Das, R. (1992) 'An SIR epidemic model with a contact rate depending on population density'. Preprint.

Grenfell, B.T. (1992) 'Chance and chaos in measles dynamics', *J. R. Statist. Soc. B.* **54**, 383–398.

Heesterbeek, J.A.P. (1992) R_0, PhD Thesis, University of Leiden.

Heesterbeek, J.A.P. and Metz, J.A.J. (1993) 'The saturating contact rate in marriage- and epidemic models', *J. Math. Biol.* **31**, 529–539.

Hethcote, H.W. (1976) 'Qualitative analysis for communicable disease models', *Math. Biosci.* **28**, 335–356.

Hethcote, H.W. (1993) 'A thousand and one epidemic models'. To appear in *Frontiers in Theoretical Biology*, S.A. Levin (ed.), Lecture Notes in Biomathematics, **100**, Springer, Berlin.

Hethcote, H.W. and Levin, S.A. (1989) 'Periodicity in epidemic models'. In *Applied Mathematical Ecology*, S.A. Levin, T.G. Hallam and L.J. Gross (eds.), Springer-Verlag, Berlin, 193–211.

Hethcote, H.W. and Thieme, H.R. (1985) 'Stability of the endemic equilibrium in epidemic models with subpopulations', *Math. Biosci.* **75**, 205–227.

Hethcote, H.W. and Yorke, J.A. (1984) *Gonorrhea Transmission Dynamics and Control*, Lecture Notes in Biomathematics, **56**, Springer-Verlag, Berlin.

Huang, W., Cooke, K.L. andCastillo-Chavez, C. (1992) 'Stability and bifurcation for a multiple group model for the dynamics of HIV/AIDS transmission', *SIAM J. Appl. Math.* **52**, 835–854.

Inaba, H. (1990) 'Threshold and stability results for an age-structured epidemic model', *J. Math. Biol.* **28**, 411–434.

Jacquez, J.A., Simon, C.P., Koopman, J., Sattenspiel, L. and Perry, T. (1988) 'Modeling and analyzing HIV transmission: the effect of contact patterns', *Math. Biosci.* **92**, 119–199.

Jacquez, J.A., Simon, C.P. and Koopman, J.S. (1995) 'Core groups and the R_0's for subgroups in heterogeneous SIS and SI models', this volume.

Jagers, P (1992) 'The deterministic evolution of general branching populations'. Preprint 1992-25, Department of Mathematics, Chalmers University Göteborg.

Kermack, W.O. and A.G. McKendrick, A.G. (1927, 1991a) 'Contributions to the mathematical theory of epidemics, part I', *Proc. Roy. Soc. Edin. A* **115**, 700–721.
[**Reprinted** (1991) as *Bull. Math. Biol.* **53**, 33–55.]

Kermack, W.O. and McKendrick, A.G. (1932, 1991b) 'Contributions to the mathematical theory of epidemics. II – The problem of endemicity', *Proc. Roy. Soc. Edin. A* **138**, 55–83.
[**Reprinted** (1991) as *Bull. Math. Biol.* **53**, 57–87.]

Kermack, W.O. and McKendrick, A.G. (1933, 1991c) 'Contributions to the mathematical theory of epidemics. III – Further studies of the problem of endemicity', *Proc. Roy. Soc. Edin. A* **141**, 94–122.
[**Reprinted** (1991) as *Bull. Math. Biol.* **53**, 89–118.]

Kretzschmar, M. and Adler, F.R. (1993) 'Aggregated distributions in models for patchy populations', *Theor. Pop. Biol.* **43**, 1–30.

Kuznetsov, Yu.A. and Piccardi, C. (1992) 'Bifurcation analysis of periodic SEIR and SIR epidemic models', *J. Math. Biol.*, to appear.

Lajmanovich, A. and Yorke, J.A. (1976) 'A deterministic model for Gonorrhea in a nonhomogeneous population', *Math. Biosci.* **28**, 221–236.

Lin, X. and So, J.W.-H. (1990) 'Global stability of the endemic equilibrium in epidemic models with subpopulations'. Preprint.

Liu, W.M. (1992) 'Models of recurrent outbreaks of infectious diseases'. To appear in *Proceedings 3rd International Conference on Mathematical Population Dynamics*, Pau, 1992.

May, R.M., Anderson, R.M. and McLean, A.R. (1988a) 'Possible demographic consequences of HIV/AIDS epidemics: I. Assuming HIV infection always leads to AIDS', *Math. Biosci.* **90**, 475–505.

May, R.M., Anderson, R.M. and McLean, A.R. (1988b) 'Possible demographic consequences of HIV/AIDS epidemics: II. Assuming HIV infection does not necessarily lead to AIDS'. In *Mathematical Approaches to Problems in Resource Management and Epidemiology*, C. Castillo-Chavez, S.A. Levin, C.A. Shoemaker (eds.), Lecture Notes in Biomathematics **81**, 220–248.

Mena-Lorca, J. and Hethcote, H.W. (1992) 'Dynamic models of infectious diseases as regulators of population sizes', *J. Math. Biol.* **30**, 693–716.

Metz, J.A.J. (1978) 'The epidemic in a closed population with all susceptibles equally vulnerable; some results for large susceptible populations and small initial infections', *Acta Biotheoretica* **27**, 75–123.

Metz, J.A.J. and van den Bosch, F. (1995) 'Velocities of epidemic spread', this volume.

Metz, J.A.J. and Diekmann, O. (eds.) (1986) *The Dynamics of Physiologically Structured Populations*, Lecture Notes in Biomathematics **68**, Springer, Heidelberg.

Mollison, D. (1991) 'Dependence of epidemic and population velocities on basic parameters', *Math. Biosci.* **107**, 255–287.

Mollison, D. (1995) 'The structure of epidemic models', this volume.

Morris, M. (1995) 'Data driven network models for the spread of disease', this volume.

Nåsell, I. (1995) 'The threshold concept in stochastic epidemic and endemic models', this volume.

Pugliese, A. (1990) 'Population models for diseases with no recovery', *J. Math. Biol.* **28**, 65–82.

Radcliffe, J. and Rass, L. (1984) 'The spatial spread and final size of the deterministic non-reducible n-type epidemic', *J. Math. Biol.* **19**, 309–327.

Rand, D.A. and Wilson, H. (1991) 'Chaotic stochasticity: a ubiquitous source of unpredictability in epidemics', *Proc. R. Soc. Lond. B* **246**, 179–184.

Roberts, M.G., Smith, G. and Grenfell, B. (1995) 'Mathematical models for macroparasites of wildlife'. In *Ecology of Infectious Diseases in Natural Populations*, B.T. Grenfell and A.P. Dobson (eds.), Cambridge University Press, Cambridge, to appear.

Ross, R. and Hudson, H.P. (1917) 'An application of the theory of probabilities to the study of a priori pathometry, part III', *Proc. R. Soc. Lond. A* **43**, 225–240.

Sattenspiel, L. (1987) 'Population structure and the spread of disease', *Hum. Biol.* **59**, 411–438.

Sattenspiel, L. and Castillo-Chavez, C. (1990) 'Environmental context, social interactions and the spread of HIV', *Am. J. Hum. Biol.* **2**, 397–417.

Schaffer, W.M. (1985) 'Can nonlinear dynamics elucidate mechanisms in ecology and epidemiology?', *IMA J. Math. Appl. Med. Biol.* **2**, 221–252.

Schenzle, D. (1984) 'An age-structured model of pre- and post-vaccination measles transmission', *IMA J. Math. Appl. Med. Biol.* **1**, 169–191.

Schenzle, D. and Dietz, K. (1987) 'Critical population sizes for endemic virus transmission'. In *Räuliche Persistenz und Diffusion von Krankheiten*, W. Fricke and E. Hinz (eds.), Heidelberger Geographische Arbeiten, **83**, Heidelberg, pp. 31–42.

Schwarz, I.B. (1985) 'Multiple stable recurrent outbreaks and predictability in seasonally forced nonlinear epidemic models', *J. Math. Biol.* **21**, 347–361.

Schwarz, I.B. (1988) 'Nonlinear dynamics of seasonally driven epidemic models'. In *Proc. 12th IMACS World Congress* R. Vichnevetsky, P. Borne and J. Vignes (eds.), vol. IV. pp. 166–169.

Shurenkov, V.M. (1992) 'On the relationship between spectral radii and Perron roots'. Preprint 1992-17, Chalmers Univ. of Technology, Dept. of Math.

Smith, H.L. (1983) 'Multiple stable subharmonics for a periodic epidemic model', *J. Math. Biol.* **17**, 179–190.

Taib, Z. (1992) *Branching Processes and Neutral Evolution*, Lecture Notes Mathematical Biology, **93**, Springer-Verlag, Berlin.

Thieme, H.R. (1977a) 'A model for the spread of an epidemic', *J. Math. Biol.* **4**, 337–351.

Thieme, H.R. (1977b) 'The asymptotic behaviour of solutions of nonlinear integral equations', *Math. Z.* **157**, 141–154.

Thieme, H.R. (1980) 'On the boundedness and the asymptotic behaviour of the non-negative solutions of Volterra-Hammerstein integral equations', *Manuscr. Math.* **31**, 379–412.

Thieme, H.R. (1992) 'Epidemic and demographic interaction in the spread of potentially fatal diseases in growing populations', *Math. Biosci.* **111**, 99–130.

Tuljapurkar, S.D. and John, A.M. (1990) 'Disease in changing populations: growth and disequilibrium'. Preprint

Zhou, J. and Hethcote, H.W. (1993) 'Population size dependent incidence in models for diseases without immunity'. Preprint.

Part 2
Spatial Models

Incorporating Spatial Components into Models of Epidemic Spread

Andrew Cliff

Summary

This paper reviews a series of linear and non-linear mapping methods that may be used to establish the spatial corridors followed by an infectious disease as it moves from one geographical area to another. The techniques enable the relative importance of different spread components to be determined, as well as the velocity and direction of disease propagation. The manner in which spatial corridors may change over time is also examined. The paper concludes by assessing attempts to add spatial components to both *SIR* and time series models of epidemic spread.

1   Introduction

> It is obvious that this whole approach is of considerable importance to the forecasting and control of serious epidemic diseases, both within countries and on a worldwide scale.
> *(Bailey 1975, p. 356)*

While Bailey's comment may appear to be self-evident, relatively few studies have successfully incorporated explicit spatial components into usable epidemic models; see, for example, the discussion in Bailey (1975, chapters 9 and 19). In contrast, there is a large, mainly qualitative, epidemiological literature on spatial aspects of disease spread which is summarized in Cliff and Haggett (1988). This contrast reflects in part the aspatial tradition of much work in biomathematics but also, as Bailey notes (1975, p. 171), the difficulty of devising spatial models which are both mathematically tractable and which are, at the same time, geographically and epidemiologically plausible. A current account of the difficulties is provided by Anderson and May (1991, pp. 304-15).

In view of these remarks, this paper has two main objectives. First, it illustrates the way in which space structures the corridors along which epidemics move from one geographical area to another. Second, it introduces a variety of techniques that can be used not only to identify these corridors, but also to determine the manner in which temporal changes in spatial structures can affect epidemic diffusion. Once the nature of any spatial components has been identified, it may be possible to incorporate these elements into formal models of epidemic spread. A subsidiary objective is, therefore, briefly to review the progress made to date in this task. The approach of this paper differs, therefore, from that of many others in this volume. It makes no claims that the methods to be described are especially geared to the analysis of disease transmission mechanisms as do the methods devised by those involved in disease modelling. Rather, it takes a selection of the general techniques currently used by geographers to tease out the spatial structures affecting any geo-coded data; and it seeks to show that, when applied to disease data, they yield valuable insights into disease transmission processes over space which may be subsequently incorporated into formal models of spread.

We begin in Section 2 by illustrating simple mapping techniques which may be used to identify the time-space ordering of epidemic spread. A different approach is to treat maps as graphs. Here, the nodes represent areas that are coded in some epidemiologically meaningful way, and the edges of the graphs represent the corridors of spread. Once cast as a graph, a variety of analytical methods may be employed. We illustrate one such in Section 3, the use of spatial autocorrelation techniques. Other central issues addressed that affect our understanding of spatial aspects of disease spread are the assessment of the velocity of spread (Section 4) and the spatial scale at which any analysis is conducted (Section 5).

The research described in Sections 2-5 will confirm that geographical space behaves in a non-linear way in directing the spread of disease. Accordingly, we consider the use of non-linear mapping in Section 6 to establish the nature of epidemiological links between areas. The paper is concluded in Section 7 where the issue of adding spatial components to models of spread is considered.

The work described in this review is illustrated using two viral diseases of humans: measles and influenza. Both have occupied central positions in the development of epidemiological models (Fine 1982). We also focus upon geographical scales at the city and above, and we do not consider the variety of micro-scale studies within, for example, cities, schools and families. An account of this research appears in Bailey (1975, chapter 14).

2   Lag maps

In looking at the spread of any infectious disease, particular insights into the spread process may be gained by examining the changing disease distribution over time. Thus, in Figure 1, we use proportional circles to map the cases of measles reported month by month in each Icelandic medical district for

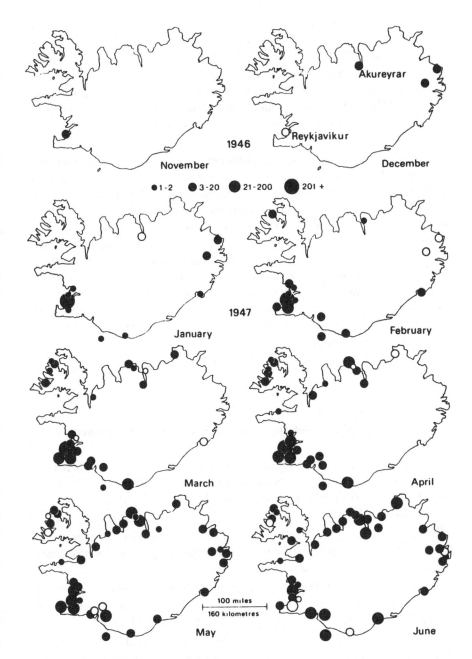

Figure 1.   Iceland, November 1946-June 1947: map sequences. Monthly sequence of measles cases by medical district. Open circles denote districts reporting on an earlier map that failed to report cases on the current map. *(From Cliff and Haggett 1988)*

the time interval from November 1946 to June 1947. This period covers part of one of the major epidemics of measles that affected Iceland in the post-1945 period. The epidemic started in the largest urban area, Reykjavík in November. The map sequence illustrates the way in which the epidemic subsequently spread rapidly to, and intensified in, the Reykjavík region and in the towns of the southwest corner of Iceland (January-April, 1947). Wholesale diffusion to settlements in the north, northwest, and on the east coast followed later (May-June, 1947).

By itself, the map sequence for a single epidemic wave may make relatively little sense. But, when several sequences of such epidemic maps are placed together, we can begin to pick out the main threads of the ways in which measles spreads. So the picture outlined above for the specific 1947 wave is seen in Figure 2A to be typical of a general pattern. This shows, for the eight measles epidemics that hit Iceland from 1945 to 1970, the average time (in months) from the start of an epidemic before each settlement was reached. We define the average time as follows. Let t_{ij} denote the month in which cases were first reported in settlement i in epidemic j. In each epidemic, t is coded as an integer with reference to $t = 1$, the month in which cases were first reported anywhere in Iceland. Then the average time to infection in settlement i, $\overline{t_i}$ is given by

$$\overline{t_i} = \sum_j t_{ij}/n, \tag{2.1}$$

where n is the number of epidemics.

The diagram reveals four phases:

(i) Originating phase (less than three months); measles confined to the capital city, Reykjavík.

(ii) Localized spread phase (third to fifth months); measles spreads locally in a neighbourhood fashion to communities around the capital and by long-range diffusion to regional centres (for example, Akureyri, 5.8 months) in the northern half of the island.

(iii) Generalized spread (sixth to eighth months); measles becomes established in all the other parts of the island, with the exception of the two zones identified in the fourth phase.

(iv) Remote outliers (nine and more months); measles is delayed in getting into two inaccessible parts of Iceland - the northwest fjords (for example, Djúpavikur, 16.0 months; Flateyjar, 17.0) and the eastern fjords.

Comparison of these four phases with the circle sizes used in Figure 2A to represent population totals appears to support the idea of a spread model for measles epidemics down the hierarchy of urban size from larger settlements to smaller, and the contagious spread of epidemic waves out from the initial centres of introduction. However, this interpretation is complicated by the high inverse correlation between population size of settlements and distance

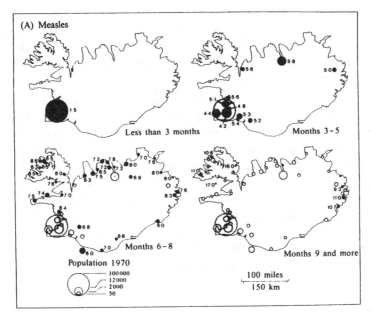

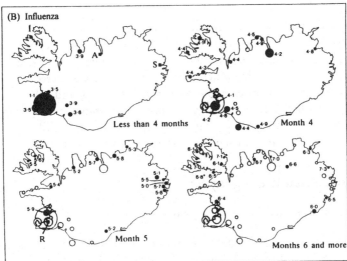

Figure 2.   Iceland, 1945-70: average times to infection for measles and influenza epidemics.

(A)   Mean time in months from the start of eight measles epidemics occurring between 1945 and 1970 before medical districts were reached. Stipple indicates districts shown as reached on earlier maps. Area of circles proportional to population size of districts in 1970.

(B)   As (A), but for influenza.

(From Cliff and Haggett 1988)

from Reykjavík. Many smaller settlements are generally distant from the source areas, and so it is difficult, even with partial correlation analysis, to disentangle the size and distance effects. As we shall see in the next subsection, hierarchical effects frequently dominate the early stages in the spread of epidemics, and contagious effects become more important later.

If the analysis is repeated for a second viral disease, influenza, then Figure 2B indicates that the same general spatial sequencing of events is found as with measles, but the timing is compressed into eight rather than seventeen months. Taken together, Figures 2A and 2B lead to the general points that (i) the spatial heterogeneities caused by variations in the geographical distribution of population have a profound effect in defining the channels followed in the spread of disease from area to area and (ii) these heterogeneities may define similar corridors for different infectious diseases. Differences in the time taken to propagate through the spatial system may be directly related, *inter alia*, to the serial intervals of the diseases (c.14 days for measles and 3 days for influenza, leading to faster transmission for influenza).

3   Maps as graphs

One useful approach to mapping the spatial spread of an infectious disease like measles is to treat the area over which spread is occurring as a graph (Haggett 1976, Cliff and Haggett 1980). The methodology is illustrated here by tracing the processes by which measles has been transferred from one region to another using an example from Southwest England. We look first at the ways in which autocorrelation on space-time graphs can be measured (3.1.1). Using this approach, we can build up different types of graphs and employ them to test different models of the spatial spread of epidemics (3.2).

3.1   Correlation on graphs

3.1.1   Southwest England as a graph

As suggested above, the geographical spread of common transmissible diseases like measles in urbanised societies frequently exhibits two components. Relatively long-distance diffusion occurs by spread from city to city and from town to town, often leap-frogging the intervening countryside between urban areas. The second component consists of the in-filling of the space between towns by localised spread outwards from each infected urban centre into the surrounding countryside which falls within its sphere of influence. In less urbanized regions, the component of spread between urban areas is often reduced, so that diffusion is much more wave-like from the initial points of introduction of the disease.

Link distance	General Register Office (GRO) areas		
	Bristol CB	Plymouth CB	Penzance UD
Total	1,090	1,141	2,576
Mean	6.12	8.02	14.47
Maximum	16	15	22
Percent of all GRO areas within three links	24	11	6

Table 1. Southwest England, 1966-70: relative location of the three major measles centres on a graph of the region.
(From Cliff and Haggett 1988)

To illustrate these generalizations using a graph-theoretic approach, we consider the spread of two measles epidemics which affected Southwest England between October 1966 and December 1970 (Cliff *et al.* 1975). The main units used by the General Register Office (GRO) for gathering disease data in the United Kingdom are the local authority administrative areas of county boroughs, municipal boroughs, urban districts and rural districts. The six counties of Southwest England, namely Cornwall, Devon, Somerset, Glouces-ter, Dorset and Wiltshire, are divided into 179 such areas. If we ignore the Scilly Isles, the remaining 178 areas comprise a contiguous network that may be represented as a graph. Each GRO area forms a node or vertex on the graph, while the existence of a common boundary between any pair of areas is indicated by a link. The number of links in the shortest route between any pair of GRO areas is referred to as the spatial lag between the two areas.

For the 151 vertices relating to GROs not located at the junction of the Southwest with adjacent regions of England, the average number of links with other vertices is 5.22. This is slightly less than the 5.79 expected for a random set of contiguous areas (Dacey 1963) and reflects the strongly peninsular and linear form of the graph in Devon and Cornwall. The linear nature of the graph also produces 22 links in the shortest route through the graph from the extreme southwest to the extreme northeast. Table 1 gives the relative location of the three main diffusion centres for measles in the Southwest in relation to the rest of the graph. The greater connectedness of the largest centre, Bristol, is evident.

3.1.2 Space-time correlograms

The 179 GRO areas permit a large number (15,842) of pairwise comparisons to be made between their time series of reported measles cases. The data analysed consist of the reported number of cases of measles in each GRO

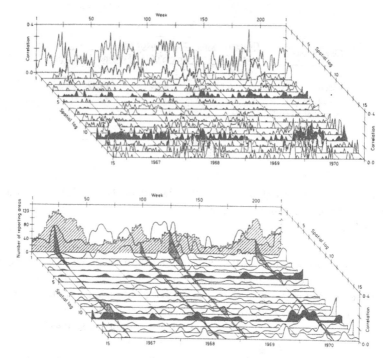

Figure 3. Southwest England, 1966-70: correlograms.
Upper: Space-time correlogram for areas at spatial lags up to 15 for weekly measles records.
Lower: Smoothed version of upper block, generated by a three-point running average, with cross-sectional slices at the peaks of measles epidemics. Number of reporting areas shown as a histogram on the back plane.
(From Cliff and Haggett 1988)

area in each week of the time series from 1966 (week 40) to 1970 (week 52). If the average correlation for reported cases between all pairs of time-series which are 1, 2, .. spatial lags apart on the graph is computed for each of the 222 weeks of the study period, the complex time-space correlogram shown in Figure 3 (*upper*) can be constructed. The average correlation is plotted on the vertical axis, while spatial lag and time form the axes of the base of the block diagram. Only positive correlations are shown. The diagram is based upon the calculated values of the correlation coefficients.

In the lower block of Figure 3, the average correlations have been smoothed using a running mean to bring out more clearly the broad space-time patterns. On the backplane of the lower block, the number of areas reporting cases in each week is plotted in the diagonally-shaded histogram. The first of the major measles epidemics which occurred in the time period studied peaked in the Southwest in February 1967 (week 20). It was characterised by a strengthening of the correlation bonds at some spatial lags (for example at one, two and eleven). The second major epidemic peaked in the summer of 1970 (weeks 186-204) and produced marked positive average correlations at spatial lags from one to four and at eleven and twelve. Other peaks appear in an irregular fashion on the correlogram in the inter-epidemic periods and reflect a scatter of small, localized outbreaks throughout the study period.

The four vertically-shaded cross-sectional slices parallel to the spatial lag axis on the lower block diagram show clearly how the average correlation falls exponentially with increasing spatial lag. This implies that, at any time, similar case levels are found in GRO areas which are close together on the graph of the Southwest and is produced by the spread of disease from urban areas into their spheres of influence.

3.1.3 Local maxima on the correlation profiles

Special interest attaches to the two local maxima in the correlation profiles, plotted in black, at around spatial lags five and twelve. These maxima imply greater than expected correlation, since, for purely contagious diffusion, the correlation should fall exponentially with increasing spatial lag (Kendall 1957). In fact, at lags five and twelve, the average correlation rises as compared with the average correlation at adjacent lags. These local maxima reflect the average spacing on the graph between the main population centres in the Southwest. As Table 1 demonstrates, the average separation between all GROs and Bristol on this graph is six links, and Bristol is the main endemic reservoir for measles in the Southwest. The separation between Bristol and Plymouth is 12 links. These centres, with their adjacent urbanized areas, had populations of one half and one quarter of a million respectively in 1970, when they made up about one fifth of the total population of the study area. The two cities were persistent centres of measles infection and recorded a continuous trace of cases over the entire study period.

The local maximum at lag five is related to the average spacing between fairly persistent pockets of infection in smaller urban centres. Apart from Bristol and Plymouth, there were, at the time, four urban areas with populations in excess of 100,000 namely Gloucester-Cheltenham (200,000), Poole (120,000), Swindon (120,000), and Torbay (100,000). Thus the spread of measles in the Southwest appears to show both the diffusion components uncovered in Iceland, namely, hierarchical spread between urban areas and contagious spread from urban areas into their hinterland regions.

3.2 Testing diffusion hypotheses on graphs

A specific way of testing for the relative importance of hierarchical and contagious elements in a diffusion process is to use spatial autocorrelation tech-

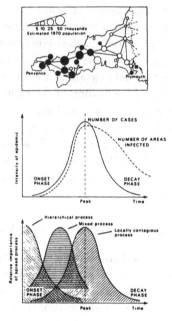

Figure 4.   Cornwall, England, 1966-70.
Upper: Cornish local authority areas shown as a graph.
Centre: Generalized pattern of intensity of a measles epidemic wave in terms
of number of cases and number of geographical areas infected.
Lower: Generalized pattern of spread processes during a measles epidemic
wave.
(From Cliff and Haggett 1988)

niques. The method is illustrated in Figure 4 and is taken from Haggett
(1976). This shows the county of Cornwall in Southwest England. The nodes
on the graph are the General Register Office (GRO) areas. The size of each
node has been drawn proportional to its population in 1970. The links in
the graph represent the contacts based on adjacency. The spread of measles
through this graph was examined for a 222-week period extending from the
autumn of 1966 to the end of 1970. Maps of Cornwall were constructed for
every week of the study period, with each of the 27 nodes coded to show
presence (black) and absence (white) of the disease. Figure 4 (*upper*) shows
one of the maps in the sequence, in which the disease was strongly concentrated in West Cornwall. In addition to the adjacency graph, six other graphs
were constructed, each linking the nodes in the Cornwall graph in different
ways to reflect hierarchical and contagious diffusion. Thus together, the seven
graphs represented different hypotheses for the ways in which measles spread
through the county during the 222-week study period.

3.2.1   Join count statistics tests for spatial autocorrelation on graphs

To discriminate between the seven graphs, the 222 weekly maps were translated into binary (outbreak/no outbreak) terms. Vertices on each of the 1,554 (that is, 222×7) graphs were coded either black (B = outbreak) or white (W = no outbreak). Then the Moran BW test for spatial autocorrelation under non-free sampling (see Cliff and Ord 1973, pp. 4-7) was computed for each graph to measure the degree of clustering of cases present on that graph in each week. The greater the degree of correspondence of a particular diffusion graph with the observed pattern of outbreaks, the greater should be the degree of spatial autocorrelation of disease incidence on the graph.

We define BW as

$$BW = \frac{1}{2} \sum_{i=1}^{n} \sum_{j=1}^{n} w_{ij}(x_i - x_j)^2, \tag{3.1}$$

where $w_{ij} = 1$ if a link existed between vertices i and j on the graph in question and $w_{ij} = 0$ otherwise; we define $w_{ii} = 0$. Additionally, $x_i = 1$ if vertex i was colour-coded B and $x_i = 0$ if the vertex was coded W. The sampling distribution of BW under the null hypothesis of no spatial autocorrelation in outbreaks on the graph is approximately Normal for the number of vertices (27) considered here, and we may test BW for significant departure from its null value as a standardised normal (z) score. The expectation and variance of BW under H_0 are given in Cliff and Ord (1973, Chapter 1). The greater the degree of correspondence between any graph and the transmission path followed by the diffusion wave, the larger (negative) should become the standardised score for BW. As Haggett (1976, p. 145) has noted, the graphs will not be independent because the same link may appear on more than one graph.

3.2.2   Results for different graphs

Figures 4 (*centre*) and 4 (*lower*) present a generalised picture of the results obtained for the seven graphs. The advance phase of a measles epidemic in Cornwall, illustrated in the centre diagram, is marked by a rapid increase in both the number of cases and, as judged by the number of GRO areas affected, the geographical extent of the disease. During the subsequent retreat phase after the peak case load has passed, the number of cases falls off rapidly. However, this is not associated with a corresponding reduction in the geographical extent of the disease; the number of areas still affected falls off much more slowly, so that the epidemic appears to decay spatially *in situ* rather than retreating in a spatially organized manner.

These onset and decay phases of the measles epidemic are critical in interpreting the autocorrelation scores on the seven graphs (see Figure 4, *lower*). A graph was deemed to be important if, at the $\alpha = 0.05$ level, it displayed significant positive spatial autocorrelation (clustering) of the GROs coloured black. As the lower diagram shows, graphs reflecting spread down the urban population size hierarchy were dominant at the start of an epidemic. They became progressively less critical as contagious spread took over. At the epidemic peak, local contagion effects dominated, setting up strong regional contrasts between the compact clusters of infected and uninfected GRO areas. In the retreat phase, the general level of autocorrelation fell steadily on almost all graphs. The one exception was a graph measuring spatial interaction arising from commuting. This graph took into account travel between urban areas and the homes of people living within their spheres of influence, and had somewhat greater sustained importance just after epidemic peaks.

3.2.3   Extension to Iceland

The results obtained for Cornwall have been tested at a much larger geographical scale by Cliff and Haggett (1988) in Iceland for both measles and influenza. Whereas in the Cornish example distinctive differences in the hierarchical and contagious diffusion components were found between the build-up and fade-out phases of epidemics, these differences were less marked in Iceland. However, it was found that similar results were obtained for the two diseases. This suggests the important possibility that, over limited periods of time, geographical space may behave in a consistent manner across different respiratory infectious diseases in defining corridors of disease spread. If this can be confirmed, it may permit, in any given geographical area, the specification of formal models with the same spatial components that may be used to characterize the diffusion processes of broad classes of disease.

4   Disease centroids

One of the most difficult aspects of the geographical spread of disease to measure is the direction and velocity of propagation of an epidemic, particularly when the spatial distribution changes rapidly from month to month. We illustrate one approach to the problem in this section.

4.1   Centroid movements

Suppose we define a centroid for each map to show its mean centre of reported disease incidence. Time changes in the position of the centroid may then be monitored to determine both direction and velocity of spread. To define an appropriate statistic, assume that data are recorded for areas. The location of the jth areal unit whose disease incidence is to be measured may be given a horizontal cartesian co-ordinate u_j and a vertical map co-ordinate v_j (say for its geographical centre). Let the reported number of cases for the jth unit be I_j. The mean centre of the reported number of cases in the set of $j = 1$, 2, ... , n regions is located at $\overline{U}, \overline{V}$, where

$$\overline{U} = \sum_{j=1}^{n} I_j u_j / \sum_{j=1}^{n} I_j, \tag{4.1}$$

and

$$\overline{V} = \sum I_j v_j / \sum_{j=1}^{n} I_j. \tag{4.2}$$

The mean is one of the simplest of a series of measure of central location, each with particular advantages and drawbacks, developed by geographers. See the literature reviewed by Haggett, Cliff and Frey (1977, pp. 312-3). One especially useful measure is the Kuhn-Kuenne centroid (Kuhn and Kuenne 1962). This is computed by choosing an initial location for the centroid at a map co-ordinate position $\hat{U}, \hat{V}$. This might be, for example, the spatial mean given in equations (3) and (4). The centroid of the distribution is now located by an iterative search procedure based upon repeated solution of the equations

$$\hat{U}_{k+1} = \sum_{j=1}^{n} I_j u_j d_{j(k)} / \sum_{j=1}^{n} I_j d_{j(k)} \tag{4.3}$$

and

$$\hat{V}_{k+1} = \sum_{j=1}^{n} I_j v_j d_{j(k)} / \sum_{j=1}^{n} I_j d_{j(k)}, \tag{4.4}$$

until

$$\hat{U}_{k+1} - \hat{U}_k \text{ and } \hat{V}_{k+1} - \hat{V}_k < \epsilon, \tag{4.5}$$

where ϵ is a pre-specified convergence error level. In these equations, d_j is the distance between the latest centroid and the jth area. The new centroid is denoted by the subscript $(k + 1)$.

By plotting centroids for successive periods and linking them in sequence, the general direction of movement can be captured. As an illustration, Figure 5 plots the successive locations of the Kuhn-Kuenne centroid of outbreaks for the eight measles epidemics that affected Iceland between 1945 and 1970. The diagrams show the trajectories for each of the waves. The first (wave 1) had the simplest structure, moving from Reykjavikur to Dalvíkur. Note the contrast between waves 3 and 4; the former was a large outbreak of over 6,000 cases concentrated in the western part of Iceland, whereas the latter was smaller (fewer than 1,900 cases). It followed rapidly after wave 3 and

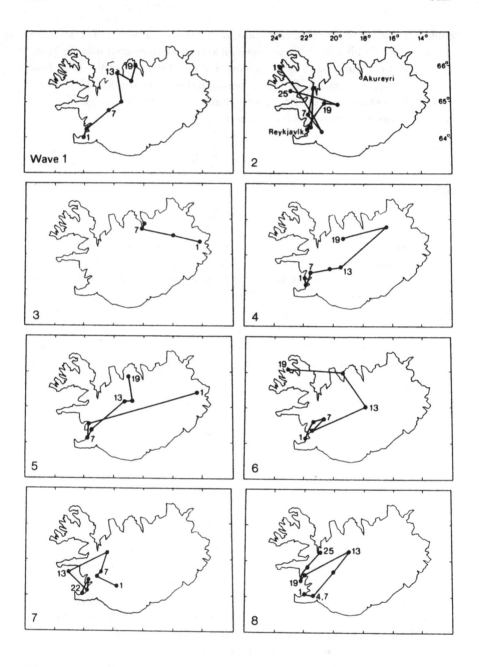

Figure 5. Centroids for measles epidemics in Iceland, 1945-70. Tri-monthly trajectory of the geographical centroid of reported cases for eight measles waves.

(From Cliff, Haggett, Ord and Versey 1981)

was confined to the eastern half of the island. Arguably, wave 4 exhausted the susceptible population missed by wave 3.

As we noted in Section 2, measles outbreaks in Iceland seem either to start in the Reykjavík area or to reach it very quickly. A general north-easterly drift tended to occur after the seventh month of each wave in the period, 1945-70. With the exception of wave 7, the trajectories of centroids plotted in Figure 5 terminate at the end of each epidemic in the north or northwest corner of the country.

The location of the geographical centre of an outbreak at any point in time obviously captures only one limited aspect of the spread of disease. For example, if we imagine a wave spreading in two dimensions, and take the ideal case of rotationally symmetric spread, the centroid stays at the centre over time, yet there is clearly an expanding wave. This illustrates how difficult the notion of movement is to capture, and temporal changes in the variance and other higher order moments may yield further insights. What the centroid does tell us, however, is where the action is concentrated at any particular moment in time.

4.2 Epidemic velocity

The concept of epidemic velocity has attracted theoretical attention because of its importance for possible preventive measures; the spread of slow-moving waves may be simpler to check than that of rapidly moving waves. Basic references are Mollison (1991) and van den Bosch, Metz and Diekmann (1990). If we are dealing with a simple spatial process where the epidemic spreads with a well-defined wavefront (as in the case of the studies by Mollison 1977), then the physical concept of distance travelled over time may be appropriate. However, where the wavefront is not a well-defined line, and where the susceptible population through which the epidemic moves is both discontinuous in space and has sharp variations in density, then alternative definitions of velocity must be sought. One possibility would be to express the total distance travelled by the centroid defined in the preceding subsection as a distance per unit time. Another is to use the moments of the frequency distribution of cases measured in the time domain.

Compared with an epidemic curve in which the frequency distribution of reported cases against time in a given area is Normally distributed, fast waves will peak early, implying small values for both the mean time to infection, $\bar{t}$, and the standard deviation, s; see the upper part of Figure 6. An early concentration of cases would also result in a large value for for the Pearson kurtosis coefficient, b_2, and a positively skewed frequency distribution. These features would reflect an early peaking of cases. A slow-moving wave might be expected to peak late in time (large $\bar{t}$) and to have cases more evenly

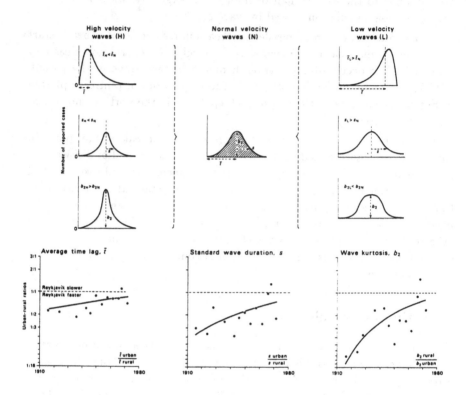

Figure 6.   Measles wave velocity in Iceland.

Upper: Definitions of epidemic velocity based upon the moments of a frequency distribution.

Lower: Average time, $\bar{t}$, in months when cases occurred for each of 14 measles waves between 1916 and 1975 for Reykjavíkur and the rest of Iceland. The sample kurtosis coefficient, b_2, for Iceland for each wave, 1896-1975, is also shown.

(From Cliff et al. 1988)

spread over the duration of the wave (large s, small b_2).

To illustrate these ideas, we show in the lower part of Figure 6 the ratios of $\bar{t}$, s and b_2 calculated for the 14 measles epidemics which passed through Iceland from 1916 to 1974; to define the ratios, a simple twofold geographical division of Iceland into urban and the rural rest of Iceland has been employed. This is not unreasonable geographically. Reykjavíkur has contained something like a half of the total Icelandic population throughout the twentieth century. In 1970, its population was 95,000. The next largest place had a population of 15,000, and medical districts ranged down in size to the smallest, Flateyjar, with only 50 people.

The plotting of the ratios has been done so that movement up the charts implies a relative slow-down in epidemic velocity in urban as compared with rural Iceland. All the ratios have approached unity over the study period, implying increasing similarity in the rates of propagation of measles epidemics through urban and rural Iceland. This is the result of two countervailing trends; (1) a decreasing velocity for Reykjavíkur, and (2) an increasing velocity for the rest of the country. It would be tempting to associate the increased velocity within the rest of Iceland with improved internal transport links, while the relative slowdown in Reykjavíkur itself might be seen in terms of improved public health control within the urban community.

5 Spatial scale

A series of modelling issues revolve around the concept of geographical scale. How do epidemics in families tie together to produce epidemics in cities, cities in regions, regions in countries, and so on? Do results at one geographical scale nest within those at another? And how can models designed to operate at different geographical scales be integrated? Analytical methods are sensitive to spatial scale, and we explore some aspects of this topic here using the concept of geographical coherence.

5.1 Geographical coherence

We define geographical coherence as the degree to which the behaviour of a time series (for example the monthly reported morbidity of a disease) in one geographical area corresponds with the time series behaviour in another, as measured by the Pearson product moment correlation coefficient. For any given geographical unit, the coherence may be external or internal. External (or between area) coherence measures the time-series comparison with another geographical unit at the same spatial scale. Alternatively, the coherence may be internal (or within area), where the time series comparison is an average of the $\frac{1}{2}(n^2 - n)$ different correlation coefficients among the n spatial units which comprise the reference area, and are therefore at a smaller spatial scale. We illustrate the coherence concept using the epidemiological time series for reported monthly measles cases in the United States over a 27-year period from January 1962 to December 1988, and at the spatial scales of states, regions and divisions (Cliff *et al.* 1992). Over the time period studied, the incidence of measles in the United States decreased substantially due to a series of major vaccination programmes.

5.2   Levels of geographical area

As a prelude to the analysis, the long time series of 324 months in all the
geographical units at a particular spatial scale were first cut into a set of 24-
month segments to yield 26 overlapping biennial windows starting with the
period, January 1962-December 1963, and ending with the period, January
1987-December 1988.

Within each biennial time segment, the monthly measles morbidity records
were correlated for all pairs of neighbouring geographical areas. Because
the time windows overlap, correlations will not be independent. The basic
data were available at four geographical levels: for the United States as a
whole and for the three divisions (defined below), nine standard regions and
51 conterminous areas (the conterminous states plus New York City and
Washington D.C.). All the areas are standard statistical units apart from the
three divisions. These are termed here North (comprising the Mid Atlantic,
New England, West North Central and East North Central standard regions),
South (West South Central, East South Central, South Atlantic standard
regions), and West (Mountain and Pacific standard regions).

5.3   Spatial coherence at different geographical levels

The change in coherence for the United States as a whole (based on the
average internal coherence between its three geographical divisions) is graphed
in Figure 7A.This plots, over time, the average correlation coefficent for each
biennial window over the 27-year period 1962-88. The graph shows three
features: (a) the secular trend of falling coherence from over $r = 0.95$ at the
start of the period to around $r = 0.60$ at the end, (b) minor cyclic variations
about that trend and (c) a major discontinuity in 1981-2 and 1982-3. The
cause of this discontinuity is discussed below.

The remaining three graphs show comparable results for the three major
divisions of North (Figure 7B), South (Figure 7C) and West (Figure 7D). Each
diagram has two line traces. The external coherence, based on the average
intercorrelation of the reference division with other divisions, is plotted as
a pecked line. Internal coherence, based on the average intercorrelations
between the standard regions which comprise each division, is illustrated as
a solid line. In all three divisions, the external coherence generally runs at a
slightly higher level than the internal. Otherwise the graphs reflect the overall
United States pattern, but with higher variability. The sharp downturn in
the early 1980s is a feature of all three graphs.

The contrast between external and internal coherence becomes still more
marked when the analysis is repeated at the standard region level.

Figure 8 plots both internal and external coherence for the nine regions
arranged in a broadly east-to west sequence from New England (Figure 8A)

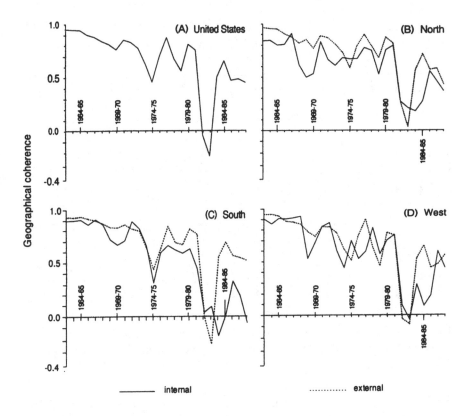

Figure 7. United States measles epidemics, 1962-88. Internal and external coherences by biennial periods at the geographical scale of regional divisions. *(From Cliff et al. 1992)*

to the Pacific (Figure 8I). Again, external coherence generally runs at a higher level than internal. The difference is particularly marked in the case of the South Atlantic (Figure 8C), West South Central (Figure 8G) and Mountain (Figure 8H) regions. The cyclic patterns are more strongly marked than at the divisional level, with both New England (Figure 8A) and West North Central (Figure 8F) showing strong pulses in coherence. The most unusual traces are provided by the internal coherences of the Mid Atlantic (Figure 8B) and East North Central(Figure 8D) regions, which register a collapse in 1980-1981 and fail to recover thereafter.

Plots for the individual states are too numerous to show. However, their external coherences showed the same general decline over the study period, but with much stronger cyclic effects. The marked reduction in cohesion, 1962-1988, is mapped in Figure 9. This gives coherence at the state level for the first 24-month window (1962-1963), and again for the last biennial

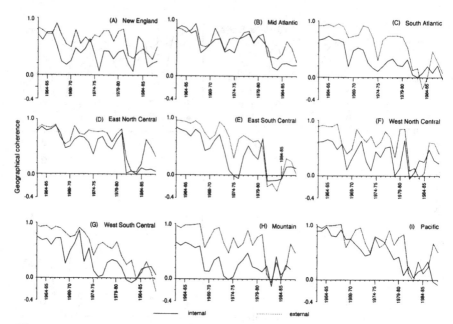

Figure 8.   United States measles epidemics, 1962-88. Internal and external coherences by biennial periods at the geographical scale of standard regions. *(From Cliff et al. 1992)*

window in 1987-1988. The same categories of shading have been used for both to emphasize the contrast between the opening and closing biennia. On the 1962-1963 map (upper), no state has a value less than $r = 0.4$; on the 1987-1988 map (lower), only two states (Missouri, New Hampshire) still have values above this level.

Cliff *et al.* (1992) have related changes in coherence both to changes in the levels of reported cases following mass vaccination programmes in the United States, and to changes in the seasonal distribution of cases. They concluded that any forcing of coherence patterns came principally through a lowered number of cases over time, rather than through a changing seasonal distribution. Geographical structure waxes and wanes with the rise and fall of epidemics.

It is change in levels which probably accounts for the virtual disappearance of both internal and external geographical coherence at all spatial scales in the early 1980s. Reported cases were then at their lowest level, with less than 100 cases recorded in some months for the United States as a whole. In terms of the scale problem, Figures 7 and 8 illustrate the scale dependence of findings; external coherences (which are at a coarser scale) are generally stronger than internal coherences (the aggregation problem of Yule and Kendall 1950, pp. 310-13).

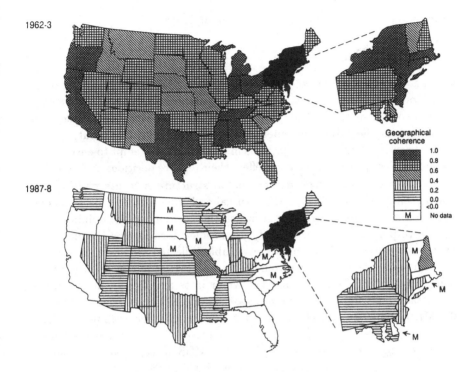

1962-3

1987-8

Geographical
coherence

1.0
0.8
0.6
0.4
0.2
0.0
<0.0

M   No data

Figure 9. United States measles epidemics, 1962-88. Temporal changes in the external geographical coherences of states between 1962-63 and 1987-88. *(From Cliff et al. 1992)*

6   Non-linear mapping

So far, we have examined the spread of disease over space, treating the map base in an conventional atlas-like fashion. However, it is evident from the preceding sections that the disease diffuses in spatially and temporally non-linear and non-stationary ways. Thus, in this section, we turn to a consideration of maps which are unconventional in that they deal with events in geographical spaces that are not measured in a distance metric (for example, miles or kilometres), but are transformed into an epidemiological metric (for example, epidemic lags in weeks or cross-associations between between morbidity time series as measured by correlation coefficients). Unlike geographical space,the relationships between events in this more complex space will generally not be linear. The general class of problems falls under the heading of non-linear mapping and the main solution method is that of multidimensional scaling (MDS). We look first at the principles of MDS methods, and then illustrate their use with reference to an Australasian example of measles mortality and an Icelandic example using influenza morbidity data.

6.1   Principles

When a conventional map of a portion of the earth's surface is drawn, some distortion inevitably results in translating a curved segment of the globe onto a flat (two-dimensional) piece of paper. The particular map projection used will determine the nature and extent of the distortion introduced but, subject to this proviso, all the map projections in common use attempt to ensure that the locations of points on the map reflect their relative positions on the globe.

An alternative way of examining spatial structure is to use multidimensional scaling (Kendall 1971, 1975, Kruskal and Wish 1978). This technique enables a map to be constructed in which the positions of the points on the map correspond not to their (scaled) geographical locations on the globe but to their degree of similarity on some variable collected for them. So, for example, points may be mapped from geographical space into a 'disease space'; then places which display similar behaviour in terms of, say, the frequency and attack rates for an infectious disease are located close to each other on the MDS map even though they may be far removed geographically. The greater the degree of similarity between the places on the variable measured, the closer together the places will be in the MDS space. Conversely points which are dissimilar on the variable measured will be widely separated in the MDS space, irrespective of their geographical location on the globe.

Transformations to other metrics are possible. For example, we might wish to map geographical space into a travel cost space. Then places which are 'near' to each other in travel cost characteristics will be located in close proximity on the MDS map; places with very different characteristics will be widely separated.

6.2   Technical description

Broadly stated, the problem of MDS is to find a configuration of n points in m-dimensional space such that the interpoint distances in the configuration reflect the experimental dissimilarities of the n objects (points); we use δ_{ij} to denote the dissimilarity between points i and j. The problem may be viewed as one of statistical fitting. The dissimilarities are fixed given quantities and we wish to find the m-dimensional configuration of objects whose inter-object distances 'fit them best'. The ultimate locations of the points in the configuration are selected to preserve the rank ordering of the relative distances of the experimental dissimilarities. Thus the final distance metric may be regarded as a monotone transformation of the rank ordering.

By adopting as our central goal the requirement of a monotonic relationship between the observed dissimilarities and the distances in the configuration, the accuracy of a proposed solution can be judged by the degree to which this condition is approached. For a proposed configuration, we perform a monotonic regression of distance upon dissimilarity and use the residual sum of squares, suitably Normalised, as a quantitative measure of fit, known as the stress. The configuration we seek is that with minimum stress.

The interpretability of the coordinates is of obvious importance so that, for geographical problems, our analysis is carried out in two dimensions ($m = 2$). Denote the n points in the configuration by $x_1, \ldots, x_n$ and let $x_i = [x_{i1}, x_{i2}]^T$, where the second subscript denotes the space dimension. Let d_{ij} be the (euclidean) distance between the points x_i and x_j. Then we define the stress, S, of the fixed configuration $x_1, \ldots, x_n$ to be

$$S_{(x_1, \ldots, x_n)} = \min_{\hat{d}_{ij} \text{ satisfying } M} \left[\sum_{i<j} \left(d_{ij} - \hat{d}_{ij} \right)^2 / \sum_{i<j} d_{ij}^2 \right], \qquad (6.1)$$

where M is the monotonicity condition. The exact form of M depends on how we deal with ties in the dissimilarities. Commonly, M is the condition whenever

$$\delta_{ij} < \delta_{rs} \text{ then } \hat{d}_{ij} \leq \hat{d}_{rs}, \qquad (6.2)$$

and whenever

$$\delta_{ij} = \delta_{rs} \text{ then } \hat{d}_{ij} = \hat{d}_{rs}, \qquad (6.3)$$

The configuration with minimum stress is found iteratively and computational details are given in Kruskal (1964). At each stage of the iterative procedure, the monotone regression to find the $\{\hat{d}_{ij}\}$ from the fixed known values $\{d_{ij}\}$ of the distances in the current configuration is also computed to yield two-dimensional plots which can be represented as maps.

6.3 An Australasian example

Our first illustration of the use of multidimensional scaling is by an application to the measles mortality records for six Australian states and New Zealand, 1860-1949. The general background to measles introduction into this area is discussed in Cliff *et al.* (1993, chapter 6).

The locations of the seven areas are plotted on a conventional map in Figure 10A. We can, however, plot their locations on other 'maps' more relevant to their history of measles mortality. For example, if we calculate the matrix of inter-correlations between the seven time series, we obtain the values given in Table 2. This shows that measles deaths in the adjacent states of Victoria and Tasmania are closely intercorrelated ($r = 0.893$). But the time series for Western Australia and Tasmania have little in common ($r = 0.040$). The last row in the table gives the average correlation between each state and all the

State (colony)	NSW	Vic	Qld	SA	WA	Tas	NZ
New South Wales	1.000	0.809	0.773	0.431	0.118	0.751	0.700
Victoria		1.000	0.666	0.433	0.134	0.893	0.628
Queensland			1.000	0.337	0.181	0.650	0.695
South Australia				1.000	0.320	0.267	0.600
Western Australia					1.000	0.040	0.119
Tasmania						1.000	0.567
New Zealand							1.000
Average over all states	0.597	0.594	0.550	0.398	0.152	0.528	0.551

Table 2.   Australia and New Zealand, 1860-1949: matrix of Pearson correlation coefficients between seven measles mortality time series. *(From Cliff et al. 1993)*

six other states. New South Wales (0.597) has the highest average correlation, while Western Australia (0.152) has the lowest. Despite the separation afforded by the Tasman Sea, New Zealand, with the third highest average (0.551), is closely tied to the eastern Australian states.

We can convert the concept of correlation into distance by taking the reciprocal of the coefficient. Thus the highly correlated Victoria-Tasmania series ($r = 0.893$) yields a reciprocal distance of 1/0.893 or 1.12 units; in contrast, the weakly-correlated Western Australia-Tasmania series ($r = 0.040$) have a longer distance of 25 units. Using these distances in place of the original correlation coefficients, multidimensional scaling produces the map that appears in Figure 10B. Four of the Australian states, plus New Zealand, form a cluster; conversely, South Australia and Western Australia stand apart from the rest. The size of each circle is drawn proportional to the average correlation, and the closest bond for each state is plotted as a vector.

The map in Figure 10B reflects average links over the whole period from 1860 to 1949. However, there is no reason to think that epidemiological associations have remained temporally constant. The individual states grew rapidly over the 90 years, and internal transport connections were greatly improved. So, in the next two maps of Figure 10, we explore the spatial pattern in the first and second halves of the period. Map (C) illlustrates the MDS plot from 1860 to 1904. Over these 45 years, the links between the five-state cluster were slightly stronger than in map (B). This earlier period stands in sharp contrast with the second half (1905-49) mapped in (D). Here the average correlation between states has nearly halved (from 0.502 to 0.286); the MDS map shows that the tight cluster has now broken up, and all seven geographical units are more scattered.

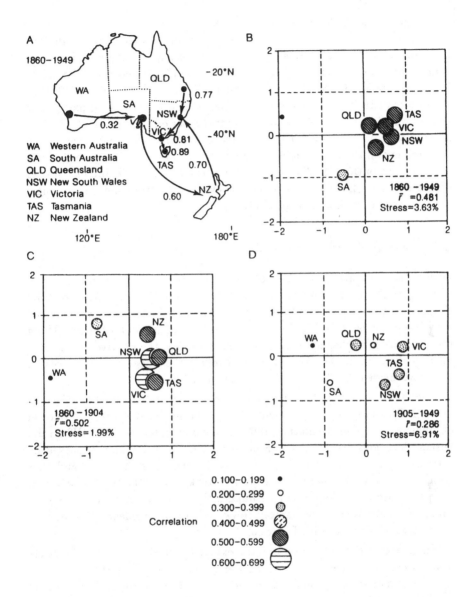

Figure 10. Australia and New Zealand: non-linear mapping of measles mortality.

(A) Conventional map of the states (colonies) for which measles mortality records are available over the period, 1860-1949. Non-linear MDS maps of cross-correlations (product moment correlation coefficient) between the measles mortality time series for the periods **(B)** 1860-1949, **(C)** 1860-1904, and **(D)** 1905-49.

(From Cliff et al. 1993)

One plausible epidemiological interpretation of the contrast between the two maps is that it reflects a coming-of-age in measles endemicity. Bearing in mind Bartlett's (1957, 1960) population threshold of 250,000 for measles endemicity, New South Wales crossed this line in 1850 and was followed by Victoria in 1880. By the close of the first half of our study period in 1904, all the other Australian states (except Tasmania) and New Zealand had passed the threshold. Thus, in the second half of the period, almost all states were large enough to have sustained and independent measles epidemics, rather than relying on the import of measles infectives from reservoir states to initiate their own outbreaks. This independence is reflected in the broader scatter of states in map (D). The epidemiological events that lie behind these changes are discussed in Cliff and Haggett (1985).

6.4   An Icelandic example

Our second illustration uses the monthly time series of influenza morbidity for Iceland, available for some 50 medical districts from 1945 to 1970. To study the space-time dynamics of the districts, the monthly time series were divided into four periods, namely: 1945-52, 1953-60, 1961-68 and 1969-70. Using the correlation coefficient as a measure of similarity, the relative locations of medical districts in the MDS space will reflect their degree of similarity in influenza incidence. The results are mapped in Figure 11.

The upper and lower left plots show the locations of the medical districts in the MDS spaces for 1945-52 and 1969-70. From 1945-52, the H1N1 strain of influenza A was in circulation; 1969-70 was dominated by the H3N2 strain. District locations are plotted as a point pattern, with Reykjavík marked by a triangle. The plots show Reykjavík at the centre of the space and that districts are clustered more closely around Reykjavík in the later time period than they are in the earlier. This implies that medical districts have, over time, become more like the capital, Reykjavík, in the incidence of influenza, a result which accords with Figure 6.

The maps in Figure 11 examine the extent to which (1) medical districts have, over time, have converged on Reykjavík in terms of their influenza time series (*upper right*) and (2) medical districts have similarly converged on their nearest regional centres (*lower right*). Those medical districts which either moved consistently nearer to (converging) or farther from (diverging) Reykjavík in terms of their point locations in the four MDS spaces, have been differently shaded on the upper right map. Most districts in the west and north of Iceland have moved closer to Reykjavík. Only the remotest districts in the northwestern and eastern fjords and on the south coast where the permanent icecap, Vatnajökull, reaches the sea, do not exhibit this trend.

The lower right map examines the behaviour of medical districts with

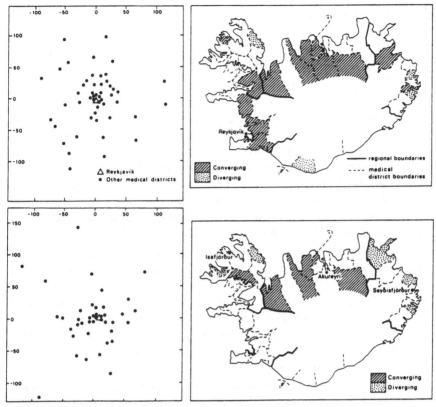

Figure 11. Iceland: non-linear mapping of morbidity in Icelandic influenza epidemics, 1945-70. Location of medical districts in MDS spaces for 1945-52 (*upper left*) and 1969-70 (*lower left*). The choropleth maps show which districts consistently converged on or diverged from Reykjavik (*upper right*) or their nearest regional centres (*lower right*) in MDS space over the period from 1945 and 1970.
(*From Cliff and Haggett 1988*)

respect to their regional capitals (named) in each of the regions delimited by the solid lines. In the north, there is a fairly consistent convergence of districts on Akureyri. In contrast, in the east, medical districts have become increasingly dissimilar to Seyðisfjörður.

Overall the maps imply an increased bonding of medical districts in their time series behaviour to the larger towns, a trend which reflects the growing internal cohesiveness of Iceland since 1945, brought about by the development of the country's internal airline network.

7   Conclusion

This paper has illustrated a series of mapping and statistical methods whereby the channels through which disease spread from one area to another is directed. The uneven distribution of population brought about by urban-rural contrasts frequently results in both wave-like and city-to-city spread of disease, and the channels are frequently similar for diseases of the same broad type. Viewing space as a graph upon which correlations are assessed may often help to determine the relative importance of the two components. Nor is the behaviour of space time-stationary. The use of multidimensional scaling and inter-area correlation techniques has shown that the cohesiveness of space may change in response to changes in, for example, transport technology, seasonal features of a disease and patterns of vaccination. The spatial scale of any analysis is also important in pattern detection.

Given that space has such a profound impact upon disease spread, it seems likely that models of spread which include explicit spatial components will show marked improvements in goodness-of-fit as compared with models that omit such features. In Table 3, we summarize the results of our own experience obtained by applying a variety of models with spatial components to Icelandic data for both measles and influenza morbidity in the period, 1945-70. The models used are formally defined in Cliff et al. (1993, Chapters 14 and 15). As implied by the names in the first column of Table 3, they include linear and non-linear regression formulations, as well as models of a disease transfer mechanism such as the Hamer-Soper and chain binomial.

The conclusions that may be drawn on the basis of our experience are:

(1) No model has yet been found that gives reasonable projections of both epidemic recurrences and epidemic size. Generally, if a model is devised which will forecast recurrences acceptably, then size is over-estimated. To forecast recurrences adequately, the model has to be made sensitive to changes signalling the approach of an epidemic, with the result that it overshoots when the epidemic is in progress.

(2) Models which are based only on the size of the infective population in previous time periods consistently fail to detect the approach of an epidemic. Instead, they provide reasonable projections of cases reported, but tend to run in arrears.

(3) Time series models with parameters fixed through time have a tendency to smooth through the highs and lows of an epidemic because they are unable to adapt to the changes between build-up and fade-out phases of an outbreak. Time-varying parameter models are better at avoiding this problem.

(4) Epidemic recurrences can be reasonably anticipated only by incorporating into the model information on the size of the susceptible population and/or properly identifying the lead-lag structure among geographical areas.

Model	Application format		Principal data inputs		Temporal parameter structure		Comments
	Single region	Multi-region	S	I	Fixed	Varying	
Hamer–Soper	To all medical districts		x	x	x		Good at forecasting epidemic recurrence years ahead; average to poor on estimating epidemic size
Chain binomial	Reykjavik		x	x	x	x	Initial one month lag effect; able to lock onto course of epidemic; reasonable estimates of epidemic size
		Northwest Iceland ($n = 5$)	x	x	x		Use of regional centre as epidemic lead indicator produces good estimates of epidemic starts in other medical districts; poor estimates of epidemic size
Autoregressive	Reykjavik			x	x		One month lag effect; consistently misses epidemic statrts; reasonable estimates of epidemic size
	Reykjavik			x		x	Initial one month lag effect; adapts to changing phases characteristics; overestimates epidemic size
GLIM		Northwest Iceland ($n = 5$)	x	x	x		As fixed in time parameter chain binomial
Kalman filter	Reykjavik			x		x	Initial lag effect, but locks on to epidemic course at expense of over estimates of epidemic size
Bayesian entropy	Reykjavik		x	x		x	Despite separate epidemic/no epidemic models, one month lag effect in predicting epidemic curve; probability forecasts of epidemic/no epidemic good; model switches states in correct month
Simultaneous equation		Multi-region chains	x			x	Areas studied as causal chains; good phase characteristics guarenteed by formulation of model; non-registration of serial interval and data recording interval restricts use in forecasting
Logistic transformation		Multi-region chains	x			x	Good probability forecasts of epidemic/no epidemic states; slow state switching

Table 3. Characteristics of models applied to Icelandic measles data, 1945-70.
(From Cliff et al. 1993)

Incorporation of spatial interaction information markedly improves an ability to forecast recurrences in lagging areas. Information on susceptible population levels also serves to prime a model to the possibility of a recurrence, as is made clear by the various threshold theorems. Models based on susceptible populations, but which are single- rather than multi-region, tend to miss the start of epidemics but rapidly lock on to the course of an epidemic thereafter. Models which are dominated by spatial transmission information at the expense of information on the level of the susceptible population in the reference region, produce estimates of epidemic size which reflect the course of the epidemic in the triggering regions rather than in the reference region.

These conclusions all highlight the need to identify precisely the costs and gains to be made for each extra element of complexity added to our models. It is all too easy to specify statistically sophisticated models which often achieve little more than simple trend predictors. But by adding in time-varying parameters, spatial lead-lag structures, and local small-area data on susceptible populations, it may be possible to edge closer to one of the epidemiological goals set out by William Farr (1840) a century and a half ago when, in his second Registrar General's report for England and Wales, he expressed his hope that empirical laws could be discovered underlying the waxing and waning of epidemics.

Acknowledgements

The work described in this paper has resulted from collaborative research with Professor P. Haggett, Department of Geography, University of Bristol, England, stretching back over a decade. Our principal funding body is the Wellcome Trust.

References

Anderson, R.M. and May, R.M. (1991) *Infectious Diseases of Humans: Dynamics and Control*, Oxford University Press, Oxford.

Bailey, N.T.J. (1975) *The Mathematical Theory of Infectious Diseases and its Applications*, Griffin, London.

Bartlett, M.S. (1957) 'Measles periodicity and community size', *J. R. Statist. Soc. A* **120**, 48–70.

Bartlett, M.S. (1960) 'The critical community size for measles in the United States', *J. R. Statist. Soc. A* **123**, 37–44.

Cliff, A.D. and Haggett, P. (1980) 'Geographical aspects of epidemic diffusion in closed communities'. In *Statistical Applications in the Spatial Sciences*, N. Wrigley (ed.), Pion, London, 5–44.

Cliff, A.D. and Haggett, P. (1988) *Atlas of Disease Distributions: Analytic Approaches to Epidemiological Data*, Blackwell Reference, Oxford.

Cliff, A.D., Haggett, P., Ord, J.K., Bassett, K. and Davies, R.B. (1975) *Elements of Spatial Structure: a Quantitative Approach*, Cambridge University Press, Cambridge.

Cliff, A.D., Haggett, P., Ord, J.K. and Versey, G.R. (1981) *Spatial Diffusion: an Historical Geography of Epidemics in an Island Community*, Cambridge University Press, Cambridge.

Cliff, A.D., Haggett, P., Stroup, D.F. and Cheney E. (1992) 'The changing geographical coherence of measles morbidity in the United States, 1962–88', *Statist. in Med.* **11**, 1409–24.

Cliff, A.D., Haggett, P. and Smallman-Raynor , M. (1993) *Measles: an Historical Geography of a Major Human Viral Disease from Global Expansion to Local Retreat, 1840-1990*, Blackwell Reference Books, Oxford.

Cliff, A.D. and Ord, J.K. (1973) *Spatial Autocorrelation*, Pion, London.

Dacey, M.F. (1963) 'Order neighbor statistics for a class of random patterns in multidimensional space', *Ann. Assoc. Amer. Geog.* **53**, 505–15.

Farr, W. (1840) 'Progress of epidemics', Second Report of the Registrar General of England, 91–8.

Fine, P.E.M. (1982) 'Applications of mathematical models to the epidemiology of influenza: a critique'. In *Influenza Models: Prospects for Development and Use*, P. Selby (ed.), MTP Press, Lancaster, 15–85.

Haggett, P. (1976) 'Hybridizing alternative models of an epidemic diffusion process', *Econ. Geog.* **52**, 136–46.

Haggett, P., Cliff, A.D. and Frey, A.E. (1977) *Locational Analysis in Human Geography* (2nd edition), Arnold, London.

Kendall, D.G. (1957) 'La propagation d'une épidémie ou d'un bruit dans une population limitée', *Publications de l'Institute de Statistique de l'Université de Paris* **6**, 307–11.

Kendall, D.G. (1971) 'Construction of maps from odd bits of information', *Nature* **231**, 158–9.

Kendall, D.G. (1975) 'The recovery of structure from fragmentary information', *Phil. Trans. R. Soc. Lond. A* **279**, 547–82.

Kruskal, J.B. (1964) 'Multidimensional scaling', *Psychometrika* **29**, 1–42.

Kruskal, J.B. and Wish, M. (1978) *Multidimensional Scaling*, Sage, Beverly Hills, CA.

Kuhn, H.W. and Kuenne, R.E. (1962) 'An efficient algorithm for the efficient solution of the generalized Weber problem in spatial economics', *J. Reg. Sci.* **4**, 21–33.

Mollison, D. (1977) 'Spatial contact models for ecological and epidemic spread', *J. R. Statist. Soc. B* **39**, 283–326.

Mollison, D. (1991) 'Dependence of epidemic and population velocities on basic parameters', *Math. Biosci.* **107**, 255–87.

van den Bosch, F., Metz, J.A.J. and Diekmann, O. (1990) 'The velocity of spatial population expansion', *J. Math. Biol.* **28**, 529–65.

Yule, G.U. and Kendall, M.G. (1950) *An Introduction to the Theory of Statistics* (14th edition), Griffin, London.

Velocities of Epidemic Spread

J. A. J. Metz
F. van den Bosch

Summary

The main aspect singling out geography from among other potential hetero-geneities, is that a local invariance under translations allows the construction of intermediate asymptotic solutions which describe how an epidemic expands in between the initial stage of exponential increase and the final stage when the front runs into the boundary of the spatial domain. During that interme-diate period, the infected area expands at a constant rate; as a consequence the size of the epidemic increases according to a power of time equal to the dimension of the domain (usually 1 or 2).

Except when contacts are extremely local, the speed at which the infected area expands is essentially determined by the deterministic linear process which results from keeping the density of susceptibles fixed at its disease free value. That process can be specified quite generally by means of the spatial analog of Lotka's equation from demography. Two recent papers (Mollison (1991), Van den Bosch et al. (1990a)) already gave a thorough review of the ins and outs. In the first part of this paper we give a short description of these ideas emphasizing the biological intuitions involved, and detailing a number of conjectures which still need proof.

Our main concrete examples in this paper are various fungal epidemics in agricultural crops. These examples also provide the motivation for two special topics treated in the second part of the paper, viz. (i) the rationale behind a quick procedure for calculating the asymptotic shape of the infested area from the Laplace transform of the infection kernel in case dispersal is not rotationally symmetric, e.g. owing to a prevailing wind direction, and (ii) an approximate, but effective, way of dealing with multiple dispersal mecha-nisms. The reason for considering (ii) is that in many fungal crop diseases most spores are dispersed in the canopy over only short distances, giving rise to local patches of high infestation called foci or hot spots. These foci are sep-arated spatially from other such hot spots deriving from the few spores which managed to get carried out of the canopy. As a result the local depletion of susceptibles already makes itself felt inside the foci before the effects of demo-graphic stochasticity are ironed out sufficiently for a deterministic model to apply to the epidemic as a whole. But the existence of a range of disease den-sities in between the stochastic and the susceptible depletion regimes formed

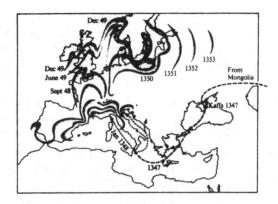

Figure 1: The spread of the Black Death in Europe, 1347–1353
(*From McEvedy and Jones (1978)*)

part and parcel of the 'linear conjecture' which was basic to the applications discussed earlier. The solution is to consider the foci as generalized diseased individuals. Field observations moreover force us to distinguish in addition between a further within field, and a long distance dispersal term, roughly corresponding respectively to spores staying within and leaving the boundary layer.

We end by discussing a number of open mathematical problems, the solution of which would be very helpful in various applied contexts.

1   What is so special about space?

At the highest level of epidemiological abstraction geographical position is just a special heterogeneity variable of the host population, to be treated on an equal footing to, for example, age, sex, social status, office, or commuter train. There are however a number of properties which make space stand out as rather special.

First and foremost, the spatial aspect of epidemics naturally lends itself to graphical presentations of considerable immediate appeal, as illustrated beautifully by Cliff and Haggett's (1988) Atlas of Disease Distributions. An example is the picture of the advancing wave of the Black Death as it circled the more sparsely populated and/or less well travelled southeastern parts of medieval Europe, eventually reaching Moscow by way of St. Petersburg (Figure 1).

A second reason for the popularity of space as a stratifying variable is that contact patterns are more easy to discern than for any other grouping of the host population. (After all, a respondent probably will give a more reliable answer to the question when he last visited a certain city than when he last sneezed near a 58 year old.) Good examples of modelling and of empirical research in this tradition are the big Russian computer simulations of the spread of influenza through the major cities of Russia (where traffic was both restricted and well monitored) or the world (see e.g. Rvachev and Longini (1985)) and the field work of Sattenspiel and Powell (1993) on the island of Dominica.

The third reason for paying special attention to the spatial aspect of epidemics is that the, local, translation invariance of the contact structure allows the construction of intermediate asymptotic solutions for the time range between the, usually short, initial stage of exponential increase and the final stage when epidemic expansion comes to a halt against the boundary of the spatial domain. The main result is that a local infection gives rise to an infected area which soon starts expanding at a constant rate, with a shape determined only by the nature of the infection process and not by the initial infection. Applied to an SIR epidemic in $\mathbf{R}^n$ this implies that there will be a longish period during which the total score of victims increases as t^n. In the remaining sections of our paper we shall concentrate on this intermediate domain, basing ourselves almost from the start on the assumption that space extends in a translationally invariant manner infinitely far in all directions.

Clearly the assumption of local translation invariance will not hold true for modern city-dwelling humans. It often will apply, though, as a good enough first approximation, in the case of plant epidemics as well as for many species of wildlife, and probably also for rural societies. Figure 2 shows all three phases of the spread of an unintentionally imported parasitic fungus over a hitherto clean continent. Unfortunately this is only one out of many such examples. A second scenario for the intermediate asymptotics game derives from the fact that many plant diseases are, as it is called, focal, i.e., most propagules of the disease organism disperse over only short distances, giving rise to local patches of high infestation called foci or hot spots. These foci are separated spatially from other hot spots deriving from the few propagules which managed to get transported over longer distances. As it turns out, the growth of such foci conforms well to the predictions from our models based on translationally invariant local contacts. The intermediate regime comes to an end when the foci start colliding.

As a final point we note that, though geographical dispersion undoubtedly is the prime candidate for letting us assume a locally translation invariant contact structure, it is the abstract nature of that structure that matters, not the semantic rule tying it to geographical space. If there would, for instance, exist examples of social space, as expressed in a contact structure, which happen to be isomorphic to $\mathbf{R}^n$, the same intermediate asymptotics would obtain. (We offer this, tongue in cheek, as an alternative explanation of the increase of the number of AIDS cases in the USA as t^3, postulated by Hyman and Stanley (1988)).

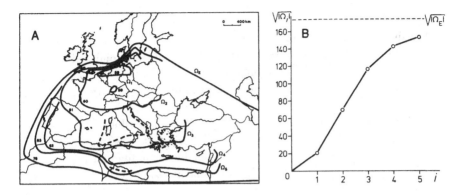

Figure 2: The spread of the tobacco blue mold (*Peronospora tabacina*) in Europe, 1959–1976.
A: $\Omega_E \equiv$ eventual endemic region, $\Omega_i \equiv$ the region covered by year i, the broken lines indicate intermediate late winter situations.
B: The square root of the area covered by year i, in units of approximately 20km.
(*From Heesterbeek and Zadoks (1987)*).

2 A short refresher on the spatial variant of the Kermack and McKendrick integral equation

In this section we concentrate on the epidemic with removal in a demographically closed situation, as this is the only case for which to this date firm mathematical results are available. Models for spatial epidemics of this type were first considered by Kendall (1957, 1965), who, however, only considered the special case where the time dependence can be represented through a differential equation (see Diekmann *et al.* 1995), though he formulated the spatial dependence in terms of a convolution integral representing the jump transport of infectivity over a longer distance. The existence and uniqueness of wave solutions for this model was investigated by Mollison (1972a), Mollison (1972b), Atkinson and Reuter (1976), Brown and Carr (1977), Barbour (1977). We shall start here immediately, in the wake of Diekmann (1978), Diekmann (1979), Thieme (1977a), Thieme (1977b), Thieme (1979a), with the most general model formulated as an integral equation in the spirit of Kermack and McKendrick (1927). Extensions to the n-type and vector borne cases are covered by Radcliffe *et al.* (1982), Radcliffe and Rass (1983, 1984a, 1984b, 1984c, 1984d, 1985, 1986, 1991), who also give the most general conditions for the occurrence of wavelike behaviour. The connection with the underlying individual-based stochastic model is considered by Mollison (1977),

Mollison (1991).

We shall use the following notation

$v(t,x)$	$\equiv$	local density of accumulated victims,
$\lambda(t,x)$	$\equiv$	local instantaneous infectivity, or 'force of infection'
$s(t,x) = s_0(x) - v(t,x)$	$\equiv$	local density of susceptibles,
$\Lambda(\tau,x,\xi)$	$\equiv$	mean infectivity at position x contributed by an individual infected τ time units ago at position ξ,
$h(t,x)$	$\equiv$	contribution to the local force of infection by the inoculum, or produced by victims infected before $t = 0$.

We assume that Λ is continuous and that both Λ and h are such that all the objects that we consider below are well defined.

Given the local force of infection individuals get infected independently. Therefore we may write

$$\frac{\partial v}{\partial t}(t,x) = s(t,x)\lambda(t,x)$$

$$= (s_0(x) - v(t,x))\left(\int_0^t \left(\int_\Omega \frac{\partial v}{\partial t}(t-\tau,\xi)\Lambda(\tau,x,\xi)d\xi\right)d\tau + h(t,x)\right), (2.1)$$

where the last expression results from adding all possible contributions to the infectivity at x (compare Diekmann *et al.* (1995)).

In the rest of this paper we assume that $\Omega = \mathbf{R}^n$, that s_0 is independent of x, and that Λ is invariant under translation, that is,

$$\Lambda(\tau,x,\xi) = A(\tau,x-\xi). \tag{2.2}$$

Within this context we define

$$\gamma := \int_0^\infty \int_\Omega A(\tau,\zeta)d\zeta d\tau, \quad R_0 := \gamma s_0, \tag{2.3}$$

$$B_0(\tau,\zeta) := s_0 A(\tau,\zeta), \tag{2.4}$$

and, provided $R_0 < \infty$,

$$a(\tau,\zeta) := \gamma^{-1} A(\tau,\zeta), \tag{2.5}$$

(so that $B_0 = R_0 a$). R_0 is the basic reproduction ratio (see e.g. Diekmann *et al.* 1995), B_0 the basic reproduction kernel of the disease, i.e., the reproduction kernel in an as yet disease free territory, and a the probability density of the $(1 + n)$-variate random variable: (infectors disease age at infecting, relative position of produced infection).

We assume everywhere that $R_0 > 1$.

The final assumption that we shall make everywhere, except in section 7, is that A is rotationally symmetric around $\zeta = 0$.

We start by considering the asymptotic behaviour for the case $\Omega = \mathbf{R}$. Any asymptotic solutions to (2.1), for $\Lambda(\tau, x, \xi) = A(\tau, x - \xi)$ and s_0 independent of x, should satisfy the time invariant equation

$$\frac{\partial v}{\partial t}(t, x) = (s_0 - v(t, x)) \int_0^\infty \int_\Omega \frac{\partial v}{\partial t}(t - \tau, \xi) A(\tau, x - \xi) d\xi d\tau. \qquad (2.6)$$

The translation invariance of (2.6) in both time and space suggests trying self-similar solutions

$$v(t, x) = \tilde{v}(x - ct). \qquad (2.7)$$

These solutions are naturally interpreted as waves travelling at speed c. By substituting (2.7) in (2.6) and rearranging the result, we find the equation for the wave shape

$$\frac{d\tilde{v}}{dy}(y) = (s_0 - \tilde{v}(y)) \int_{-\infty}^\infty \frac{d\tilde{v}}{dy}(\eta) K_c(y - \eta) d\eta, \qquad (2.8)$$

with

$$K_c(\eta) = \int_0^\infty A(\tau, \eta + c\tau) d\tau. \qquad (2.9)$$

Result 1 (Diekmann 1978; see also Diekmann and Kaper 1978 and Radcliffe and Rass 1983, 1984b) *If for a given c there exists a solution to (2.8) strictly confined between zero and s_0, then this solution is unique up to translation. The wave front is exponential, and moving from the front to the tail the density of victims monotonically increases from 0 to*

$$\tilde{v}(-\infty) = p(R_0)s_0, \qquad (2.10)$$

where p satisfies

$$\log(1 - p) = -R_0 p, \quad p(\infty) = 1 \qquad (2.11)$$

(as in the homogeneously mixed case, compare e.g. Diekmann et al. (1995)).

Whether or not (2.8) has a positive solution can be decided by considering the linearized equation

$$\frac{d\tilde{v}}{dy}(y) = s_0 \int_{-\infty}^\infty \frac{d\tilde{v}}{dy}(\eta) K_c(y - \eta) d\eta. \qquad (2.12)$$

(2.8) has a solution strictly confined between 0 and s_0 iff (2.12) has a positive solution (Diekmann 1978, Radcliffe and Rass 1983).

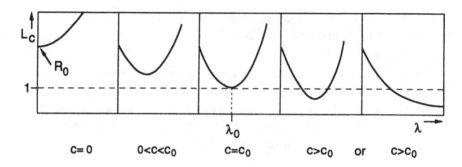

Figure 3: Shape of the function L_c defined in (2.16).

The positive solutions to (2.12) necessarily have the form

$$\tilde{v}(y) = \alpha \exp(-\lambda y) \qquad (2.13)$$

(we put in the minus sign since we are thinking of waves moving to the right). Substituting (2.13) into (2.12) gives the characteristic equation

$$L_c(\lambda) = 1, \qquad (2.14)$$

where

$$L_c(\lambda) \;:=\; s_0 \int_{-\infty}^{\infty} e^{-\lambda \eta} K_c(\eta) d\eta \qquad (2.15)$$

$$= \int_0^{\infty} \left(\int_{-\infty}^{\infty} e^{-\lambda(\zeta + c\tau)} B_0(\tau, \zeta) d\zeta \right) d\tau = \overline{B}_0(\lambda c, \lambda), \qquad (2.16)$$

where $\overline{B}_0(q, z)$ is the Laplace transform of $B_0(\tau, \zeta)$, one-sided with respect to τ, and two-sided with respect to ζ. λ^{-1} characterizes the steepness of the wave front. Using the various properties of the Laplace transform it is easy to show that $L_c(\lambda)$ has the kind of properties depicted in Figure 3. From this we deduce that there exists a c_0 such that (2.14) allows real solutions for all $c \geq c_0$, and none for $c < c_0$, where c_0 can be calculated from

$$\frac{\partial L_{c_0}}{\partial \lambda}(\lambda_0) = 0, \quad L_{c_0}(\lambda_0) = 1. \qquad (2.17)$$

As it turns out, c_0 is the only wave speed that matters. To see why, consider a line of firepots, where each subsequent one has a slightly longer length of fuse attached to it. On igniting the fuses we see a wave of flares progressing at a speed dependent on the increment in fuse length between subsequent pots. However, when the firepots can also be set alight by a neighbouring flare, there will be a minimal speed. Any slower wave will be overtaken by the autonomous one generated by the mutual ignition.

Van den Bosch *et al.* (1990a) give graphs of the solutions of (2.17) for various kernels of practical interest. They moreover give approximate explicit formulas in terms of the cumulants of a, derived from a perturbation expansion in $\epsilon = \log(R_0)$, as well as a, numerically derived, indication of their domain of applicability.

Remark

Of the authors to whom we refer for the proof of result 1, Radcliffe and Rass (1984b) make the weakest assumptions about the infection kernel. The only properties of the kernel that really seem to matter are that its Laplace transform should be well defined on at least some open set in the (q, z)-plane and that λ_0 does not coincide with the upper boundary of the interval of definition of L_{c_0}. No need to say that the exceptions will be exceedingly rare as the domain of definition of L_c is usually bounded by the occurrence of a pole. (For some reason both Diekmann 1978 and Radcliffe and Rass 1983, 1984b, restricted themselves to the case where the infection kernel can be written as a product $A(\tau, \zeta) = A_1(\tau)A_2(\zeta)$, but this assumption does not appear to play any special role in their proofs.)

We are now ready for the case $\Omega = \mathbf{R}^n$, $n > 1$. (In most applications n will be two.) Of course we have the possibility of plane waves in which at any one time the density of victims is constant along an $n - 1$ dimensional subspace, moving with speed $c \geq c_0$ in the direction orthogonal to that subspace. Now consider the more realistic case of an epidemic started from a localized initial infection. As the infected area expands, its contours, as seen by a local observer moving along with the expansion, will become flatter and flatter, and the outgoing wave of infection will become ever more akin to a plane wave with speed c_0. At present only a slightly weaker result has been proven though, following a line of investigation initiated by Aronson and Weinberger (1975), Aronson and Weinberger (1978) and Aronson (1977) for reaction diffusion equations, resp. the simple epidemic:

Result 2 (Diekmann 1979, Thieme 1979a, Radcliffe and Rass 1986): *Let c_0 and λ_0 be calculated from the model for one dimensional epidemic spread based on the, marginal, basic reproduction kernel*

$$B_{0m}(\tau, \zeta_1) = \int_{-\infty}^{\infty} \cdots \int_{-\infty}^{\infty} B_0(\tau, \zeta_1, \zeta_2, \ldots, \zeta_n) d\zeta_2 \ldots d\zeta_n. \qquad (2.18)$$

Suppose the epidemic in n dimensions gets started by an initial infection h such that for all $u \in \mathbf{R}^n$ with Euclidean norm $\|u\| = \langle u, u \rangle = 1$

$$\int_0^{\infty} \left(\int_{\Omega} e^{\lambda \langle u, x \rangle} h(t, x) dx \right) dt < K(\lambda) < \infty \text{ for all } 0 < \lambda < \lambda_0, \qquad (2.19)$$

then an observer moving out at a speed $c > c_0$, will outrun the epidemic, i.e., see $v \to 0$, and an observer moving at a speed $c < c_0$ will see $v \to p(R_0)s_0$,

Remarks

1. A simple sufficient condition for (2.19) is that
   (a) the total initial infection is finite and
   (b) far away the total starting infection at any one place,

$$h_{tot}(x) = \int_0^\infty h(t, x)dt, \qquad (2.20)$$

is $O(e^{-\lambda_0 \|x\|})$, i.e., there exist constants d and k such that $h_{tot}(x) < ke^{-\lambda_0 \|x\|}$ for $\|x\| > d$.

2. Radcliffe and Rass (1986), who in other respects made the weakest assumptions possible, once more assumed that $A(\tau, \zeta) = A_1(\tau)A_2(\zeta)$. Moreover they broke down h in terms of possible component processes, and expressed their conditions on h in terms of conditions on its components. However, their proof appears to go through almost without change for the slightly more general assumptions considered here.

3 Some applications: foci in fungal crop diseases

To apply the results from the previous section, we have to construct specific submodels telling us the nature of the infection kernel A. In this section we elaborate on this idea, using the expansion of foci of fungal crop diseases as an example (see Van den Bosch *et al.* 1988a, 1988b, 1988c, 1990b, and Zadoks and Schein 1979 for background information).

Focus formation occurs when by far the largest fraction of disease propagules stay in a close neighbourhood of the parent disease organism, while the remaining fraction of propagules is dispersed over much larger distances. In the case of fungal plant diseases the distinction is most often coincident with spores staying within, or being lifted above, the canopy, In the remainder of this section we ignore any long distance dispersal. In section 6 we shall investigate how the various dispersal processes combine in the speed at which an epidemic spreads over, say, a continent.

The spreading of spores in the canopy takes a very short time, in the order of minutes in the case of wind dispersed spores and in the order of hours for splash dispersed ones, compared to the lifetime of a single fungal lesion, which is in the order of weeks. Therefore we can write

$$a(\tau, \zeta) = a_1(\tau)a_2(\zeta). \qquad (3.1)$$

The next step is to find expressions for a_1 and a_2. In the case of a_2 it is fairly easy to devise a mechanistic model for the dispersal process. In the case of

a_1 the best we can do is a curve fitting job. To this end we chose the delayed gamma family:

$$a_1(\tau) = \begin{cases} 0 & \text{if } 0 < \tau \leq \alpha \\ \frac{\beta(\beta(\tau-\alpha))^{k-1}e^{-\beta(\tau-\alpha)}}{\Gamma(\beta)} & \text{if } \alpha \leq \tau \end{cases} \qquad (3.2)$$

(α is the length of the latency period), as it both encompasses in a parameter sparse way the range of shapes one would expect to occur and has a simple Laplace transform.

To derive a_2, or rather its Laplace transform, we start from the observation that, in the canopy, spores essentially perform a Brownian random walk, moved by either air turbulence or splashing rain drops, except that they may randomly stay put. Therefore the probability density $p(t, \zeta)$ of the position of a spore which is still on the move satisfies

$$\frac{\partial p}{\partial t} = \frac{1}{2}\sigma^2\left(\frac{\partial^2 p}{\partial \zeta_1^2} + \frac{\partial^2 p}{\partial \zeta_2^2}\right) - \mu p, \quad p(0, \zeta) = \delta(\zeta_1)\delta(\zeta_2), \qquad (3.3)$$

and

$$a_2(\zeta) = \int_0^\infty \mu p(t, \zeta)dt, \qquad (3.4)$$

where σ^2 is the variance increment per unit of time and μ the rate at which spores get trapped. Laplace transforming (3.3) and (3.4) yields

$$q\overline{p}(q, z) - 1 = \frac{1}{2}\sigma^2(z_1^2 + z_2^2)\overline{p} - \mu\overline{p}, \quad \overline{a}_2(z) = \mu\overline{p}(0, z). \qquad (3.5)$$

From (3.5) we find that

$$\overline{a}_2(z) = \frac{1}{1 - \omega^2(z_1^2 + z_2^2)}, \text{ and } \overline{a}_{2m}(z_1) = \overline{a}_2(z_1, 0) = \frac{1}{1 - \omega^2 z_1^2}, \qquad (3.6)$$

where $\omega^2 = \sigma^2/2\mu$. The corresponding marginal distribution a_{2m} is a double exponential one, and the distance bridged follows a so-called Bessel distribution (Broadbent and Kendall 1953, Williamson 1961).

Data to calibrate the model are provided by two sorts of experiments done on various occasions in the past: (i) Spores about to disperse are collected every day with a little vacuum cleaner from experimentally induced infections. (ii) First generation lesions are counted at various distances from an infected plant put in an otherwise clean field. For most published data sets which we looked at, the fit of our submodels turned out to be surprisingly good. In fact the Bessel distribution overall gave a better fit than any of the various published empirical families, which were devised specifically with the purpose of fitting this type of data!

To predict the rate of focus expansion we also need the value of R_0. This quantity cannot be obtained from the vacuum cleaner data, as most spores fail to reach favourable spots, or fail to successfully germinate due to lack of moisture at the right moments. If a_1 shows a sharp peak after a long latency period, R_0 can be estimated from the size of the first generation after the sharply timed introduction of a uniformly sparse initial infection in an otherwise clean field. When the generations show considerable overlap already from the start we may use the observed intrinsic rate of epidemic increase, r_0, (provided of course that the exhaustion of susceptibles does not make itself felt before the exponential phase is reached) to calculate R_0 from the characteristic equation of the well mixed case

$$1 = R_0 \int_0^\infty e^{-r_0\tau} a_1(\tau)d\tau. \tag{3.7}$$

Unfortunately, as published the available data sets almost uniformly fall short of giving the full details needed for testing the theoretical developments. In particular estimates of R_0 are found wanting; of all the quantities involved, R_0 is most intricately dependent on local environmental circumstances, and only the value of R_0 pertaining to the precise environmental circumstances of the focus expansion will do. Therefore in 1985 Professor Jan Carel Zadoks of Wageningen Agricultural University and the second author performed a set of additional experiments to estimate both R_0 and c_0 for two fungus-host systems about which already a good amount of basic data were available in the Wageningen archives, stripe rust (*Puccinia striiformis*) race 232E137 on wheat cultivar Clement, and downy mildew (*Peronospora farinosa*) race 3 on spinach cultivar Noorman (Van den Bosch *et al.* 1988c). Estimates for the parameters α, k, β and ω^2 were derived from earlier experiments on different but similar race-cultivar combinations. The observed values of c_0 were resp. $9.4 \pm 0.8 \, \mathrm{cm\,day}^{-1}$ and $2.3 \pm 0.2 \, \mathrm{cm\,day}^{-1}$, compared to predicted values of $8.0 \pm 1.5 \, \mathrm{cm\,day}^{-1}$ and $3.0 \pm 2.4 \, \mathrm{cm\,day}^{-1}$, an altogether satisfying result.

Remark

Given all the special precautions that should be taken to get at least the potential for a good correspondence between theory and data, one might well ask about the value of such experiments. The answer to this is that (i) the theory still makes a large number of simplifying assumptions, such as neglecting host plant growth during the growing season or the three dimensional architecture of the canopy, (ii) the problems cropping up when trying to get a good match helped to clarify our own mental picture of the disease transmission process, and (iii) the sensitivity analysis on the calculation of the speed from the primary data gave clear indications about the weakest links in any attempt at a mechanistically based prediction of, say, loss of harvest due to focal fungal disease outbreaks.

A final outcome from the modelling exercise was that for the particular family of kernels under consideration the dependence of R_0 on c_0 over largish regions of the parameter space turns out to be well fitted by

$$c_0 \approx f + g \log(R_0), \qquad (3.8)$$

with f and g dependent on α, k, β and ω^2 (Van den Bosch *et al.* (1988b); from the characteristic equation (2.13) this relation can easily be seen to apply for R_0 very large, but it also applies, with different, eyeballed, values of f and g, at fairly small values of R_0). One use of (3.8) is to give a relation between focus sizes at harvest time and (i) the fraction of resistant hosts in host dilution experiments, for which R_0 is proportional to the fraction of nonresistant hosts, or (ii) the degree of resistance of a host. An experiment specifically designed for the purpose (Van den Bosch *et al.* 1990b) amply confirmed the applicability of (3.8) in practical situations. Our present view is that formula (3.8) may well turn out to be the most directly useful result of the developments presented in this section!

4 Conjectures about generalizations, and the connection to Fisher's equation

4.1 Some preliminary remarks about the integral equation representation of the density dependent dynamics of well mixed populations

The birth rate b of a, non-spatial, general structured population model with everybody born equal, necessarily satisfies the integral equation

$$b(t) = \int_0^t B(\tau, t - \tau; y_b | E) b(t - \tau) d\tau + \int_Y B(t, 0; y | E) N_0(\{dy\}) \qquad (4.1)$$

with corresponding equation for the population state N

$$N(t) = \int_0^t U(\tau, t - \tau; y_b | E) b(t - \tau) d\tau + \int_Y U(t, 0; y | E) N_0(\{dy\}) \qquad (4.2)$$

In this expression $B(\tau, t - \tau; y | E)$ is the rate at which an individual having state y at time $t - \tau$ ($\tau \geq 0$) and exposed to an environment E, gives birth a time interval of length τ later, at time t. Here $\mathbf{Y}$ denotes the set of possible physiological states in which an individual may reside, or *i*-state space, and y_b the birth state. $N(t)$ and $N_0 = N(0)$ are measures on $\mathbf{Y}$. Finally $U(\tau, t - \tau; y | E)$ is a measure on $\mathbf{Y}$ giving the probabilities that an individual is still alive at time t and resides in certain subsets of $\mathbf{Y}$, conditional on it being alive and in state y at time $t - \tau$, and it being exposed to the environment E. Of course

(i) $B(\tau, t - \tau; y|E)$ and $U(\tau, t - \tau; y|E)$ depend on E over the interval $[t - \tau, t]$ only, and

(ii) for constant E, say $E(t) = E^*$, B and U do not depend on their second arguments.

In the non-spatial variant of the epidemic model of the previous sections $b(t) = dv/dt$, $E(t) = s(t) = s_0 - v(t)$, and $B(\tau, t - \tau; y_b|E) = E(t)A(\tau)$.

Remarks

1. The interpretation makes clear that B and U should satisfy the consistency relations

$$B(\tau, t; y|E) = \int_Y B(\tau - \tau', t + \tau'; y'|E)U(\tau', t; y|E)(\{dy'\}), \qquad (4.3)$$

$$U(\tau, t; y|E) = \int_Y U(\tau - \tau', t + \tau'; y'|E)U(\tau', t; y|E)(\{dy'\}), \qquad (4.4)$$

2. If we wish to be completely general we should work with the once integrated form of (4.1), as there exist cases, and not even very exceptional ones, in which the cumulative number of births is well defined, but the birth rate is not. A more detailed, but still heuristic, exposition of the ensuing formalism can be found in Diekmann *et al.* (1995) and Diekmann and Metz (in press). Metz and de Roos (1992) discuss in general heuristic terms the connection of (4.1) and (4.2) with the underlying individual-based stochastic formulations. If $E = E^*$, a constant, (and if some slight additional conditions are fulfilled) Feller's renewal theorem (see e.g. Jagers 1975) guarantees that for large time

$$b(t) \sim e^{r(E^*)t}, \qquad (4.5)$$

where the intrinsic rate of population increase $r(E^*)$ can be calculated from the usual characteristic equation

$$1 = \int_0^\infty e^{-r(E^*)\tau} B(\tau, 0; y_b|E^*)d\tau, \qquad (4.6)$$

while the corresponding normalized stable *i*-state distribution $N_d(E^*)$ can be written as

$$N_d(E^*) = \frac{\int_0^\infty e^{-r(E^*)\tau} U(\tau, 0; y_b|E^*)d\tau}{\int_Y (\int_0^\infty e^{-r(E^*)\tau} U(\tau, 0; y_b|E^*)d\tau)(\{dy\})} \qquad (4.7)$$

In the general autonomous case the environment is determined directly by the population according to

$$E = F(HN), \qquad (4.8)$$

H a linear operator. Still more generally the environment may itself be the output of some dynamical system having the population output HN and possibly some external driver, like the weather, as inputs.

This formalism can be immediately extended to the case where individuals may differ in their states at birth, but general existence and uniqueness results are only available, yet, when the number of possible states at birth is finite.

Below we shall consider the extension of this formalism to the spatially distributed case, again under the additional assumptions that space is homogeneous and infinitely extended, and that all movement is isotropic.

4.2 The 'linear conjecture'

The essential ingredients of the Diekmann/Thieme/Radcliffe and Rass results were

1. homogeneity of the virgin environment: $E(0,x) = E_0 \ (= s_0)$, or more generally, $E(0,x) \to E_0$ for $\|x\| \to \infty$ sufficiently fast (and the initial environmental conditions, $E(0,\cdot)$, are not that bad near to $x = 0$, and the initial population state, N_0, that localized, that the population is driven to an early extinction),

2. 'sublinearity' of the birth process: individuals should perform uniformly less well in non-virgin environments than in the virgin one:

$$\forall \tau, t \ B(\tau, t, \zeta, x; y_b | E) \le B(\tau, 0, \zeta, x; y_b | E_0) =: B_0(\tau, \zeta; y_b) \qquad (4.9)$$

   for all E that can develop from E_0 over the course of time,

3. the influence of individuals on the environment should be sufficiently localized around their place of birth, and the influence of the environment on $B(\tau, t, \zeta, x; y_b | \cdot)$ should be sufficiently localized around x (or, equivalently, $x + \zeta$).

Conjecture 1 *As soon as (1)–(3) (and some appropriate continuity conditions) are fulfilled and*

$$R_0 := \int_0^\infty \int_\Omega B_0(\tau, \zeta; y_b) d\zeta d\tau > 1, \qquad (4.10)$$

asymptotic spread results analogous to result 1 apply: let c_0 and λ_0 be calculated from (2.16) and (2.17) with the marginal expected reproduction kernel in the virgin environment

$$B_{0m}(\tau, \zeta_1; y_b) = \int_{-\infty}^\infty \cdots \int_{-\infty}^\infty B_0(\tau, \zeta_1, \zeta_2, \ldots, \zeta_n; y_b) d\zeta_2 \ldots d\zeta_n \qquad (4.11)$$

substituted for the one dimensional basic reproduction kernel B_0. Suppose that for all $u \in \mathbf{R}^n$, with $\|u\| = 1$,

$$\int_0^\infty \int_\Omega e^{\lambda \langle u,x \rangle} h(t,x) dx dt < K(\lambda) < \infty \text{ for all } 0 < \lambda < \lambda_0, \qquad (4.12)$$

where

$$h(t,x) = \int_\Omega \int_{\mathbf{Y}} B_0(t, x - \xi; y) N_0(\xi, \{dy\}) d\xi \qquad (4.13)$$

then (1) an observer who runs faster than c_0 will see b as well as N decline to zero, and (2) there exist a number $b_{cr} > 0$ (cr for 'crest') and a Borel measure $N_{cr} > 0$, such that an observer who runs at a speed $c_- < c_0$ ends up in places where in the past there has at least once occurred a birth peak of size b_{cr} or larger, and the local supremum over $(0,t)$ of N has a value of N_{cr} or larger, i.e. for all $u \in \mathbf{R}^n$, with $\|u\| = 1$, and all measurable $Y \subset \mathbf{Y}$

$$\lim_{t \to \infty} \sup_{\tau \in (0,t)} b(\tau, c_- tu) \geq b_{cr}, \qquad (4.14)$$

and

$$\lim_{t \to \infty} \sup_{\tau \in (0,t)} N(\tau, c_- tu)(Y) \geq N_{cr}(Y). \qquad (4.15)$$

The idea behind this conjecture is that the wave is pulled by its forward tail, where the environment still looks sufficiently virgin. Below we shall refer to c_0 calculated from (4.11), (2.16) and (2.17) as the 'linear speed of spread'.

Remark

If we wish to apply the previous conjecture in concrete situations we have to watch out for cases where the deterioration of the environment makes itself felt already before the local number of individuals is sufficiently large to iron out the effects of demographic stochasticity. In situations where this is the case we may expect the linear speed of spread, calculated from the expected reproduction kernel in a perpetually virgin environment, to overestimate the rate of spread for the stochastic model (see also Mollison 1991, Mollison and Levin 1995).

Thieme (1979b) proved an asymptotic spread result of roughly this kind for the special case of juvenile dispersal combined with nursery competition. (We only characterize his mathematical assumptions by one of the biological mechanisms which lead to them. The class of biological mechanisms considered by Thieme was considerably larger. In fact even the epidemic equations from section 2 can by an appropriate change of variables be recast in a 'nursery competition cum juvenile dispersal' form.) A good survey of the many results that are available for the discrete time case can be found in Kot (1992); see also Lui (1989a, 1989b).

4.3 Connection with the Fisher/KPP equation

The model for spatial spread usually encountered in the population dynamical literature is phrased as a diffusion equation,

$$\partial n / \partial t = D \Delta n + f(n) n \qquad (4.16)$$

(see Skellam 1951, 1973, Okubo 1980). This equation is the differential equation analog of our, more general, integral equation for the dynamics of a spatially distributed population. The main advantage of (4.16), and its close kin, over our integral equation models is that a lot more is known about its solutions. Good general references are Fife (1979), Okubo (1980), Britton (1986), Murray (1989), Grindrod (1991).

In accordance with the sublinearity assumption (2) from the previous subsection we shall assume that f decreases monotonically from a positive value at $n = 0$ to negative values at high n. The fulfilment of assumptions (1) and (3) comes as an immediate consequence of the fact that we let f depend on n only, and not, for example, on x as well.

The speed of spatial spread corresponding to (4.16),

$$c_0 = 2\sqrt{Df(0)}, \qquad (4.17)$$

was already calculated in 1937 by Fisher and independently by Kolmogorov *et al.* (1937), who also proved the convergence of the fronts in the one dimensional case for a particular class of initial conditions. Bramson (1983) gives full necessary and sufficient conditions for convergence to the various wave solutions for the one dimensional case.

It can be deduced from (2.17) that the linear speed of spread of any structured population in which the individuals move according to a Brownian motion with i-state independent diffusion coefficient D, is given by (4.17), with r_0, the intrinsic rate of population increase in the virgin environment, substituted for $f(0)$ (Van den Bosch *et al.* 1990a, Mollison 1991). For more general movement patterns (4.17) corresponds to the lowest order term in the perturbation expansion for c_0 in terms of $\epsilon = \log(R_0)$ for ϵ small, if we make the identifications

$$D = \frac{1}{2} \mu_0^{-1} \sigma_0^2, \quad f(0) = \mu_0^{-1} \log(R_0), \qquad (4.18)$$

with μ_0 the mean age at childbearing and σ_0^2 the mean squared displacement of childbearing, both in the virgin environment (Van den Bosch *et al.* 1990a). (This expression may get a little more intuitive appeal from the observation that the lowest order term in the perturbation expansion for r_0 in terms of $\epsilon := \log(R_0)$, ϵ small, in the non-spatial case also equals $\mu_0^{-1} \log(R_0)$.)

Conjecture 2 *Any model for the autonomous spatial dynamics of a structured population in which (a) all individuals are born equal, and for which (b) there exists environment-independent, Laplace transformable (in space and time) U° and B°, with corresponding $R^\circ = 1$, mean age at reproduction μ° and dispersal variance per generation $\sigma^{\circ 2}$, such that*

$$|B(\tau, t, \zeta, x; y|E) - B^\circ(\tau, \zeta; y)| \ll 1 \qquad (4.19)$$

$$\|U(\tau, t, \zeta, x; y|E) - U^\circ(\tau, \zeta; y)\| \ll 1 \qquad (4.20)$$

can be approximated by Fisher's equation with

$$f(n) = r(F(nHN_d^\circ))n \text{ and } D = \frac{1}{2}\mu^{\circ - 1}\sigma^{\circ 2}, \qquad (4.21)$$

with N_d° the normalized stable population state corresponding to the spatially integrated version of the pair (B°, U°),

$$N_d^\circ = \frac{\int_0^\infty \int_\Omega U^\circ(t, \zeta; y_b) d\zeta dt}{\int_Y \int_0^\infty \int_\Omega U^\circ(t, \zeta; y_b) d\zeta dt(\{dy\})}, \qquad (4.22)$$

and $r(E^*)$ the intrinsic rate of natural increase corresponding to

$$\int_\Omega B(\tau, 0, \zeta, 0; s_0|E^*) d\zeta, \qquad (4.23)$$

provided we look at correspondingly large time and space scales. [N.B. $r(E^*)$ can again be approximated by $\mu(E^*)^{-1} \log(R(E^*))$.]

The non-spatial variant of this conjecture is considered in Greiner *et al.* (in press). Some more insight in the spatial variant may be gained from the consideration of the case $B = B^\circ$: in that case every individual on average produces one offspring, independent of the condition of the environment. The, linear, integral equation for b is the same as the integral equation for the probability density of a cumulative process defined on a renewal process (Cox 1962, Smith 1956, 1958). Therefore convergence of the population process to the solution of (4.16) with $f = 0$ is guaranteed by the central limit theorem. This tells us the correct time and space scales for looking in the large at the population models under consideration. When we only let B be near to B° (assumption (4.19) we have to guarantee that $r(E^*)$ should, for all relevant E^*, match with the time scale set by the diffusion limit for the case $B = B^\circ$.

Remark

Just as the diffusion limit for $B = B^\circ$ has the central limit theorem as its probabilistic counterpart, so has the linear speed of spread result as its counterpart the results from large deviation theory. The seamless meshing of the two classes of probabilistic results is visible in the fact, already mentioned above, that $c_0 = (\sigma_0/\mu_0)\sqrt{2\log(R_0)}(1 + O(\log(R_0)))$ for small $\log(R_0)$.

If we try to apply conjecture 2 to the epidemic with removal from section 2 we find that to get a non-degenerate limit we have to rescale the victim density v to keep $\tilde{v}(-\infty) = p(R_0)s_0$ equal to, say, K. If we do this, and rescale time such that $\mu^{-1}\log(R_0)$, μ the mean disease age at infecting, is made equal to, say, r_0, we end up with Fisher's equation with

$$f(n) = r_0(1 - n/K). \qquad (4.24)$$

4.4 Conjectures about the convergence of the wave shapes

All our remaining conjectures refer to the model for the epidemic with removal from section 2. We start with a conjecture for the case that $\Omega = \mathbf{R}$:

Conjecture 3 *For the one dimensional epidemic with removal a true convergence of fronts occurs, in the sense that an observer who rides with the wave sees a constant shape appearing, provided of course that $h(t, x)$ satisfies the conditions necessary to guarantee the usual asymptotic spread result.*

Figure 4 shows an example of such convergence as it is generally observed in numerical simulations.

Our final two conjectures deal with the convergence to planar waves in the case that $\Omega = \mathbf{R}^n$.

Conjecture 4 *If $h(t, x)$ satisfies the conditions necessary to guarantee the usual asymptotic spread result, then an observer riding with the wave along a radius from the origin will see around him the appearance of a constant wave shape which is flat in all directions orthogonal to his direction of movement.*

The phrasing of our last conjecture is considerably more vague:

Conjecture 5 *Wiggly fronts have a strong tendency to straighten.*

The rationale behind conjecture 5 is that we expect invaginations to receive a greater spill of infectious particles from adjacent areas so that they fill up, or equivalently lobes to erode as a result of the lesser spill of infectious particles immediately in front.

The reason for explicitly formulating conjecture 5 is that it leads us to indeed expect the presence of fairly well defined fronts in nature, despite all the distorting effects of, for example, local variations in terrain.

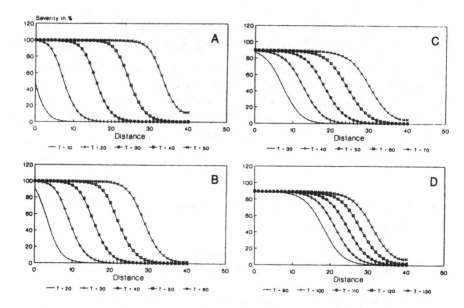

Figure 4: Convergence to a fixed wave shape in a simulation model for the two dimensional expansion of an epidemic with infectivity kernel $A(\tau, \zeta) = \int_0^\infty A_1(\tau')a_2(\tau - \tau', \zeta)d\tau'$, with A_1 a block between τ_0 and τ_1, and a_2 satisfying (3.3), with high values of μ and σ^2.
A: $R_0 = 5$, $\tau_1/\tau_0 = 8/3$.   **B**: $R_0 = 5$, $\tau_1/\tau_0 = 10/3$.
C: $R_0 = 2.5$, $\tau_1/\tau_0 = 8/3$.   **D**: $R_0 = 2.5$, $\tau_1/\tau_0 = 12/7$.
(From Zawolek and Zadoks 1989)

5   Some further applications

Thanks to the linear conjecture we can provisionally apply our speed of spread calculations to a much larger range of practical problems. Figure 5 shows the results of the efforts at predicting speeds in which we ourselves took part (Van den Bosch *et al.* 1988c, 1990a, 1992). It should be said, however, that in all cases but one, the approximate speeds calculated from (4.17) with (4.18) did an about equally good job on the scale of the figure. The one exception is striped rust on wheat, which had the immensely high R_0 of 55.

Other attempts at predicting speeds of population spread, all based on the diffusion model, were made by Skellam (1951) (oaks), Ammerman and Cavalli-Sforza (1984) (early farmers), Lubina and Levin (1988) (sea otters), and Andow *et al.* (1990) (muskrats, cereal leaf beetle, small cabbage white). (Skellam also analysed the range expansion of muskrats in Europe, but did not yet have access to the data on individual behaviour necessary for an *a priori* prediction.) Most of those predictions also turned out to be very good, considering the acts of faith involved in using measured individual parameters

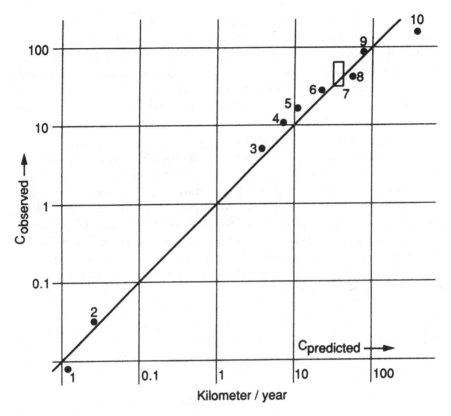

Figure 5: Observed and predicted speeds of population expansion. 1: Downy mildew foci on spinach ($R_0 = 3.2$). 2: Stripe rust foci on wheat ($R_0 = 55$). 3: Muskrat, Europe after 1930 ($R_0 = 1.6$). 4: Muskrat, Europe before 1930 ($R_0 = 3.1$). 5: House sparrow, North America ($R_0 = 1.8$). 6: House sparrow, Europe ($R_0 = 4.2$). 7: Rabies, Europe. 8: Collared Dove, Europe ($R_0 = 1.3$). 9: Starling, North America ($R_0 = 1.6$). 10: Cattle egret, South America ($R_0 = 1.45$). (Notice that some of the predictions are still off by, at most, 50%.)
(Data from Van den Bosch et al. 1988c, 1990a, 1992)

out of their original context, with the oaks and cereal leef beetles as notable exceptions. However, as pointed out already by Skellam, given the quality of the predictions in other cases, those predictions that are way off are often the most interesting ones, as they provide strong evidence for the presence of other dispersal mechanisms than the ones accounted for in the model. (A good general dicussion of these and other issues involved in linking models for distributed populations to reality can be found in Mollison (1991).)

The three main animal diseases that have been the subject of attempts at quantitatively predicting their patterns of spatial spread, are the Black Death, in essentially a one off undertaking by Noble (1974), Murray (1989), nuclear polyhedrosis virus in Douglas-fir tussock moths (Dwyer 1992, 1994) and rabies, all with fair results. (However, in the case of Black Death, and also of some of the many published rabies models, it has not been made clear beyond doubt that the parameter estimates were indeed obtained from independent sources.)

In the remaining part of this section we shall summarize our own trick for modelling rabies spread on the cheap (Van den Bosch *et al.* 1990a) – not so much that we take those efforts very seriously, but rather to illustrate that a little consideration of the empirical interpretation of the model constituents can still lead to unexpected results. Good general discussions about rabies modelling can be found in Bacon (1985). Murray (1989) surveys the alternative deterministic spatial approach taken by his own group, which in our opinion is certainly not less misguided than our own. Mollison (1991) provides a well reasoned antidote against the considerable naivities perpetrated both by ourselves and the Murrayans.

The primary hosts for rabies in Europe are foxes. Transmission takes place only in direct contacts (c.q. biting). Foxes have roughly fixed home ranges. The few radio-tracking data available suggest that home range use by rabid and uninfected foxes does not differ extensively (Andral *et al.* 1982). Therefore we may write

$$a(\tau, \zeta) = a_1(\tau) a_2(\zeta). \tag{5.1}$$

Radio-tracking data suggest moreover that the relative presence over the home range can be described roughly by a Gaussian density, with covariance matrix, say, $\theta^2 I$. Therefore we took a_2 to be a Gaussian density with mean zero and covariance matrix $\sigma^2 I$, with $\sigma^2 = 2\theta^2$, on the assumption that the movement of foxes in different home ranges is independent, and that the infection rate is proportional to the fraction of the time that they happen to be in close proximity. Rabies has a long latency period and a relatively short infectious period. For kernels which are Gaussian in space and very concentrated in time, around a mean μ, we may to a very good approximation set (Van den Bosch *et al.* 1990a, Mollison 1991)

$$c_0 \approx \frac{\sigma}{\mu} \sqrt{2 \log(R_0)}. \tag{5.2}$$

The main interest is in the dependence of c_0 on the properties of the local fox community. Here remarkable things start to happen: R_0 and σ are clearly not independent! Lower fox densities correspond to larger home ranges (if the densities are regulated by the quality of the terrain and not by shooting). Our earlier assumption about the infection process now forces us to set

$$\sigma^2 \propto \text{ area of home range } \propto s_0^{-1} \propto R_0^{-1}. \tag{5.3}$$

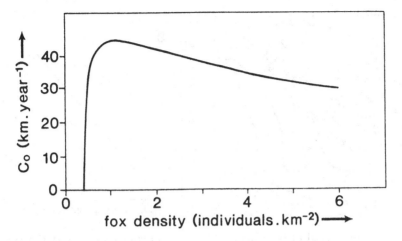

Figure 6: Predicted speed of spread of rabies in Europe as a function of the local fox density.

Substituting (5.3) into (5.2) gives

$$c_0 = \alpha\sqrt{\frac{\beta + \log s_0}{s_0}}, \quad \alpha \text{ and } \beta \text{ unknown constants.} \tag{5.4}$$

The resulting relation between the predicted speed of the rabies front and the range of feasible local fox densities (using independently derived estimates of α and β gleaned from the literature for calibration; Van den Bosch *et al.* 1990a) is depicted in figure 6. A striking feature is that intermediate velocities occur only in a very narrow interval of population densities: Effectively there is either an epidemic wave travelling at a, more or less, constant velocity, or no epidemic at all.

6 Multiple dispersal: one possible approach to the large scale spread of focal plant epidemics

Figure 7 shows the spread of a focal epidemic, late blight of potatoes, over part of Europe. When trying to predict the speed of such large scale spread we run into a problem. Before we can safely neglect the demographic stochasticity in the front part of the wave, inherent in the initiation of the especially important new infections outside the few foci which already got started, a non-negligible depletion of susceptibles already occurs inside those older foci. Therefore focal epidemics fail to satisfy the restriction on the practical applicability of the linear conjecture voiced in the remark at the end of subsection 4.2.

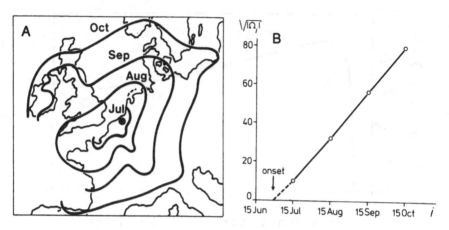

Figure 7: The spread of late blight of potato (*Phytophthora infestans*) over Europe in 1843.
A: Disease contours.
B: The square root of the area covered at different dates, in units of approximately 20 km.
(From Heesterbeek and Zadoks 1987)

The approximate solution which we shall pursue is to consider the foci as generalized diseased individuals.

Before we plunge into the calculations a few more observations on the modelling of this type of plant epidemic are in order (compare Heesterbeek and Zadoks 1987).

1. Field observations force us to distinguish between a further within field, and a long distance dispersal term, roughly corresponding to spores staying within resp. leaving the boundary layer, in addition to the within canopy dispersal which underlies its focal nature. Below the somewhat unexpected numerical effects of the partitioning of the spores between these two dispersal routes will be our major concern.

2. The distribution of the long range dispersed spores should in principle be derived from models for the dispersal of air-borne particles (smog, fall-out). A problem is that it is next to impossible to estimate the parameters using for example spore traps, as we did in the case of within canopy dispersion. This is of course the usual problem with rare but important events. The best we can hope for is a mechanistically based framework for the comparison of different diseases (Van den Bosch *et al.* 1994).

3. Often we shall be interested in the spread over a number of years. Here we are more lucky: winter mortality, m, may be expected to act roughly

by just pushing the wave back over a distance $\lambda_0^{-1}\log(1-m)$ (Van den Bosch *et al.* (1994)).

4. The peculiar local nature of the non-linearity inherent in the collision and subsequent merging of foci does preclude the construction of a deterministic limit model based on mass action considerations of the type discussed in its most general form in subsections 4.1 and 4.2. However, it is possible to produce a coupling argument (see Ball 1995) by constructing the spatial stochastic process under consideration from a spatial branching process. Since the sample functions of the focal epidemic lie below the corresponding sample functions of the branching process, the asymptotic speed of spread of the epidemic cannot be above the linear one. The two speeds will moreover presumably be close when the number of foci in the front of the wave can become fairly large before the effects of the local non-linearities (interaction of foci and interception of distantly dispersed spores by foci) becomes too noticeable.

Remark

A more precise phrasing of (4) would amount to presenting a stochastic version of the linear conjecture from subsection 4.2. We allowed ourselves a little less precision here on the pretext that we are only reviewing the deterministic theory. We shall make the following modelling assumptions:

$$B_0(\tau, \zeta) = \int_0^\infty B_1(\tau')B_2(\tau - \tau', \zeta)d\tau' \tag{6.1}$$

$$B_1(\tau) = \alpha\tau \tag{6.2}$$

$$B_2(\tau, \zeta) = \psi\kappa\delta(\tau)\delta(\zeta_1)\delta(\zeta_2) + \psi\phi(1 - \kappa)a_3(\tau, \zeta), \tag{6.3}$$

with

B_1	$\equiv$	the rate of spore production by a focus,
ψ	$\equiv$	the probability that a spore once landed in a host field produces a focus,
κ	$\equiv$	the fraction of spores that stays fairly close by,
ϕ	$\equiv$	the fraction of the country covered with host fields,
a_3	$\equiv$	the (normalized) long distance spore dispersal kernel.

For a_3 we shall only consider two, rotationally symmetric, limiting cases, derived from a more general long distance dispersal model,

$$a_{3a}(\tau, \zeta) = \delta(\tau)[\text{Bessel}]_\omega(\zeta), \tag{6.4}$$

$$a_{3b}(\tau, \zeta) = \delta(\tau)[\text{rotated exponential}]_\omega(\zeta). \tag{6.5}$$

Both distributions have but a single scale parameter ω. The corresponding

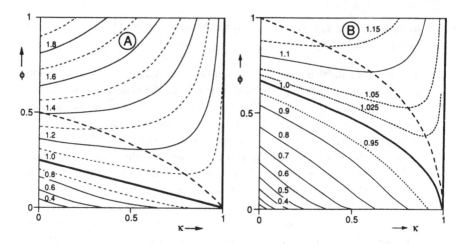

Figure 8: The effect γ, defined in equation (6.7), of the fraction of the spores that stays close to the mother focus, κ, and the fraction of the country covered by host fields, ϕ, on the rate of long distance spread of a focal epidemic.
$- - - -$: maximum of γ in the κ direction.
A: transport Bessel distributed.
B: transport rotated exponentially distributed.

Laplace transforms of the one-dimensional marginal distributions are

$$\bar{a}_{3am}(z_1) = \frac{1}{1 - \omega^2 z_1^2}, \quad \bar{a}_{3bm}(z_1) = \frac{1}{\sqrt{1 - \omega^2 z_1^2}} \tag{6.6}$$

(compare also section 3). The scale parameter ω has been chosen such that the convergence interval of the Laplace transform of a_3 is bounded by poles at $\pm\omega^{-1}$.

The interpretation makes clear that α and ψ always appear together as the product $\psi\alpha$. Dimensional considerations furthermore dictate

$$c_0(\alpha, \psi, \kappa, \phi, \omega) = \gamma(\kappa, \phi)\sqrt{(\psi\alpha)}\,\omega, \quad \lambda_0(\alpha, \psi, \kappa, \phi, \omega) = \rho(\kappa, \phi)\omega^{-1} \tag{6.7}$$

with γ and ρ still depending on whether we are dealing with model a or b. Substituting (6.7) into the (2.17) gives an equation for γ and ρ. The resulting contour plots of γ are shown in Figure 8.

The intriguing observation is that for sufficiently small ϕ, the curve of c_0 against κ shows a maximum. For models a and b the borderline is $\phi = 0.5$ resp. $\phi = 1$. For most crop species ϕ is well below 0.2, corresponding to maxima of c_0 at values of $\kappa > 0.8$ resp. $\kappa > 0.95$.

A little fiddling with the equation for γ and ρ, exploiting the properties of the Laplace transform of (6.3), shows that the last result is robust, at least for the probably practically most relevant case of fast rotationally symmetric dispersal. To this end one writes

$$L_c(\lambda) = \overline{B}_0(\lambda c, \lambda) = \frac{\phi(1 - \kappa)\psi\alpha}{(\lambda c)^2 - \kappa\psi\alpha} \frac{1}{g((\omega\lambda)^2)} \quad \text{with } g(y) := [\overline{a}_{3m}(\sqrt{\omega y})]^{-1}.$$

(6.8)

The scale parameter ω is is chosen such that $\overline{a}_{3m}$ has its poles at $z_1 = \pm\omega^{-1}$ and is well defined for $-\omega^{-1} < z_1 < \omega^{-1}$, so that $g(y) > 0$ for $0 \leq y < 1$, and $g(1) = 0$, (2.17) with (6.8) is equivalent to

$$\phi(1 - \kappa) = [(\gamma\rho)^2 - \kappa]g(\rho^2), \quad g(\rho^2) = -[(\gamma\rho)^2 - \kappa]g'(\rho^2)/\gamma^2. \quad (6.9)$$

(6.9) loses its meaning as an equation for a wave speed when $\kappa = 1$ or $\phi = 0$ but the solutions are continuous on the closed square $0 \leq \kappa \leq 1$, $0 \leq \phi \leq 1$. This allows us to conclude (just solve (6.9) for $\kappa = 0, 1,$ or $\phi = 0$) that

$$\lim_{\kappa \to 1} \gamma(\kappa, \phi) = 1, \quad \lim_{\phi \to 0} \gamma(\kappa, \phi) = \sqrt{\kappa}, \quad \gamma(0, \phi) = \eta\sqrt{\phi}, \quad (6.10)$$

with η still depending on the shape of the dispersal distribution. Therefore the contour line for $\gamma = 1$ in the (κ, ϕ)-plane consists of the vertical line $\kappa = 1$ in combination with a curve starting on the ϕ-axis at $\phi = \eta^{-2} > 0$, to the lower right hand corner of the square given by $(\kappa, \phi) = (1, 0)$. Above and to the right of this curve γ is larger than 1, only to decrease again to 1 when $\kappa \to 1$.

A final observation is that we expect that in most practical cases κ will be large, making γ roughly equal to one, independent of the dispersal model!

7 Relaxing the assumption of rotational symmetry

The use of self-similarity arguments in characterizing the intermediate asymptotics of deterministic epidemic spread is in no way dependent on the spreading mechanism being rotationally symmetric. We only made the isotropy assumption for pragmatical reasons, as it (i) considerably simplified the arguments, and (ii) is as least as good a modelling approximation in most applications as is the assumption of translation invariance. In this section we shall heuristically consider the extension to the non-isotropic case. Both for completeness sake and since we know of at least one important practical example where the isotropy assumption fails, viz. the dispersal of fungal spores in areas with a prevailing wind direction. We shall confine ourselves to the 2-dimensional case, since (i) it is the only case of clear practical interest, and (ii) it allows an exceedingly simple algorithm for calculating and plotting asymptotic disease contours. A rigorous underpinning of our arguments for the discrete time case can be found in Weinberger (1978, 1982) and Lui (1989a), 1989b).

If the wind blows sufficiently hard, even an exponentially growing population of finitely lived wind dispersed plants may eventually be blown off to infinity without leaving any trace of its passing. In other cases, the passing of the population leaves a visible trail. Think for example of the devastation caused by a fungal crop disease. Apparently we should distinguish between the spatial behaviour of a population (or rather of its birth rate) and possibly the aftermath of population growth. For the sake of definiteness we shall concentrate on two specific models, to wit the SIR epidemic model from section 2,

$$\frac{\partial v}{\partial t}(t,x) = [s_0 - v(t,x)]\left(\int_0^t \left(\int_\Omega \frac{\partial v}{\partial t}(t-\tau,\xi)A(\tau,x-\xi)d\xi\right)d\tau + h(t,x)\right), \quad (7.1)$$

and the corresponding linear model

$$b(t) = \int_0^t \left(\int_\Omega b(t-\tau,\xi)B_0(\tau,x-\xi)d\xi\right)d\tau + h(t,x), \quad (7.2)$$

$B_0 = s_0 A$, with h satisfying condition (2.19), but with λ_0 now depending on the direction $u = (\cos\phi, \sin\phi)^T$, $\phi \in \mathbf{R}/2\pi$, (see below).

To define our asymptotic contours we first introduce the limit contours corresponding to (7.1) and (7.2). To this end imagine that we observe the epidemic/population expansion from high up in a balloon which rises in such a manner that Ω in our perception is multiplied by t^{-1}. The curve in our field of vision outside of which v goes to zero, and inside of which v goes to $p(R_0)s_0$, we call V_E, and the curve outside of which b goes to zero, and inside of which b goes to infinity, we call V_L. The functions which map t into tV_E and tV_L will be called asymptotic contours.

V_E and V_L are connected in the following manner. Let P_E denote the set bounded on the outside by V_E, and P_L the set bounded on the outside by V_L. The considerations spelled out below imply that P_E is convex (we construct P_E as the intersection of infinitely many half planes). Combining this fact with the interpretation of P_E as the area of devastation left in the wake of the epidemic (remember that we look from sufficiently high up not to notice any small irregularities at its margins) shows that P_E can be constructed as the convex hull of $P_L \cup \{0\}$. Therefore we shall from now on concentrate on V_L. To simplify the notation we shall moreover drop the L.

It is technically more convenient to express V in terms of polar coordinates:

$$V =: \left\{r(\phi)\begin{bmatrix}\cos\phi \\ \sin\phi\end{bmatrix} \mid 0 < \phi \le 2\pi\right\}. \quad (7.3)$$

To calculate r we once more start with the consideration of plane waves. The difference from the isotropic case is that now the velocity c_0 of a plane

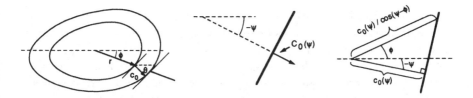

Figure 9: **A**: In the non-isotropic case different directions, ψ, support different speeds of plane waves, $c_0(\psi)$.
B: The speed of spread in a direction ϕ from the origin versus the normal speed, in the direction θ, of a disease contour.
C: When moving out in a direction ϕ while keeping inside the asymptotic contour we may never overtake a plane wave travelling in the direction ψ.

wave depends on its direction of movement, to be indicated as ψ ($\psi \in \mathbf{R}/2\pi$, see Figure 9A; the recipe for calculating $c_0(\psi)$ will be detailed below). When $c_0(\psi) > 0$ for all ψ, the relation between the functions c_0 and r can be deduced from the consistency conditions:

1. Where r is smooth the local speed of the asymptotic contour in the normal direction is $c_0(\theta)$, θ the direction of the outward normal (Figure 9B).

2. If we run in a direction ϕ at speed r we may never overtake any plane wave (Figure 9C). Therefore

$$\text{for all } \psi \quad r(\phi) \le F_\phi(\psi) := \frac{c_0(\psi)}{\cos(\psi - \phi)}. \tag{7.4}$$

Together conditions (1) and (2) imply that at points where r is smooth

$$r(\phi) = \min\{F_\phi(\psi) \mid \phi - \pi/2 < \psi < \phi + \pi/2\}. \tag{7.5}$$

Therefore in all points of smoothness the pairs (ϕ, r) should satisfy

$$\frac{dF_\phi}{d\psi}(\psi) = 0, \quad r(\phi) = F_\phi(\psi). \tag{7.6}$$

$F_\phi(\psi) \to \infty$ when $\psi \to \phi \pm \pi/2$. Therefore F_ϕ has at least one local minimum in the interval $(\phi - \pi/2, \phi + \pi/2)$. In solving (7.6) in dependence on ϕ we should of course follow the lowest local minimum. As long as c_0 depends smoothly on ϕ, r can be non-smooth only for those ϕ for which a second local minimum collides with the lowest one. In that case the full solution set of (7.5) will be larger than the graph of r by at least some 'leaves verging on abcission'. However, we haven't yet found examples of such leaves, or any loose ones, even though we tried.

Whenever $c_0(\psi)$ is negative we have to apply the previous arguments in reverse, while running backwards we should not be overtaken by any backward wave. Therefore also in this case r corresponds to the minimum of $F_\phi(\psi)$ for $\psi \in (\phi - \pi/2, \phi + \pi/2)$. However, c_0 can only be negative for a limited set of ψs. The end result is an r which is negative for one interval of ϕ-values, positive for the interval of ϕ-values corresponding to the opposite directions, and undefined for all other ϕ. The stretches of V corresponding to positive and negative r join smoothly at $\phi = \phi_\pm$, bounding the interval of angles ϕ for which $c_0(\psi) > 0$ for all ψ between $\phi - \pi/2$ and $\phi + \pi/2$, resp. $\phi'_\pm = \phi_\pm + \pi$ bounding the interval of angles ϕ for which $c_0(\phi \pm \pi/2) > 0$ (so that $F_\phi(\psi) \to +\infty$ when $\psi \to \phi \pm \pi/2$) and $c_0(\psi) < 0$ for some ψ in $(\phi - \pi/2, \phi + \pi/2)$. Those two intervals of ϕ-values are separated by intervals in which $c_0(\phi - \pi/2)$ and $c_0(\phi + \pi/2)$ have different signs. The boundary angles $\phi_\pm$ and $\phi'_\pm$ satisfy $c_0(\phi_+ + \pi/2) = c_0(\phi_- - \pi/2) = c_0(\phi'_+ - \pi/2) = c_0(\phi'_- + \pi/2) = 0$.

$r(\phi)$ can be calculated in parametric form, with parameter ψ, through the following algorithm:

1. Solve $c_0(\psi)$ and $\lambda_0(\psi) < 0$ from

$$\overline{B}_0(c_0\lambda_0, -\lambda_0 \boldsymbol{v}) = 1 \qquad (7.7)$$

$$c_0\lambda_0\partial_1\overline{B}_0(c_0\lambda_0, -\lambda_0 \boldsymbol{v}) - \lambda_0\langle\partial_2\overline{B}_0(c_0\lambda_0, -\lambda_0 \boldsymbol{v}), \boldsymbol{v}\rangle = 0 \qquad (7.8)$$

where $\overline{B}_0$ is the 3-dimensional Laplace transform of the basic reproduction kernel B_0, and

$$\boldsymbol{v} = \begin{bmatrix} \cos\psi \\ \sin\psi \end{bmatrix}. \qquad (7.9)$$

2. Calculate

$$\theta = \frac{\langle\partial_2\overline{B}_0(c_0\lambda_0, -\lambda_0 \boldsymbol{v}), \boldsymbol{v}'\rangle}{\langle\partial_2\overline{B}_0(c_0\lambda_0, -\lambda_0 \boldsymbol{v}), \boldsymbol{v}\rangle} \quad \text{with } \boldsymbol{v}' = \begin{bmatrix} -\sin\psi \\ \cos\psi \end{bmatrix} \qquad (7.10)$$

3. Finally calculate ϕ and r as

$$\phi = \psi + \arctan\theta, \quad r = (1 + \theta^2)c_0. \qquad (7.11)$$

The following result due to Van den Bosch *et al.* (1990a) hopefully gives some feeling for what all this amounts to: when $\log R_0$ is small the limit contour V corresponds, up to a correction factor $1 + O(\log R_0)$, to the ellipse

$$(x - \mu^{-1}m)^T S^{-1}(x - \mu^{-1}m) = 2\log R_0 \qquad (7.12)$$

deriving from the diffusion approximation (compare subsection 4.3). In this formula μ is the mean disease age at the birth of a daughter infection and m its mean displacement relative to its mother, and

$$s_{ij} = \frac{\sigma_{ij}^2}{\mu^2} + \left[\frac{\nu}{\mu}\right]^2 \frac{m_i}{\mu}\frac{m_j}{\mu} - \left[\frac{\phi_i}{\mu^2}\frac{m_i}{\mu} + \frac{\phi_j}{\mu^2}\frac{m_j}{\mu}\right] \qquad (7.13)$$

with (σ_{ij}), i, $j = 1$, 2, the covariance matrix of the displacement of a daughter infection, ν^2 the variance of the disease age at its birth, and ϕ_i the covariance between the disease age at the birth of a daughter infection and its mean displacement.

8 Further open problems

We have now come at the end of our review of what is known mathematically, or can be firmly conjectured, about the deterministic spread of epidemics over space. In this final section we shall indicate what important open questions remain. Most of these questions are concerned with various ways in which the assumption of translation invariance may be relaxed. However, our first question derives from a closer look at the convergence problem, as this convergence is the cornerstone of all applications.

A good way to look at the rate at which the asymptotic speed of spread is attained is to write out in full conjecture 3 from subsection 4.4 about the convergence of the wave shape. There we conjectured that there exists a function $C: \mathbf{R}^+ \to \mathbf{R}$ such that

$$v(t, x + C(t)) \to \tilde{v}(x) \quad \text{for } t \to \infty. \tag{8.1}$$

From the asymptotic speed of spread result (result 2 from section 2) we already know that necessarily

$$\frac{dC}{dt}(t) \to c_0. \tag{8.2}$$

Can anything stronger be said about C?

For the scaled one-dimensional Fisher equation (4.16), Bramson (1983) found that, for sufficiently concentrated initial conditions, $C(t)/c_0 - t = -\frac{3}{4} \log t + O(1)$. For the corresponding linear diffusion model one easily finds for the furthest position $y(t)$ at which the population density exceeds a certain level, that $y(t)/c_0 - t = -\frac{1}{4} \log t + O(1)$. Apparently the ceiling to the population density comes in crucially in slowing down the population expansion, if only slightly!

No real habitat is translationally invariant in the strict sense, not even locally. One way to relax the assumption of translational invariance, and yet keep to the idea of an intermediate asymptotics based on such an invariance, is to assume that the invariance only applies 'on average'. In mathematical terms this amounts to the assumption that the spatial environment is an ergodic random function, and in biological terms, that one deals with a mixed environment of intermediate grain. (Remember that according to our definitions in subsection 4.1, the susceptible density was considered to be just one component of the environment of the disease population.)

For the one dimensional Fisher equation, Shigesada *et al.* (1986), Shigesada *et al.* (1987) found that

$$c_0 \approx 2\sqrt{\langle D \rangle_H \langle f(0) \rangle_A},\qquad(8.3)$$

where $\langle \cdot \rangle_H$ and $\langle \cdot \rangle_A$ stand for respectively the harmonic and arithmetic spatial mean. It would be extremely useful if their results could be in some way extended to the integral equation framework.

In reality focus shapes are a lot less regular than predicted by the theory; usually they have a somewhat 'lobed' appearance. The likely explanation is that these lobes derive from somewhat more extended periods in which the wind blew from one or another direction. Simulations with a diffusion model for spore dispersal incorporating a random convection term, coupled with a delay differential term for spore production, indeed showed lobed patterns analogous to the observed one (Zawolek and Zadoks 1989).

Splash dispersal generally is isotropic, but even more irregular in time than wind dispersal. Other types of randomness are changes in temperature, affecting speed of lesion development, and humidity, affecting spore germination.

The difference between the randomness in for example our earlier micro-models for spore dispersal and this global randomness is that in the latter the spores no longer can be assumed to move independently. (To be consistent we also should have accounted for such a dependency in our discussion of long distance spore dispersal in section 6, had we not assumed in the end that spores dispersed infinitely fast. Without this assumption equation (6.3) makes little sense!)

Taking all this into account it becomes rather surprising that our simplified picture of focus formation did such a terrific job, based as it was on submodels using averaged data on individuals, not taking account of any dependency between these individuals. It would be of interest if at least some insight could be gained into the process of epidemic spread under simple ergodic temporal regimes.

The example with which we introduced our subject, the picture of the spreading of the Black Death in Europe, brings out yet another way of looking at the intermediate asymptotics game. What if the environment locally is effectively translationally invariant, but its parameters change very slowly? Of course we expect that in that case we shall see everywhere locally a convergence to a neatly shaped wave front, moving in the normal direction at a speed dictated by the local environment.

This leads us to the following mathematical problem. Assume that there is given a sufficiently well behaved set W_0 in $\mathbf{R}^2$ and a sufficiently smooth function $c_0 : \mathbf{R}^2 \to \mathbf{R}^+$. W_0 stands for the initially infected area, and c_0 for the local speed of epidemic expansion. Construct a map W from $\mathbf{R}^+$ to the subsets of $\mathbf{R}^2$ such that (i) $W(0) = W_0$, and (ii) for all $t, h > 0$,

$$\text{for all } x \in \partial W(t), \; \lim_{h \to 0} \frac{d[x, \{x + \alpha n(x) \mid \alpha > 0\} \cap \partial W(t + h)]}{h} = c_0(x),$$
(8.4)

where $n(x)$ denotes the outward normal of $W(t)$ at x, $d[\cdot, \cdot]$ stands for the Euclidian distance, and $\partial W(t)$ denotes the boundary of the set $W(t)$ in $\mathbf{R}^2$.

A further question is whether we may indeed abstract in as simple a manner as we did in the previous paragraph. And maybe it is possible to do an intermediate job which at some points still accounts for the surmized smoothing of the front when it gets too wrinkled, for example when two sections of it collide.

A final point on which we wish to touch is the sublinearity assumption (see subsection 4.2) which was so basic to all our deliberations. Relaxing this assumption leads to a whole new range of unexplored problems. A good source for the special case embodied in the Fisher equation, with constant diffusion coefficient but non-monotone per capita growth rate, is Lewis and Kareiva (1993). The discrete time case with general density independent movement is covered by Lui (1983), Lui (1989a, 1989b) and Creegan and Lui (1984). General references for the diffusion case are Murray (1989) and Grindrod (1991).

Acknowledgements

The figures were drawn by Peter Hock. We thank Odo Diekmann and Hans Heesterbeek for their comments, Odo Diekmann, Denis Mollison, Marek Zawolek, Jan Carel Zadoks, Rob Hengeveld and John Val for useful discussions on various occasions, and Hans Heesterbeek for his detailed comments on the manuscript. Horst Thieme put the first author on this course during a workshop he organized in Heidelberg in 1979.

References

Ammerman, A.J. and Cavalli-Sforza, L.L. (1984) *The Neolithic Transition and the Genetics of Populations in Europe*, Princeton University Press.

Andow, D.A., Kareiva, P.M., Levin, S.A. and Okubo, A. (1990) 'Spread of invading organisms', *Landscape Ecology* **4**, 177–188.

Andral, L., Artois, M., Aubert, M.F.A. and Blancou, J. (1982) 'Radio-pistage de renards enragés', *Comp. Immunol. Microbiol. Infect. Diseases* **5**, 284–291.

Aronson, D.G. (1977) 'The asymptotic speed of propagation of a simple epidemic'. In *Nonlinear Diffusion*. Research Notes in Mathematics 14 W.E. Fitzgibbon and H.F. Walker (eds.), Pitman, London, 1–23.

Aronson, D.G. and Weinberger, H.F. (1975) 'Nonlinear diffusion in population genetics, combustion and nerve pulse propagation'. In *Partial Differential Equations and Related Topics*, J.A. Goldstein (ed.), Lecture Notes in Mathematics 466, Springer, Berlin, 5–49.

Aronson, D.G. and Weinberger, H.F. (1978) 'Multidimensional nonlinear diffusion arising in population genetics', *Adv. Math.* 30, 33–76.

Atkinson, C. and Reuter, G.E. (1976) 'Deterministic epidemic waves', *Math. Proc. Camb. Phil. Soc.* 80, 315–330.

Bacon, P.J. (ed.) (1985) *Population Dynamics of Rabies in Wildlife*, Academic Press, London.

Ball, F. (1995) 'Coupling methods in epidemic theory', this volume, 31–50.

Barbour, A.D. (1977) 'The uniqueness of Atkinson's and Reuter's epidemic waves', *Math. Proc. Camb. Phil. Soc.* 82, 127–130.

Bramson, M. (1983) 'Convergence of Solutions of the Kolmogorov Equation to Travelling Waves', *AMS Memoirs* 44, no. 285. Amer. Math. Soc., Providence, R.I.

Britton, N.F. (1986) *Reaction-Diffusion Equations and their Applications to Biology*, Academic Press, London.

Broadbent, S.R. and Kendall, D.G. (1953) 'The random walk of *Trichostrongylus retotaeformis*', *Biometrics* 9, 460–465.

Brown, K.J. and Carr, J. (1977) 'Deterministic epidemic waves of critical velocity', *Math. Proc. Camb. Phil. Soc.* 81, 431–433.

Cliff, A.D. and Haggett, P. (1988) *Atlas of Disease Distributions: Analytical Approaches to Epidemiological Data*, Blackwell, Oxford.

Cox, D.R. (1962) *Renewal Theory*, Methuen, London.

Creegan, P. and Lui, P. (1984) 'Some remarks about the wave speed and travelling wave solutions of a nonlinear integral operator', *J. Math. Biol.* 20, 59–68.

Diekmann, O. (1978) ' Thresholds and travelling waves for the geographical spread of infection', *J. Math. Biol.* 6, 109–130.

Diekmann, O. (1979) 'Run for your life', *J. Differential Equations* 33, 58–73.

Diekmann, O. and Kaper, H.G. (1978) 'On the bounded solutions of a nonlinear convolution equation', *Nonlin. Anal. Theory Appl.* 2, 721–737.

Diekmann, O., Gyllenberg, M., Metz, J.A.J. and Thieme, H.R. (1994) 'The 'cumulative' formulation of (physiologically) structured population models'. In *Evolution Equations, Control Theory and Biomathematics*, P. Clément and G. Lumer (eds.), Marcel Dekker, Amsterdam, New York, 145–154.

Diekmann, O. and Metz, J.A.J. (in press) 'On the reciprocal relationship between life histories and population dynamics'. In *Frontiers of Mathematical Biology*, S.A. Levin (ed.), Lecture Notes in Biomathematics 100, Springer, New York.

Diekmann, O., Metz, J.A.J. and Heesterbeek, J.A.P. (1994) 'The legacy of Kermack and McKendrick', this volume, 93–112.

Dwyer, G. (1992) 'On the spatial spread of insect pathogens: theory and experiment', *Ecology* **73**, 479–494.

Dwyer, G. (1994) 'Density-dependence and spatial structure in the dynamics of insect pathogens', *Am. Nat.* **143**, 533–562.

Fife, P.C. (1979) *Mathematical Aspects of Reacting and Diffusing Systems*, Lecture Notes in Biomathematics **28**, Springer, Berlin.

Greiner, G., Heesterbeek, J.A.P. and Metz, J.A.J. (in press) 'A singular perturbation problem for evolution equations and time-scale arguments for structured populations', *Can. Appl. Math. Quart.*

Grindrod, P. (1991) *Patterns and Waves: the Theory of Reaction-Diffusion Equations*, Clarendon Press, Oxford.

Heesterbeek, J.A.P. and Zadoks, J.C. (1987) 'Modelling pandemics of quarantine pests and diseases: problems and perspectives', *Crop Protection* **6**, 211–231.

Hyman, J.M. and Stanley E.A. (1988) 'Using mathematical models to understand the AIDS epidemic', *Math. Biosci.* **90**, 415–473.

Jagers, P. (1975) *Branching Processes with Biological Applications*, Wiley, London.

Kato, H. and Kozaka, T. (1974) 'Effect of temperature on lesion enlargement and sporulation of *Pyricularia oryzae* in rice leaves', *Phytopath.* **64**, 828–830.

Kendall, D.G. (1957) In discussion on Bartlett, M.S.: 'Measles periodicity and community size'. *J. R. Statist Soc. A* **120**, 48–70.

Kendall D.G. (1965) 'Mathematical models of the spread of infection'. In *Mathematics and Computer Science in Biology and Medicine*, HMSO, London, 213–225.

Kermack, W.O. and McKendrick A.G. (1927) 'A contribution to the mathematical theory of epidemics', *Proc. R. Soc. Lond. A* **115**, 700–721.

Kolmogorov, A., Petrovski, I. and Piscounov, N. (1937) 'Étude de l'équation de la diffusion avec croissance de la quantité de la matière et son application à un problème biologique', *Bull. Univ. Mosc. Ser. Int.* **A1**, 1–25.

Kot, M. (1992) 'Discrete-time travelling waves: ecological examples', *J. Math. Biol.* **30**, 413–436.

Lewis, M.A. and Kareiva, P. (1993) 'Allee dynamics and the spread of invading organisms', *Theor. Pop. Biol.* **43**, 141–158.

Lubina, J. and Levin, S.A. (1988) 'The spread of a reinvading organism: range expansion in the Californean sea otter', *Am. Nat.* **131**, 526–543.

Lui, R. (1983) 'Existence and stability of a non-linear integral operator', *J. Math. Biol.* **16**, 199–220.

Lui, R. (1989a) 'Biological growth and spread modeled by systems of recursions. I Mathematical theory', *Math. Biosci.* **93**, 269–295.

Lui, R. (1989b) 'Biological growth and spread modeled by systems of recursions. II Biological theory', *Math. Biosci.* **93**, 297–312.

McEvedy, C. and Jones, R. (1978) *Atlas of World Population History*, Penguin, London.

Metz, J.A.J. and Roos, A.M. de (1992) 'The role of physiologically structured population models within a general individual-based modelling perspective'. In *Individual-Based Models and Approaches in Ecology*, B.L. DeAngelis and L.J. Gross (eds.), Chapman and Hall, London, 88–111.

Mollison, D. (1972a) 'Possible velocities for a simple epidemic', *Adv. Appl. Prob.* **4**, 233–257.

Mollison, D. (1972b) 'The rate of spatial propagation of simple epidemics', *Proc. Sixth Berkeley Symp. Math. Statist. and Prob.* **3**, 579–614.

Mollison, D. (1977) 'Spatial contact models for ecological and epidemic spread', *J. Roy. Stat. Soc. B.* **39**, 283–326.

Mollison, D. (1991) 'Dependence of epidemic and population velocities on basic parameters', *Math. Biosci.* **107**, 255–287.

Mollison, D. (1995) 'The structure of epidemic models', this volume.

Mollison, D. and Levin, S. (1995) 'Spatial dynamics of parasitism'. In *Ecology of Infectious Diseases in Natural Populations*, B.T. Grenfell and A. Dobson (eds.), Cambridge University Press, Cambridge, to appear.

Murray, J.D. (1989) *Mathematical Biology*, Springer, Berlin.

Okubo, A. (1980) *Diffusion and Ecological Problems: Mathematical Models*, Springer, Berlin.

Rvachev, L.A. and Longini, I.M. (1985) 'A mathematical model for the global spread of influenza', *Math. Biosci.* **75**, 3–22.

Radcliffe, J. and Rass, L. (1983) 'Wave solutions for the deterministic non-reducible *n*-type epidemic', *J. Math Biol.* **17**, 45–66.

Radcliffe, J. and Rass, L. (1984a) 'The spatial spread and the final size of models for the deterministic host-vector epidemic', *Math. Biosci.* **70**, 123–146.

Radcliffe, J. and Rass, L. (1984b) 'The uniqueness of wave-solutions for the deterministic non-reducible *n*-type epidemic', *J. Math. Biol.* **19**, 303–308.

Radcliffe, J. and Rass, L. (1984c) 'The spatial spread and final size of the deterministic non-reducible *n*-type epidemic', *J. Math. Biol.* **19**, 309–327.

Radcliffe, J. and Rass, L. (1984d) 'Saddle point approximations in *n*-type epidemics and contact-birth processes', *Rocky Mount. J. Math.* **14**, 599–617.

Radcliffe, J. and Rass, L. (1985) 'The rate of spread of infection in models for the deterministic host-vector epidemic', *Math. Biosci.* **74**, 257–273.

Radcliffe, J. and Rass, L. (1986) 'The asymptotic spread of propagation of the deterministic non-reducible *n*-type epidemic', *J. Math. Biol.* **23**, 341–359.

Radcliffe, J. and Rass, L. (1991) 'Effect of reducibility on the deterministic spread of infection in a heterogeneous population'. In *Mathematical Population Dynamics; Proceedings of the second international Conference*, O. Arino, D.E. Axelrod and M. Kimmel (eds.), Marcel Dekker, New York, 93–114.

Radcliffe, J., Rass, L. and Stirling, W.D. (1982) 'Wave solutions for the deterministic host-vector epidemic', *Math. Proc. Camb. Phil. Soc.* **91**, 131–152.

Sattenspiel, L. and Powell, C. (1993) 'Geographic spread of measles on the island of Dominica, West Indies', *Hum. Biol.* **65**, 107–129.

Shigesada, N., Kawasaki, K. and Teramoto, E. (1986) 'Traveling periodic waves in heterogeneous environments', *Theor. Pop. Biol.* **30**, 143–160.

Shigesada, N., Kawasaki, K. and Teramoto, E. (1987) 'The speed of travelling frontal waves in heterogeneous environments'. In *Mathematical Topics in Population Biology, Morphogenesis and Neurosciences*, E. Teramoto and M. Yamaguti (eds.), Lecture Notes in Biomathematics **71**, Springer, Berlin, 88–97.

Skellam, J.G. (1951) 'Random dispersal in theoretical populations', *Biometrika* **38**, 196–218.

Skellam, J.G. (1973) 'The formulation and interpretation of mathematical models of diffusionary processes in population biology'. In *The Mathematical Theory of the Dynamics of Biological Populations*, M.S. Bartlett and R.W. Hiorns (eds.), Academic Press, New York, 63–85.

Smith, W.L. (1956) 'Regenerative stochastic processes', *Proc. R. Soc. Lond.* A **232**, 6–31.

Smith, W.L. (1958) 'Renewal theory and its ramifications', *Proc. R. Statist. Soc.* B **20**, 243–302.

Thieme, H.R. (1977a) 'A model for the spread of an epidemic', *J. Math. Biol.* **4**, 337–351.

Thieme, H.R. (1977b) 'The asymptotic behaviour of solutions of nonlinear integral equations', *Math. Z.* **157**, 141–154.

Thieme, H.R. (1979a) 'Asymptotic estimates of the solutions of nonlinear integral equations and asymptotic speeds for the spread of populations', *J. Reine Angew. Math.* **306**, 94–121.

Thieme, H.R. (1979b) 'Density-dependent regulation of spatially distributed populations and their asymptotic speed of spread', *J. Math. Biol.* **8**, 173–187.

Van den Bosch, F., Zadoks, J.C. and Metz, J.A.J. (1988a) 'Focus expansion in plant disease. I: The constant rate of focus expansion', *Phytopath.* **78**, 54–58.

Van den Bosch, F., Zadoks, J.C. and Metz, J.A.J. (1988b) 'Focus expansion in plant disease. II: Realistic parameter-sparse models', *Phytopath.* **78**, 59–64.

Van den Bosch, F., Frinking, H.D., Metz, J.A.J. and Zadoks, J.C. (1988c) 'Focus expansion in plant disease. III: Two experimental examples', *Phytopath.* **78**, 919–925.

Van den Bosch, F., Metz, J.A.J. and Diekmann, O. (1990a) 'The velocity of spatial population expansion', *J. Math. Biol.* **28**, 529–565.

Van den Bosch, F., Verhaar, M.A., Buiel, A.A.M., Hoogkamer, W. and Zadoks, J.C. (1990b) 'Focus expansion in plant disease. IV: Expansion rates in mixtures of resistant and susceptible hosts', *Phytopath.* **80**, 598–602.

Van den Bosch, F., Hengeveld, R. and Metz, J.A.J. (1992) 'Analyzing the velocity of animal range expansion', *J. Biogeog.* **19**, 135–150.

Van den Bosch, F., Zadoks, J.C. and Metz, J.A.J. (1994) 'Continental expansion of plant disease: a survey of some recent results'. In *Predictability and Nonlinear Modelling in Natural Science and Economics*, J. Grasman and G. van Straten (eds.), Kluwer, Dordrecht, 274–281.

Weinberger, H.F. (1978) 'Asymptotic behaviour of models in population genetics'. In *Nonlinear Partial Differential Equations and Applications*, J.M. Chadam (ed.), Lecture Notes in Mathematics **648**, Springer, Berlin, 47–98.

Weinberger, H.F. (1982) 'Long-time behaviour of a class of biological models', *SIAM J. Math. Anal.* **13**, 353–396.

Williamson, E.J. (1961) 'The distribution of larvae of randomly moving insects', *Aust. J. Biol. Sci.* **14**, 598–604.

Zadoks, J.C. and Schein, R.D. (1979) *Epidemiology and plant disease management*, Oxford University Press, Oxford.

Zawolek, M.W. and Zadoks, J.C. (1989) 'A Physical Theory of Focus Development in Plant Disease'. *Wageningen Agricultural University Papers* **89-3**. Agricultural University, Wageningen.

Spatial Epidemic Models

Richard Durrett

Introduction

In this paper we will consider a spatial version of the standard SIRS epidemic model and indicate how it differs from its nonspatial analogue. We begin by defining and defending the spatial model (for its ancestry, see Bailey 1965, Mollison 1977, Cox and Durrett 1988). Space is represented by a grid of sites $\mathcal{Z}^2$, which we think of as an array of houses, each of which is occupied by exactly one individual. One could complicate the model by allowing families of various sizes to live at these sites but to do so would miss one of the points of modelling with interacting particle systems. We do not attempt to fit the quantitative characteristics of the system, but instead seek to understand what features of the system are responsible for its observed qualitative behavior. To do this, we build the simplest possible model that reproduces the behavior of interest and we rely on the idea of 'universality' from statistical mechanics. This principle asserts, for example, that the Ising model, a very simple model that represents the local magnetic states of iron atoms as up or down instead of vectors of unit length in $\mathcal{R}^3$ and that allows atoms to feel the presence of only the nearest neighboring spins, is adequate to capture the desired qualitative properties of magnets. Here, we use the notion of universality to assert that if we replace our single individuals by families or allow our individuals to interact with persons other than their nearest neighbors, the qualitative features of the model will not change. In defense of this assertion we would like to say that Zhang (1990) has proved Theorem 1 below for a model that has one individual per site but allows an arbitrary finite interaction neighborhood $\mathcal{N}$ that is symmetric, i.e. if $x \in \mathcal{N}$ then $-x \in \mathcal{N}$. Recent advances in percolation theory (see Bezuidenhout and Grimmett 1991) make it possible to prove Theorem 2 in this generality but we doubt if anyone has the patience to write down all the details.

1 Description of the model

The state of the process at time t is a function $\xi_t : \mathcal{Z}^2 \to \{0, 1, 2\}$. Here $\xi_t(x)$ gives the state of the individual at x at time t with $0 =$ susceptible, $1 =$ infected, and $2 =$ removed. In this paper we will think of nonfatal diseases such as measles or influenza, so removed means that the individual has had the disease and is immune to further infection. One can, however, think of fatal diseases such as fox rabies and interpret removed as vacant. To formulate the dynamics we let

$$\mathcal{N} = \{(1,0),(0,1),(-1,0),(0,-1)\}$$

be the four points in $\mathcal{Z}^2$ that are the closest to 0, and declare that y is a neighbor of x if $y - x \in \mathcal{N}$. Having defined the interaction neighborhood we can formulate the dynamics as follows.

(a) A susceptible individual at x becomes infected at a rate equal to the fraction of the neighbors y that are infected.

(b) An infected individual becomes healthy at rate δ.

(c) A removed individual becomes susceptible at rate $\alpha \geq 0$.

Here, we say something happens at rate r if the probability of an occurrence between times t and $t + h$, $\sim rh$ as $h \to 0$, i.e., the actual probability when divided by rh converges to 1 as $h \to 0$. One could generalize the model by allowing the infection rate in (a) to be λ times the number of infected neighbors, but then by redefining the units in which time is measured, we can set $\lambda = 1/4$ and return to formulation above.

Assumption (b) implies that the duration of the disease T has an exponential distribution with mean $1/\delta$, i.e., $P(T > t) = \exp(-\delta t)$. In the case of measles we would thus have $\delta \approx 1/14$. The duration of measles does not follow an exponential distribution (otherwise a fraction $1/e^2$ of infecteds would have the disease for four weeks) but this assumption is needed to avoid keeping track of how long each infected individual has been sick. Again, we rely on universality to claim that models that treat the infection period in a more realistic fashion will have similar qualitative behavior. In support of this we would like to observe that Cox and Durrett (1988) proved Theorem 1 below for a general infection period distribution with $ET^2 < \infty$.

To explain assumption (c), we note that if we want to model the short time behavior of a measles or flu epidemic we would set $\alpha = 0$. On the other hand, if we want to understand the behavior of measles or flu epidemics over several decades we would have a small positive value of α. Our model has a fixed population size since it insists that there is always one person at each site, so we combine the death of removed individuals and the birth of new susceptibles into one transition.

2   Results with no regrowth of susceptibles

To explain the behavior of the model we begin with the case $\alpha = 0$ and consider what happens when we start with one infected individual in an otherwise susceptible population. That is, we let

$$\xi_0^o(x) = \begin{cases} 1 & \text{if } x = (0,0) \\ 0 & \text{if } x \neq (0,0) \end{cases}$$

Here the superscript o is short for the 'origin,' a common name for the point $(0,0)$ where our initial infected individual sits. It is always possible for our initial infected individual to recover before infecting one of his neighbors. Let $\eta_t^o = \{x : \xi_t^o(x) = 1\}$ be the set of infected sites at time t and let $\tau^o = \inf\{t : \eta_t^o = \emptyset\}$. Since infected sites do not appear spontaneously we will have $\eta_t^o = \emptyset$ for $t > \tau^o$ and we say that the infection *dies out* at time τ^o.

If δ is too large then the infection always die out, i.e., $P(\tau^o = \infty) = 0$. Let $\delta_c = \inf\{\delta : P(\tau^o = \infty) = 0\}$. The value of δ_c is our first indication that the spatial model differs from its homogeneously mixing counterpart defined as follows:

(i) there are N individuals that become infected at a rate equal to the fraction of the population that is infected,

(ii) infected individuals become removed at rate δ.

In the homogeneously mixing case, $\delta_c = 1$. That is, if $\delta > 1$ the expected size of the epidemic is bounded independent of N, while if $\delta < 1$ then with probability $\geq p > 0$ the epidemic infects more than ρN individuals, where ρ is a positive constant that is independent of N.

It is easy to see that in the spatial epidemic model $\delta_c \leq 3/4$. Any infected individual at $x \neq 0$ was infected by one of his neighbors and hence has at most 3 susceptible neighbors. This means that when there are k infected sites new infecteds can arise at rate $\leq (1 + 3k)/4$ and currently infected sites will become removed at rate δk. The last bound is quite crude: numerical result suggest that $\delta_c \approx 0.22$. The moral is that since the state of a site is correlated with that of its neighbors, we need δ considerably smaller than 1 for the epidemic to persist.

The best rigorous bounds on δ_c are quite crude (see page 174 of Cox and Durrett (1988) for a description of results of Kuulasmaa (1982)) so you may be surprised to learn that it is possible to prove results about the qualitative behavior of the epidemic for all $\delta < \delta_c$. Recall that $\eta_t^o = \{x : \xi_t^o(x) = 1\}$ where ξ_t^o denotes the process starting from a single infected at $(0,0)$ in the midst of an otherwise susceptible population. Let $\zeta_t^o = \{x : \xi_t^o(x) = 2\}$ be the set of removed sites at time t, and let $\zeta_\infty^o = \cup_t \zeta_t^o$ be the set of sites that are ever infected.

Theorem 1. *Suppose $\delta < \delta_c$. Then when the epidemic does not die out, it expands linearly and has an asymptotic shape. That is, there is a nonrandom convex set D so that if $\tau^o = \infty$ then for any $\epsilon > 0$ the following holds for t*

sufficiently large

$$\zeta_\infty^o \cap t(1 - \epsilon)D \subset \zeta_t^o \subset t(1 + \epsilon)D$$
$$\eta_t^o \subset t(1 + \epsilon)D - t(1 - \epsilon)D$$

Here $sD = \{sx : x \in D\}$. In words, the infection is contained in $t(1 + \epsilon)D$, a slightly enlarged version of tD at time t, and all the sites inside $t(1 - \epsilon)D$ that will ever be infected have already been infected by time t and have become removed. In this context a picture is worth more than a hundred words, see Figure 1. It is an unfortunate feature of the proof of Theorem 1 that we do not know D or even its radius explicitly. The shape of D is roughly circular but not exactly circular since on $\mathcal{Z}^2$ the infection does not propagate in the 45 degree direction at exactly the same rate that it propagates parallel to the axes. The linear propagation of epidemics is well known. To quote Bailey (1975, p. 174):

'It was suggested by Dr. Halliday in the discussion of Soper's paper (1929) that a measles epidemic starting in September took about 24 weeks to spread over the whole of Glasgow. If, for the purposes of rough calculation we rded the latter as a circle with radius two miles, then the approximate velocity of propagation would be 1/12 of a mile per week.'

Closer to home, there is also agreement with the linear rate of spread of epidemics such as the ongoing raccoon rabies epidemic in New York state.

3   Results with regrowth of susceptibles

Turning to epidemics with $\alpha > 0$ we have the following recent result of Durrett and Neuhauser (1991).

Theorem 2. *Suppose $\delta < \delta_c$. If $\alpha > 0$ then there is a nontrivial translation invariant stationary distribution in which infected individuals have positive density.*

To explain the theorem, we recall that π is a *stationary distribution* if when the initial state ξ_0 has this distribution then the state at time t, ξ_t, has this distribution for all t, while ξ_0 is *translation invariant* if the probabilities

$$P(\xi_0(x + z_1) = i_1, \ldots, \xi_0(x + z_m) = i_m)$$

do not depend on x. In words, π is a stationary distribution if it is a possible equilibrium state for the process, and ξ_0 is translation invariant if its distribution is spatially homogeneous. When ξ_0 is translation invariant $P(\xi_0(x) = 1)$ is independent of x and is called the *density of infected individuals*.

In words, Theorem 2 says that if the epidemic is *supercritical*, i.e., has a positive probability of not dying out starting from a single infected in an otherwise susceptible population, then when reappearance of susceptibles occurs

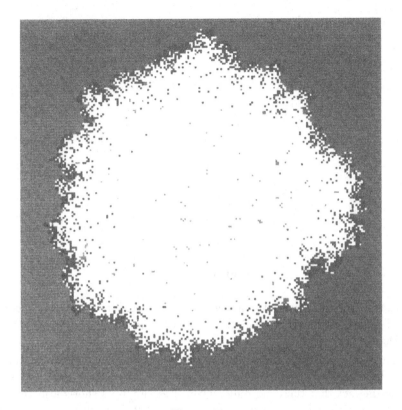

Figure 1:

at a positive rate α there is a nontrivial equilibrium distribution for the process, no matter how small α is. To get an idea of the nature of the equilibrium state we will now look at some simulations. Figure 2 shows the numbers of infected and susceptible individuals versus time in the model with $\delta = 0.1$ and $\alpha = 0.04$ for a simulation on a 100×100 lattice starting from *uniform product measure*, i.e., each site is independently designated as susceptible, infected, or removed with probability $1/3$.

When dealing with a finite set there is always the issue of what boundary conditions you choose. In the simulation pictured in Figure 2 we have used *periodic boundary conditions* in which sites on the right edge of the square are neighbors of those on the left, and those on the top row are neighbors of those of the bottom row. Identifying the sides of the square in this way turns the system into a torus. Even mathematicians are aware that the earth is not shaped like a doughnut, but these boundary conditions have the advantage of making our little universe look the same from every site. An alternative to periodic boundary conditions that we will use below is *open boundary conditions* in which we think of $[-L, L]^2$ as sitting in $\mathcal{Z}^2$ with sites

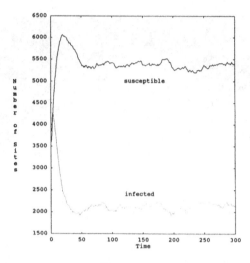

Figure 2:

outside the square immune to infection. If we changed from periodic to open boundary conditions in the simulation under consideration the behavior would not change very much.

The graph in Figure 2 shows that the densities converge exponentially rapidly to their equilibrium values, but there are fluctuations in the density due to the fact that there are only 10,000 sites. Figure 3 shows a picture of the process with these parameter values at time 200. Note that the picture is quite random but the system is not homogeneously mixed. One way to see this clearly is to compare Figure 2 with the evolution of the dynamical system that results from the limit of a large homogeneously mixing population. Writing u for the fraction of infecteds, and v for the fraction of removed individuals that well known dynamical system is

$$\frac{du}{dt} = u(1 - u - v) - \delta u \qquad (3.1)$$

$$\frac{dv}{dt} = \delta u - \alpha v \qquad (3.2)$$

Taking $\delta = 0.1$ and $\alpha = 0.04$ gives the solution drawn in Figure 4. It is easy to solve to find that for these parameter values $u = 0.257$ and $v = 0.643$ is the limiting value as $t \to \infty$. This should be contrasted with the fact that in the spatial epidemic the equilibrium level for infecteds is about 20% and for removed individuals is about 53%. The difference comes from the fact that in the spatial model (and in real life) the state of an individual has a significant correlation with the states of its neighbors.

As the graph in Figure 2 indicates, the simulation begins with an epidemic

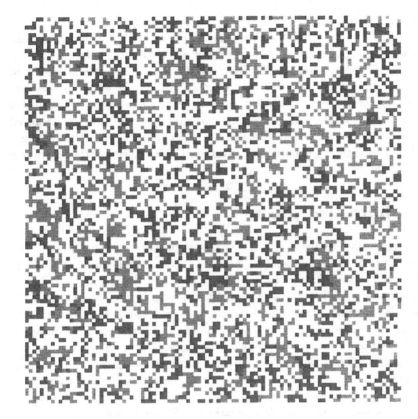

Figure 3:

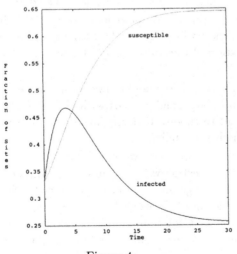

Figure 4:

that involves about 90% of the population (infected plus removed $\approx$ 9000). If we decrease α to 0.005 then the number of susceptibles will not increase to a high enough level to sustain a second epidemic wave before the initial infecteds disappear, and the epidemic will die out. If we set $\alpha = 0.01$ then the infection just barely avoids dying out and we get the graph in Figure 5. Note that there are six epidemics and the density of susceptibles oscillates in time. This occurs because the infection and recovery rates are balanced so that when the the susceptibles reach a high enough level to allow another epidemic wave there are only one or two 'pockets of infection' that start new waves of infection.

4 Finite size effects

In the epidemic literature, it is a well known phenomenon that when δ and α are fixed, if the population size, here $=L^2$, is too small then the epidemic will die out. For example, for measles, the empirical observation is that a population of roughly 250,000 is needed for measles to persist. That is, if the population is smaller than this threshold (e.g., in Iceland) then from time to time we will experience moments when no one in the population is infected. In our simulated world, it is easy to fix δ and L and vary α, so we will investigate a critical value $\alpha_c(L)$ for simulations of the epidemic on $[-L, L]^2$ so that when $\alpha/\alpha_c(L)$ is large then the epidemic will persist for a long time with high probability while if $\alpha/\alpha_c(L)$ is small then the epidemic will die out after a short time with high probability. To decide what is a long time we observe that (here and in what follows C denotes a large and c a small constant whose values depend on δ and ingeneral change from line to line)

(i) There is always a probability of at least $\exp(-CL^2)$ that all the individuals infected at time t will recover before time $t + 1$ and not infect their neighbors, so the expected duration of the infection on an $L \times L$ square is smaller than $\exp(CL^2)$.

(ii) Results of Durrett and Neuhauser (1991) can be used to show that for any α if L is sufficiently large, and we start with at least $\sqrt{L}$ infecteds (in any arrangement you want to choose) then the infection will persist for $\exp(cL^2)$ units of time with high probability.

To decide what is a short time, we note that if we start with a single infected individual the infection will take about CL units of time to spread across the system. Once we get into a situation in which the density of infected individuals is below the threshold needed for the epidemic to propagate, the epidemic will only last for $C \log L$ units of time: since this is the size of the maximum of L^2 independent exponential random variables with parameter δ.

As the last paragraph indicates, we are interested in the dependence of $\alpha_c(L)$ on L. Bak, Chen, and Tang (1989), who studied a process in which

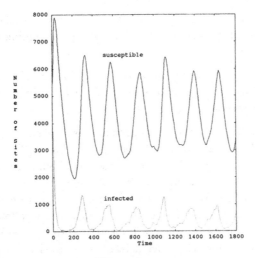

Figure 5:

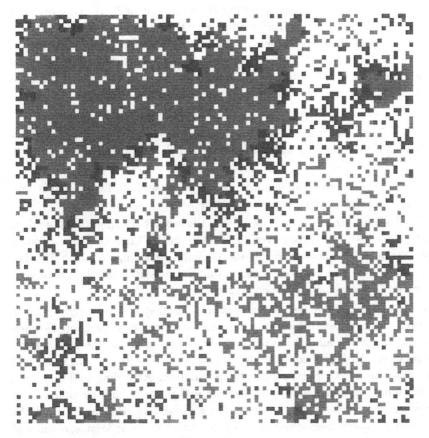

Figure 6:

infections and removals were deterministic, claimed that $\alpha_c(L) = 1/L$. We will now argue that this answer is right and wrong depending on your choice of initial configuration.

Conjecture 1. *We can choose initial conditions so that when $\alpha_c(L) = C/L$, the probability the epidemic survives for a long time, i.e., $\geq \exp(cL^2)$ units of time, converges to 1 as $L \to \infty$.*

The initial conditions we choose, supposing L is an even integer, are to have $[-L/2, L/2] \times [-L/2, L/2)$ in the removed state, $[-L/2, L, 2] \times \{L/2\}$ infected, and the other states susceptible. If we impose open boundary conditions then this initial configuration produces a wave of infection that moves along the edge of the square of removed sites. (See Figure 7.) If the recovery rate is C/L then the central square will have recovered sufficiently to allow the infection to invade it before the two waves crash into each other. (See Figure 8.) The small fragment that survives makes a larger C shaped front (see Figure 9) and the whole process repeats.

This initial condition was inspired by the band test of Fisch, Gravner, and Griffeath (1991) (see also Durrett 1992 and Durrett and Griffeath 1992) for the Greenberg-Hastings model, a discrete time deterministic system ξ_n : $\mathcal{Z}^d \to \{0, 1, \dots, \kappa - 1\}$ whose dynamics are similar to the epidemic model if we think of $0 =$ susceptible, $1 =$ infected and $2, \dots, \kappa - 1$ as a sequence of recovery states, with the following transition rules:

(i) If $\xi_n(x) = i > 0$ then $\xi_{n+1}(x) = i + 1$ where $(\kappa - 1) + 1 = 0$

(ii) If $\xi_n(x) = 0$ then we count the number of neighbors $y \in x + \mathcal{N}$ that are infected. If the number is at least θ, then $\xi_{n+1}(x) = 1$; otherwise $\xi_{n+1}(x) = 0$.

Here $\mathcal{N}$ is not just the nearest neighbors. A well studied choice is $\{x : |x_1|, |x_2| \leq r\}$, i.e., a square with side $2r + 1$.

We believe that in the limit as $L \to \infty$ the process starting from the initial state described above converges to a deterministic limit that has periodic spirals much like those found in the Greenberg-Hastings model. The few simulations we have done on a 400×400 grid indicate that this result may be easier to prove than to see on a computer.

The speculations in the last paragraph, while they may be interesting, are not relevant for applications, where we are interested in what happens when we start from a small number of infected individuals in an otherwise healthy population. To begin, consider the situation starting from a single infected individual in an otherwise susceptible population. According to Theorem 1, if the infection does not die out then we will get a roughly circular ring of infection that spreads across a system at a linear rate. Behind the front the fraction of susceptibles drops to a low level and takes at least c/α units of time to build back up above the critical density needed for another epidemic

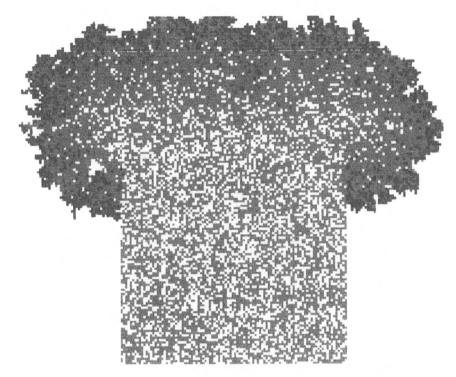

Figure 7:

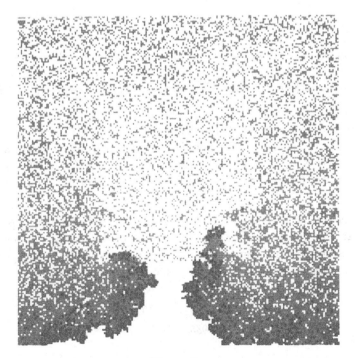

Figure 8:

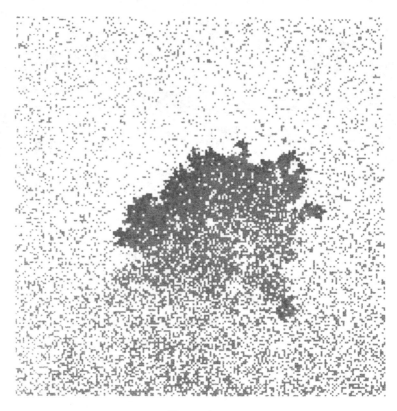

Figure 9:

wave to propagate. The probability an infected individual will stay infected long enough to start a second wave is roughly $\exp(-\delta c/\alpha)$, so the probability some individual in $[-L, L]^2$ does this is at most $(2L + 1)^2 \exp(-\delta c/\alpha)$. This leads us to

Conjecture 2. *Suppose $\alpha < c/\log L$. If we start with (i) a single infected individual in an otherwise healthy population or (ii) with a product measure in which infecteds have a positive density, then with high probability the infection will last for a short time, which means (i) CL or (ii) $C \log L$ units of time.*

While this conclusion may sound plausible, it seems to be difficult to prove. To investigate its truth, we have done simulations of the process on four different size lattices starting from 1% of the sites infected and 99% susceptible.

grid size	time	α	survivals	extinction
50 × 50	250	0.0095	27	73
		0.0120	75	25
100 × 100	250	0.0085	24	76

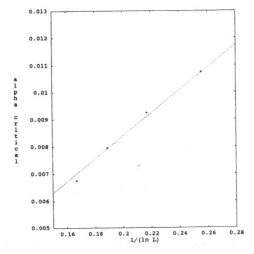

Figure 10:

		0.0100	75	25
200 × 200	250	0.0072	23	77
		0.0087	75	25
400 × 400	300	0.0060	18	82
		0.0075	82	18

Here we declare that survival occured if the epidemic was still going at the indicated time, and extinction if it died out before that time. The cutoff time was chosen based on our experience that if the epidemic survived long enough to make a second wave then the epidemic would survive for a long time.

As the reader might guess from the table we repeated the simulation 100 times for each parameter value and tried to find two values of α for each L, one where survival occurred 75% of the time and one where extinction occurred 75%. A pre-occupation with round numbers and the amount of time required for the simulation runs kept us from achieving this goal for our 400 × 400 simulations. Nonetheless when you look at a graph of α versus $1/\ln L$ and fit a line with no constant term you find

$$\alpha_c^{pm}(L) \approx \frac{0.04196}{\ln L}$$

where the superscript 'pm' indicates that we are considering the critical α starting from an initial product measure, i.e., the states of the sites in the initial configuration are independent. The good fit shown in Figure 10 $(1 - r^2 = 0.00957$ when we look at the midpoints of the intervals) supports our belief that $\alpha_c^{pm}(L) \sim C/\ln L$ as $L \to \infty$.

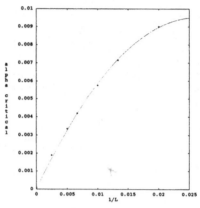

Figure 11:

We have also investigated the behavior of the epidemic model starting from the 'band test' initial condition. Using similar methods the data are as follows:

grid size	time	α	survivals	extinction
50 × 50	300	0.0080	28	72
		0.0100	72	28
75 × 75	350	0.0062	30	70
		0.0081	75	25
100 × 100	350	0.0050	27	73
		0.0065	80	20
150 × 150	500	0.0380	20	80
		0.0460	80	20
200 × 200	600	0.0030	26	74
		0.0037	74	26
400 × 400	900	0.0018	25	50
		0.0020	78	27

We have investigated more values of L in this case because our runs for $L = 50, 100, 200, 400$ suggested we should fit a curve of the form $a/L + b/L^2$, which we did to find a relationship

$$\alpha_c^{bt}(L) \approx \frac{0.72612}{L} - \frac{13.8669}{L^2}$$

Here 'bt' indicates that we are considering the band test initial configuration. Again the fit shown in Figure 11 is quite good ($1 - r^2 = 0.00172$ if we look at the midpoints of the intervals) and supports our belief that $\alpha_c^{bt}(L) \sim C/L$ as $L \to \infty$.

In closing we would like to note that even if you only care about the behavior starting from a random initial configuration the asymptotics for the band test are significant. It is only for values of α near α_c^{bt} that the densities will oscillate in time. The discrepancy between the two asymptotic formulas shows that when L is very large the process with a random start will not display oscillations. These large values of L occur only for cities with several hundred million (or billion) individuals so this asymptotic regime is probably not reached in applications. For those of you who might point out that countries (or planets) have this many individuals, we would like to reply that our spatial model is appropriate for a city while other models involving a small number of sites, one for each major city, would be appropriate for modelling epidemics on a more global scale.

References

Bailey, N.T.J. (1965) 'The simulation of stochastic epidemics in two dimensions'. In *Proc. 5th Berkeley Symp. on Math. Statist. and Prob.* **4**, 237–257.

Bailey, N.T.J. (1975) *The Mathematical Theory of Infectious Diseases and its Applications*, second edition, Griffin, London.

Bak. P., Chen, K. and Tang, C. (1989) 'A forest-fire model and some thoughts on turbulence', preprint.

Bezuidenhout, C. and Grimmett, G. (1990) 'The critical contact process dies out', *Ann. Probab.* **18**, 1462–1482.

Cox, J.T. and Durrett, R. (1988) 'Limit theorems for the spread of epidemics and forest fires', *Stoch. Proc. Applics.* **30**, 171–191.

Durrett, R. (1992) 'Some new games for your computer', *Nonlinear Science Today.* **1**(4), 1–6.

Durrett, R. and Griffeath, D. (1993) 'Asymptotic behavior of excitable cellular automata', *Experimental Math.* **2**, 182–208.

Durrett, R. and Neuhauser, C. (1991) 'Epidemics with recovery in $d = 2$', *Ann. Appl. Prob.* **1**, 189–206.

Fisch, R., Gravner, J. and Griffeath, D. (1991) 'Threshold-range scaling for excitable cellular automata', *Statist. and Comp.* **1**, 23–39.

Kuulasmaa, K. (1982) 'The spatial general epidemic and locally dependent random graphs', *J. Appl. Prob.* 745–758.

Mollison, D. (1977) 'Spatial contact models for ecological and epidemic spread', *J. R. Statist. Soc.* B **39**, 283–326.

Mollison, D. and Kuulasmaa, K. (1985) 'Spatial endemic models: theory and simulations'. In *The Population Dynamics of Rabies in Wildlife*, P.J. Bacon (ed.) Academic Press, New York, 292–309

Zhang, Y. (1990) 'A shape theorem for finite range epidemics and forest fires', *Ann. Prob.* **21**, 1755–1781.

A Perturbation Approach to Nonlinear Deterministic Epidemic Waves

Henry Daniels

Summary

The nonlinear deterministic equations of epidemic theory usually defy explicit analytic solution. Rigorous proofs of the existence of phenomena like travelling waves and investigation of their properties were provided in the pioneering work of Mollison (1972, 1977), Atkinson and Reuter (1976), Thieme (1977), Diekmann (1978). Reference may also be made, for example, to Mollison (1991) and Metz and Van den Bosch (1995) for later developments. However, in comparable situations in physics and engineering it is customary to seek approximate solutions using well established perturbation techniques. Such methods are often heuristic and difficult to rigorize but appear to capture the essence of the solution. Recently I used this approach to approximate to the variance of epidemic paths in some stochastic models (Daniels 1991).

In a paper published in a festschrift in honour of M.S. Bartlett (Daniels 1975) I obtained an approximate solution to the nonlinear equation for travelling waves in the case of a spatial simple epidemic, using what amounted to an informal perturbation approach. The present paper redevelops the solution by means of a standard perturbation technique which extends easily to the case of an epidemic with removals. For simplicity only the symmetrical one-dimensional situation is considered, though these restrictions are easily removed. However, the tails of the contact distribution are assumed to decrease at least exponentially fast, to ensure the existence of an epidemic wave with finite velocity.

Much of this paper inevitably overlaps my 1975 paper.

1   The deterministic simple epidemic

Consider a population distributed on a line with constant density N per unit length. Infectives in the population occur with density $Y(s,t)$ at a point s on the line at time t. There is a contact distribution $dV(u)$ such that an infective in the interval $(s-u, s-u-du)$ has probability $\alpha dt dV(u)$ of infecting a susceptible at s in a time interval of length dt. For convenience we take

$\alpha N = 1$, αN being the contact rate. Then the deterministic equation for the simple epidemic is

$$\frac{\partial Y(s,t)}{\partial t} = \{1 - N^{-1}Y(s,t)\} \int_{-\infty}^{\infty} Y(s - u, t)dV(u). \qquad (1.1)$$

No exact analytic solution of (1.1) is known. Our aim is to arrive at approximate solutions which describe the behaviour of the epidemic paths in a natural way. We use a perturbation technique which depends on the fact that the path is expected to change relatively slowly over the range of the contact distribution.

It is instructive to start by discussing the linear model appropriate to an unlimited number of susceptibles – essentially a simple birth process – which can be solved by standard methods. The perturbation technique will then be shown to produce equivalent results; it can, however, be applied to nonlinear models for which linear techniques are not available.

2 The linear model

When $N \to \infty$, (1.1) becomes

$$\frac{\partial Y(s,t)}{\partial t} = \int_{-\infty}^{\infty} Y(s - u, t)dV(u). \qquad (2.1)$$

The type of solution which concerns us is a travelling wave advancing at constant speed $c > 0$ with its shape unchanged. In that case $Y(s,t)$ must be a function of $z = s - ct$, and

$$Y(s,t) = f(s - ct) = f(z) \qquad (2.2)$$

satisfies

$$-c\frac{df}{dz} = \int_{-\infty}^{\infty} f(z - u)dV(u). \qquad (2.3)$$

This has an exponential solution $\exp(-\theta z)$ if $c = \Psi(\theta)/\theta$ where

$$\Psi(\theta) = \int_{-\infty}^{\infty} e^{\theta u} dV(u) \qquad (2.4)$$

exists in a non-vanishing interval containing $\theta = 0$. For a travelling wave to be possible, $c \geq c_0 = \min \Psi(\theta)/\theta$, which occurs at θ_0 satisfying (see Figure 1)

$$c_0 = \Psi(\theta_0)/\theta_0 = \Psi'(\theta_0). \qquad (2.5)$$

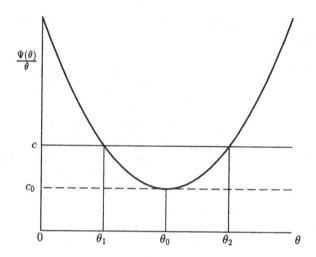

Figure 1.   Possible values of $c = \Psi(\theta)/\theta$.

When $c > c_0$ a solution exists for two values of θ, $\theta_1 < \theta_2$, and the travelling wave has the general form

$$f(z) = P_1 e^{-\theta_1 z} + P_2 e^{-\theta_2 z}; \quad P_1 \geq 0, P_2 \geq 0. \tag{2.6}$$

At the critical velocity c_0 the complete solution is $f(z) = (P + Qz)e^{-\theta_0 z}$, but Q has to vanish and $P > 0$ to avoid $f < 0$, so that $f(z) = Pe^{-\theta_0 z} = e^{-\theta_0(z-a)}$.

The development of the epidemic from a single individual is also easily found from the two-sided Laplace transform of $Y(s, t)$. The saddlepoint approximation of its inversion integral shows that as $t \to \infty$ the path settles down to a travelling wave with minimum velocity c_0. Details are given in Daniels (1975, 1977).

3   Alternative approach

The basic idea underlying this approach goes back to Daniels (1960). Because an epidemic wave is essentially a large deviation phenomenon, one seeks an approximation to $g(z) = \log f(z)$. From (2.3) the equation for $g(z)$ is

$$- cg'(z) = \int_{-\infty}^{\infty} e^{g(z-u)-g(z)} dV(u). \tag{3.1}$$

Provided $g(z)$ varies slowly over the range of the contact distribution, it is reasonable to expand (3.1) as

$$-cg' = \int_{-\infty}^{\infty} e^{-ug'} \{1 + \tfrac{1}{2}u^2 g'' - \tfrac{1}{6}u^3 g''' + \tfrac{1}{24}u^4[g'''' + 3(g'')^2] + \cdots\} dV(u),$$

i.e.

$$-cg' = \Psi(-g') + \tfrac{1}{2}\Psi''(-g')g'' - \tfrac{1}{6}\Psi'''(-g')g''' $$
$$+ \tfrac{1}{24}\Psi''''(-g')[g'''' + 3(g'')^2] + \cdots, \tag{3.2}$$

successive terms after the first being, one hopes, relatively small. Most of the information about the behaviour of the epidemic path should be contained in the first approximation g_0 which satisfies

$$-cg_0' = \Psi(-g_0'). \tag{3.3}$$

This has the solution $g_0 = -\theta z + a$ provided $c\theta = \Psi(\theta)$ so that $\theta = \theta_1$ or θ_2. Combining these solutions, we arrive at the complete solution (2.6) without further terms. Substituting g_0 and its derivatives for g in the subsequent terms of (3.2) makes them vanish, which is consistent with this fact, but a more satisfactory approach is given in the next section.

4 Simple epidemic

The technique is now applied to the nonlinear situation in a more systematic fashion. With the notation as before, the equation for the travelling wave in terms of $g = \log f$ is, from (1.1),

$$-cg'(z) = (1 - N^{-1}e^{g(z)}) \int_{-\infty}^{\infty} e^{g(z-u)-g(z)} dV(u). \tag{4.1}$$

The most satisfactory way of separating out the equations for successive terms of the approximation is to embed (4.1) in a family of models defined by

$$-cg'(z) = (1 - N^{-1}e^{g(z)}) \int_{-\infty}^{\infty} e^{\frac{1}{\epsilon}\{g(z-\epsilon u)-g(z)\}} dV(u)$$
$$= (1 - N^{-1}e^{g})\{\Psi(-g') + \tfrac{1}{2}\epsilon\Psi''(-g') \cdot g''$$
$$+ \epsilon^2\{-\tfrac{1}{6}\Psi'''(-g')g''' + \tfrac{1}{24}\Psi''''(-g')[g'''' + 3(g'')^2]\}\} + \cdots\}. \tag{4.2}$$

When $\epsilon = 0$ this reduces to the first approximation which can be solved; when $\epsilon = 1$ we have the simple epidemic model. One then writes $g = g_0 + \epsilon g_1 + \epsilon^2 g_2 + \cdots$, expands both sides of (4.2) in powers of ϵ and equates the coefficients of corresponding powers.

We shall consider only the dominant term g_0 and the first correction g_1, so the expansion is taken as far as the first power of ϵ. Thus

$$-c(g_0' + \epsilon g_1' + \cdots) = (1 - N^{-1}e^{g_0} - \epsilon N^{-1}e^{g_0}g_1 + \cdots)$$
$$\cdot\{\Psi(-g_0') - \epsilon\Psi'(-g_0')g_1 + \cdots + \tfrac{1}{2}\epsilon\Psi''(-g_0)g_0'' + \cdots\}. \tag{4.3}$$

The term g_0 satisfies the equation

$$- cg_0' = (1 - N^{-1}e^{g_0})\Psi(-g_0').$$ (4.4)

It is simplest to seek a parametric solution by writing $\theta = \theta(z) = -g_0'(z)$, so that

$$c\theta = (1 - N^{-1}e^{g_0})\Psi(\theta)$$

or

$$f_0 = N\left(1 - \frac{c\theta}{\Psi(\theta)}\right).$$ (4.5)

Then

$$g_0 = \log N + \log(\Psi(\theta) - c\theta) - \log \Psi(\theta)$$
$$-\theta = \frac{dg_0}{dz} = -c\frac{\{\Psi(\theta) - \theta\Psi'(\theta)\}}{\Psi(\theta)\{\Psi(\theta) - c\theta\}}\frac{d\theta}{dz}$$

and hence

$$z = c\int_a^\theta \frac{\{\Psi(u) - u\Psi'(u)\}du}{u\Psi(u)\{\Psi(u) - cu\}}$$ (4.6)

where a is an arbitrary constant.

The integrand has poles at 0, θ_1, θ_2, which define three possible intervals for θ (see Figure 1). The only one allowing z to range over $-\infty < z < \infty$ is $0 < \theta < \theta_1$ which is therefore chosen.

The next term g_1 satisfies the equation

$$-cg_1' = -(1 - N^{-1}e^{g_0})\Psi'(-g_0')g_1' - N^{-1}e^{g_0}\Psi(-g_0')g_1$$
$$+ \tfrac{1}{2}(1 - N^{-1}e^{g_0})g_0''\Psi''(-g_0').$$ (4.7)

Using the known expressions for g_0 and $dz/d\theta$ in terms of $\theta = -g_0'$ and the fact that $g_0'' = -d\theta/dz$, (4.7) can be reduced to

$$\frac{dg_1}{d\theta} - \frac{g_1}{\theta} = \tfrac{1}{2}\frac{\theta\Psi''(\theta)}{\{\Psi(\theta) - \theta\Psi'(\theta)\}}$$ (4.8)

which has the solution

$$g_1 = \tfrac{1}{2}\theta\int_b^\theta \frac{\Psi''(u)du}{\{\Psi(u) - u\Psi'(u)\}}$$ (4.9)

where b is an arbitrary constant.

It is characteristic of the method that the further equations for $g_2, g_3, \ldots$ all turn out to be of the form

$$\frac{dg_r}{d\theta} - \frac{g_r}{\theta} = \text{function of } g_{r-1}, g_{r-2}, \ldots$$

so that a formal series for g can be developed sequentially.

In the usual applications of the perturbation method ϵ is some small parameter. However, all that is really required is that the series for g converges or is asymptotic over the allowed range of ϵ, a fact which is not always easy to establish. The method appears to work well here because it depends on the epidemic path varying slowly over the range of the contact distribution. For that reason a suitable rescaling would presumably enable ϵ to be replaced by a small parameter.

The choice of the arbitrary constant b in (4.9) is to some extent a matter of convenience. As pointed out in Daniels (1975), a different choice of b would more or less amount to a shift in the origin of z which itself has no natural location. Thus large values of g_1 might merely arise from a lateral translation of the epidemic wave. A suitable convention is to choose $b = a$ so that g_1 vanishes when $z = a$, which is itself chosen to make $f(a) = \frac{1}{2}$.

Care is needed for values of c approaching c_0 because then θ_1 approaches θ_0 and g_1 in (4.7) becomes large for values of θ near its upper limit. This does not appear to affect the calculations over the interesting range of z even when $c = c_0$. However, in the case of the epidemic with removals discussed later, difficulties do arise near the upper limit.

5 Examples

Computations were carried out for two contact distributions with widely differing tail behaviour within the permitted range,

(i) the diffusion model with the 'improper' form $\Psi(\theta) = 1 + \frac{1}{2}\theta^2$ for which $c_0 = \sqrt{2} = 1.414$;

(ii) the double exponential model with $\Psi(\theta) = 1/(1 - \frac{1}{2}\theta^2)$ for which $c_0 = 3\sqrt{6}/4 = 1.837$.

The integrals (4.6) and (4.9) are in general most simply evaluated by numerical integration. Following Mollison (1972) the computations are performed in terms of $T = -z/c = t - s/c$, rather than z, to show the development in *time* t at a *fixed* s rather than in space at a fixed time. The critical velocity c_0 has been used. The results are shown in Figures 2 and 3.

In both cases g_1 turns out to be small. The approximation to the epidemic wave is compared to the logistic form $1/(1 + e^{-T})$ which corresponds to the nonspatial epidemic with $\Psi(\theta) = 1$. For both contact distributions the curves are close, as noted by Mollison (1972) in the double exponential case. This seems intuitively reasonable if one considers that while in the nonspatial case infections all take place at one value of s, in the spatial case infections filter in symmetrically from both sides of s. It may not be true if $\Psi(\theta)$ is not symmetrical.

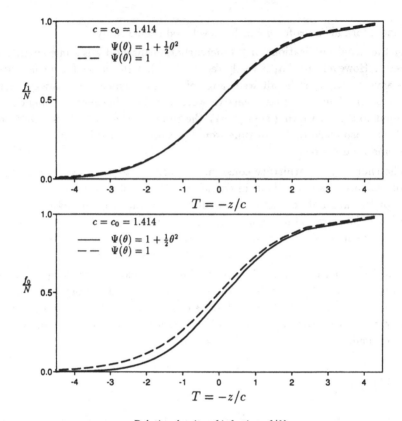

Relative density of infectives f/N.
Zeroth approximation f_0/N. With first correction f_1/N.
Non-spatial epidemic ($\Psi(\theta) = 1$) shown for comparison.

Figure 2.   Simple epidemic: waveforms for diffusion model.

The present approach can also be used for the developing epidemic, $Y(s,t)$ being replaced by $\ell(s,t) = \log Y(s,t)$ in (2.6). The method breaks down in the initial stages, but the saddlepoint approximation can be adjoined for small times. See Daniels (1975) for a discussion.

6   Epidemic with removals

We now apply the technique to the SIR model where infected individuals die or are removed from the population at a constant rate.

With population density N per unit length as before, let $X(s,t)$, $Y(s,t)$ be respectively the density of susceptibles and infectives at a point s at time t. Infectives leave the population at a relative removal rate γ. An epidemic develops provided $\gamma < 1$, and conditional on this, X and Y satisfy the equa-

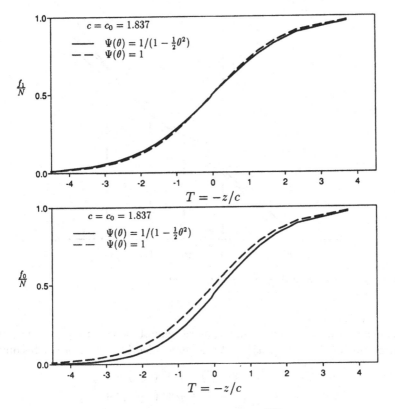

Relative density of infectives f/N.
Zeroth approximation f_0/N. With first correction f_1/N.
Non-spatial epidemic ($\Psi(\theta) = 1$) shown for comparison.

Figure 3.   Simple epidemic: waveforms for double exponential model.

tions

$$\frac{\partial X(s,t)}{\partial t} = -N^{-1} X(s,t) \int_{-\infty}^{\infty} Y(s-u,t)dV(u) \tag{6.1}$$

$$\frac{\partial Y(s,t)}{\partial t} = N^{-1} X(s,t) \int_{-\infty}^{\infty} Y(s-u,t)dV(u) - \gamma Y(s,t). \tag{6.2}$$

A travelling wave requires that

$$X(s,t) = h(z) = \exp k(z), \quad Y(s,t) = f(z) = \exp g(z) \tag{6.3}$$

with $z = s - ct$. Then

$$-cg'(z) = N^{-1} e^{k(z)} \int e^{g(z-u)-g(z)} dV(u) - \gamma \tag{6.4}$$

$$-ch'(z) = -N^{-1} e^{g(z)} \int e^{g(z-u)-g(z)} dV(u). \tag{6.5}$$

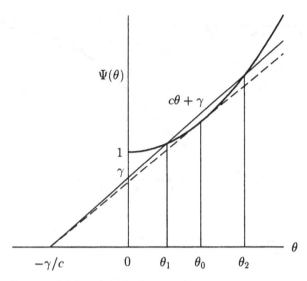

Figure 4.   Range of θ for given c *(see text)*.

As before, this is embedded in the more general model with $g(z-u)-g(z)$ replaced by $\{g(z-\epsilon u)-g(u)\}/\epsilon$. When expanded in powers of ϵ it becomes

$$-cg' = N^{-1}e^k\{\Psi(-g') + \tfrac{1}{2}\epsilon\Psi''(-g') + \cdots\} - \gamma$$
$$ck' = N^{-1}e^g\{\Psi(-g') + \tfrac{1}{2}\epsilon\Psi''(-g')g'' + \cdots\}. \qquad (6.6)$$

On putting $g = g_0 + \epsilon g_1 + \cdots$, $k = k_0 + \epsilon k_1 + \cdots$ and equating coefficients of powers of ϵ in the resulting expansion, the equations for successive approximations are obtained.

The dominant terms g_0, k_0 satisfy

$$-cg_0' = N^{-1}e^{k_0}\Psi(-g_0') - \gamma$$
$$ck_0' = N^{-1}e^{g_0}\Psi(-g_0'). \qquad (6.7)$$

Write $g_0' = -\theta$, $k_0' = \phi$. Then

$$f_0 = e^{g_0} = \frac{Nc\phi}{\Psi(\theta)}, \quad h_0 = e^{k_0} = \frac{N(c\theta + \gamma)}{\Psi(\theta)}. \qquad (6.8)$$

Since we require $0 \le h_0 \le N$, θ has to lie in the interval $-\tfrac{\gamma}{c} \le \theta \le \theta_1$ (see Figure 4), where θ_1 reduces to the previous value when $\gamma = 0$. As before, this interval for θ allows z to range from $-\infty$ to ∞. Take logs and differentiate in (6.8) to obtain

$$g_0' = -\theta = \left(\frac{1}{\phi}\frac{d\phi}{d\theta} - \frac{\Psi'(\theta)}{\Psi(\theta)}\right)\frac{d\theta}{dz}$$

$$k_0' = \phi = \left(\frac{c}{c\theta + \gamma} - \frac{\Psi'(\theta)}{\Psi(\theta)} \right) \frac{d\theta}{dz}. \tag{6.9}$$

Eliminating $d\theta/dz$ and solving for $\phi = \phi(\theta)$ gives, after some manipulation,

$$\frac{dz}{d\theta} = Q(\theta)/R(\theta), \qquad \phi = \Psi(\theta)R(\theta) \tag{6.10}$$

where

$$Q(\theta) = \frac{1}{\Psi(\theta)} \left(\frac{c}{c\theta + \gamma} - \frac{\Psi'(\theta)}{\Psi(\theta)} \right), \quad R(\theta) = \int_\theta^{\theta_1} \omega Q(\omega) d\omega. \tag{6.11}$$

The upper limit of integration θ_1 is chosen to prevent ϕ and hence f_0 taking negative values. On evaluating ϕ and z the solution can be expressed as

$$
\begin{aligned}
f_0 &= e^{g_0} = Nc \left\{ \frac{\theta_1}{\Psi(\theta_1)} - \frac{\theta}{\Psi(\theta)} - \gamma \int_\theta^{\theta_1} \frac{du}{\Psi(u)(cu + \gamma)} \right\} \\
h_0 &= e^{k_0} = N(c\theta + \gamma)/\Psi(\theta) \\
T &= -\frac{z}{c} = \int_a^\theta \{g_0(u) - g_0(\theta)\} \frac{du}{u^2}
\end{aligned} \tag{6.12}
$$

where a is an arbitrary constant.

Figure 5 shows the result of calculations of f_0 and h_0 for the double exponential case $\Psi(\theta) = 1/(1 - \frac{1}{2}\theta^2)$ with $\gamma = 0.5$, $c = c_0$ and $a = 0$ corresponding to the peak of f_0 where $g_0' = 0$. Again f_0 and h_0 are close to the nonspatial curves with $\Psi(\theta) = 1$.

7   Correction terms

The first correction terms g_1, k_1 satisfy the equations

$$
\begin{aligned}
-cg_1' &= N^{-1}e^{k_0}\{\Psi(-g_0')k_1 - \Psi'(-g_0')g_1' + \tfrac{1}{2}g_0''\Psi''(-g_0')\} \tag{7.1} \\
ck_1' &= N^{-1}e^{k_0}\{\Psi(-g_0')g_1 - \Psi'(-g_0')g_1' + \tfrac{1}{2}g_0''\Psi''(-g_0)\} \tag{7.2}
\end{aligned}
$$

which can be reduced to the inhomogeneous linear equations

$$
\begin{aligned}
\frac{dg_1}{d\theta} + \frac{k_1}{\Psi(\theta)R(\theta)} &= \tfrac{1}{2} \frac{\Psi''(\theta)}{\Psi^2(\theta)Q(\theta)} \\
\frac{dk_1}{d\theta} + R(\theta)\Psi'(\theta)\frac{dg_1}{d\theta} - \Psi(\theta)Q(\theta)g_1 &= \tfrac{1}{2}\Psi''(\theta)R(\theta)
\end{aligned} \tag{7.3}
$$

where $Q(\theta)$ and $R(\theta)$ are defined in Section 6.

The following important device enables equations like (7.3) to be solved in a straightforward way. The dominant terms g_0, k_0 contain in general two arbitrary constants α, β. Then $\left(\frac{\partial g_0}{\partial \alpha}, \frac{\partial k_0}{\partial \alpha} \right)$ and $\left(\frac{\partial g_0}{\partial \beta}, \frac{\partial k_0}{\partial \beta} \right)$ are two independent

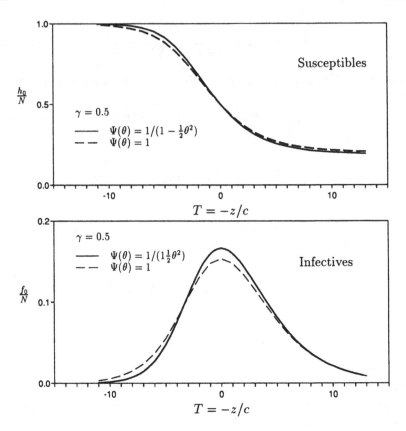

Zeroth approximation; f_0/N infectives, h_0/N susceptibles.
Non-spatial epidemic ($\Psi(\theta) = 1$) shown for comparison.

Figure 5.   Epidemic with removals: double exponential model $\Psi(\theta) = 1/(1 - \frac{1}{2}\theta^2)$.

solutions of the corresponding homogeneous equations with the right hand side zero. (To see this, expand $g_0(\alpha + \delta\alpha, \beta + \delta\beta)$ and $k_0(\alpha + \delta\alpha, \beta + \delta\beta)$ in the equations for g_0, k_0 and pick out the coefficients of $\delta\alpha, \delta\beta$.) The required solution for g_1, k_1 is then found by 'variation of parameters'. On substituting

$$g_1 = A(\theta) \frac{\partial g_0}{\partial \alpha} + B(\theta) \frac{\partial g_0}{\partial \beta}, \quad k_1 = A(\theta) \frac{\partial k_0}{\partial \alpha} + B(\theta) \frac{\partial k_0}{\partial \beta}, \qquad (7.4)$$

in (7.3), the terms in $A(\theta), B(\theta)$ disappear and the equations can be reduced to

$$A'(\theta) = \frac{\Psi''(\theta)}{2\Psi^3(\theta)Q(\theta)} \left\{ [\Psi'(\theta) + \Psi^2(\theta)Q(\theta)]R(\theta)\frac{\partial g_0}{\partial \beta} + \frac{\partial k_0}{\partial \beta} \right\},$$

$$B'(\theta) = -\frac{\Psi''(\theta)}{2\Psi^3(\theta)Q(\theta)} \left\{ [\Psi'(\theta) + \Psi^2(\theta)Q(\theta)]R(\theta)\frac{\partial g_0}{\partial \alpha} + \frac{\partial k_0}{\partial \alpha} \right\}. \quad (7.5)$$

To find $\frac{\partial g_0}{\partial \alpha}$ etc. the simplest procedure is to take g_0 and z as

$$g_0 = \log N + \log(\beta + R(\theta)) \tag{7.6}$$

$$z = \alpha + \int_a^\theta \frac{Q(\omega)d\omega}{\beta + R(\omega)} \tag{7.7}$$

leaving k_0 as before. Then use relations like

$$\frac{\partial g_0}{\partial \beta} = \left(\frac{\partial g_0}{\partial \beta}\right)_\theta - \left(\frac{\partial g_0}{\partial \theta}\right)_\beta \left(\frac{\partial z}{\partial \beta}\right)_\theta \Big/ \left(\frac{\partial z}{\partial \theta}\right)_\beta \tag{7.8}$$

where e.g. $\left(\frac{\partial g_0}{\partial \beta}\right)_\theta$ is the usual partial derivative keeping θ fixed, and put $\alpha = \beta = 0$ after evaluating the derivatives. It is found that

$$\frac{\partial g}{\partial \alpha} = \theta, \frac{\partial k_0}{\partial \alpha} = -\Psi(\theta)R(\theta),$$

$$\frac{\partial g}{\partial \beta} = \frac{1}{R(\theta)} - \theta S(\theta), \frac{\partial k_0}{\partial \beta} = \Psi(\theta)R(\theta)S(\theta) \tag{7.9}$$

where

$$S(\theta) = \int_a^\theta \frac{Q(\omega)d\omega}{R^2(\omega)}. \tag{7.10}$$

Then $A(\theta), B(\theta)$ and hence g_1, k_1 are found on integration.

Preliminary computations using these formulae for the example of Figure 5 indicate that, in the case of infectives, $f_1/N = (f_0/N)\exp g_1$ differs from f_0/N by not more than 0.005 over the effective range of T. But in the case of susceptibles, although h_1/N differs from h_0/N by about 0.01 when h_0/N is small and $T \gg 0$, it differs from h_0/N by about 0.03 when h_0/N approaches unity and $T \ll 0$, so that $h_1/N > 1$. The latter occurs when θ approaches θ_0 and the formula is clearly breaking down in this region when c has the critical value c_0.

8 Comments

No attempt has been made in this paper to justify the method rigorously. Indeed it is clear that the correction terms may become unacceptably large as the critical value θ_0 corresponding to c_0 is approached. Nevertheless, provided the epidemic path varies slowly over the effective range of the contact distribution, there is strong motivation for accepting at least the dominant term as a good approximation over the whole range of the epidemic wave. A numerical solution of (1.1) or (4.2) would help to reinforce or dispel this perception.

A similar perturbation technique could of course be used to approximate $f(z)$ directly from the untransformed equation (1.1). However, the results would appear in terms of moments and would fail to capture the critical velocity c_0 in the way the present approach succeeds in doing.

References

Atkinson, C. and Reuter, G.E.H. (1976) 'Deterministic epidemic waves', *Math. Proc. Camb. Phil. Soc.* **80**, 315–330.

Daniels, H.E. (1960) 'Approximate solutions of Green's type for univariate stochastic processes', *J. R. Statist. Soc. B* **22**, 376–401.

Daniels, H.E. (1975) 'The deterministic spread of a simple epidemic'. In *Perspectives in Probability and Statistics*, J. Gani (ed.) Applied Probability Trust, Sheffield. Academic Press, London, 373–386.

Daniels, H.E. (1977) 'The advancing wave in a spatial birth process', *J. Appl. Prob.* **14**, 689–701.

Daniels, H.E. (1991) 'A look at perturbation approximations for epidemics'. In *Selected Proceedings of the Sheffield Symposium on Applied Probability*, I.V. Basawa and R.L. Taylor (eds.) IMS Lecture Notes **18**, 48–65.

Diekmann, O. (1978) 'Thresholds and travelling waves for the geographical spread of infection', *J. Math. Biol.* **6**, 109–130.

Metz, J.A.J. and Van den Bosch, F. (1995) 'Velocities of epidemic spread', this volume.

Mollison, D. (1972) 'Possible velocities for a simple epidemic', *Adv. Appl. Prob.* **4**, 233–257.

Mollison, D. (1977) 'Spatial contact models for ecological and epidemic spread', *J. R. Statist. Soc. B* **39**, 283–326.

Mollison, D. (1991) 'Dependence of epidemic and population velocities on basic parameters', *Math. Biosci.* **107**, 255–287.

Thieme, H.R. (1977) 'A model for the spatial spread of an epidemic', *J. Math. Biol.* **4**, 337–351.

Epidemic Plant Diseases: a Stochastic Model of Leaf and Stem Lesion Growth

Lynne Billard
P.W.A. Dayananda
Zhen Zhao

1 Introduction

Although there were a few earlier studies such as the Fracker (1936) white pine blister rust and the Large (1952) potato late blight works, it was Van der Plank's (1963) landmark volume which provided the impetus to the modelling of diseases in plant sciences. Van der Plank thus established the logistic model as the basic vehicle for describing the rate of increase of infected tissue in plants.

By the 1980s, it was realized that while the basic logistic model still played an essential role, there were also many diseases and plants for which some modified form of the model was more appropriate. In this work, a brief review of the basic model and these modifications will be presented (in Section 2). Most of these models are deterministically formulated. Then, in Section 3, a closer look at a specific stochastic formulation of a modified model established to describe the spread of *anthracnose* in *Stylosanthes scabra* will be considered; this will include fitting the model to actual data generated in an experiment conducted by Chakraborty *et al.* (1987). Finally, possible further extensions and modifications are proposed in Section 4.

2 Deterministic Models

2.1 Logistic Model

In Van der Plank's (1963) fundamental logistic equation, the rate of increase in infection is proportional to the amount of susceptible or uninfected tissue, $Y(t)$, and to the amount of sporulating or infective tissue, $K - Y(t)$, where K is the total amount of tissue. [If one is dealing with proportion rather than absolute amount of tissues, then simply $K = 1$.] Thus, $Y(t) \equiv Y$ satisfies the equation

$$\frac{dY}{dt} = rY(K - Y) \tag{2.1}$$

216   *Billard* et al.

where r is the apparent infection rate.

Many researchers subsequently used this model to explain the underlying disease process for several plant epidemics. This includes Van der Plank's (1963) own analysis of the Large (1952) potato late blight data. Other examples include the study of foliar diseases (Waggoner 1986), tobacco etch virus and tobacco vein smottling virus (Madden *et al.* 1987), apple powdering mildew and apple scab (Jeger 1984), zucchini yellow mosaic virus (Marcus 1991), and yellow rust (Rapilly 1979).

2.2   Other Models

Other models can be broadly categorised into those that are still based on the logistic model formulation (see Section 2.3) and those which are not. We consider here the latter. Since many of these model categories have been reviewed in Campbell and Madden (1990), only a very brief description is included here, for completeness.

When the rate of increase in infected tissue is proportional only to the amount of susceptible, and not to the infected, tissue, the appropriate model is the so-called monomolecular model, viz.,

$$\frac{dY}{dt} = r(K - Y). \tag{2.2}$$

This situation pertains when infection is not directly transmitted from the infected tissue itself as is the case for pathogens borne by environmental factors such as rain, soil-borne pathogens, systemic diseases, etc. (as, for example, soil-borne mosaic in wheat; Madden and Campbell 1990). See, also, Campbell (1986) for a review of root and virus diseases which satisfy this model. Campbell *et al.* (1984) found that of the many models they fitted to their tobacco black shank data, this monomolecular model gave the best fit.

A Gompertz model is one for which the rate of increase of infection is given by

$$\frac{dY}{dt} = rY \ln(K/Y). \tag{2.3}$$

This model has been fitted, for example, to foliar diseases in Waggoner (1986), to cotton hypocotyl elongation data by Pegelow *et al.* (1977), and rust of coffee by Kushalappa and Ludwig (1982). The tobacco black shank data of Campbell *et al.* (1984) also seemed to follow the Gompertz process, though as noted above the Gompertz model did not fit quite as well as did the monomolecular model.

A model of a different type in which a shape parameter, m, enters the model in addition to the usual infection rate parameter, r, is the Richards

(1959) model whereby

$$\frac{dY}{dt} = rY[1 - (Y/k)^{m-1}]/(m-1). \tag{2.4}$$

Jeger (1982) applied this model to apple powdery mildew data, as did Analytis (1973) on apple scab in Germany.

In a study of noninfectious bud failure of almonds, Fenton *et al.* (1988) used a Weibull model with

$$\frac{dY}{dt} = (\gamma/\beta)[(t - \alpha)/\beta]^{\gamma-1} \exp\{- [(t - \alpha)/\beta]^{\gamma}\} \tag{2.5}$$

where γ is a shape parameter and α and β are location and scale parameters.

Behind the use of the Weibull model is the notion that randomness or stochasticity should somehow be incorporated into a model. Recognition of this fact seems to be emerging in the literature though actual studies seem to be few. These few tend to adopt a regression approach in which the amount of infection depends on time by some polynomial or nonlinear regression function; see, for example, Byrne and Drummond's (1980) regression analysis of dry matter accumulation of pasture. A few others use a regression model with infection dependent on such independent variables as temperature, humidity, or other environmental factors; see, for example, Chakraborty and Billard (1994) for a study of such factors on *anthracnose* in *S. scabra*. Jeger (1987a) replaces the constant infection rate r with a simple linear regression formulation of r as a function of time, $r(t)$, in his modelling of root disease epidemics.

2.3   Other Logistic-based Models

In recent years, it has become apparent that for some diseases, the growth of the epidemic may not be a function solely of the amounts (or proportions) of susceptible and/or infective tissue, as implied by the earlier models, but that other components play a role in the infection process. The logistic model, as used above, implicitly assumes that there is no time lag between infection and the production of secondary inoculum, and that a lesion remains infectious always. That is, there is no provision for a latent period, p, or an infectious period i. Thus, these factors are accommodated into the logistic model according to

$$\frac{dY(t)}{dt} = R[Y(t - p) - Y(t - p - i)][1 - Y(t)] \tag{2.6}$$

where R is the basic infection rate. Surprisingly perhaps given its relative lack of use until the 1980s, this modification was actually developed by Van der

Plank (1963) himself, but presumably Van der Plank (1982) later provided the necessary stimulus to its more general acceptance. Madden and Campbell (1990) applied this model to a tobacco virus disease. Gessler and Blaise (1992) also used this model for data collected in earlier experiments on yellow rust in wheat by Zadoks (1961), *septoria* leaf blotch on wheat by Bronnimann (1968), apple scab by Analytis (1973), powdery mildew on Californian grapes by Delp (1953), and downy mildew on Swiss grapes by Goidanich (1982). More recently, Dayananda *et al.* (1993) considered this model for *anthracnose* in *S. scabra*; while earlier, Fleming (1983) used it for a cereal rust epidemic.

Other investigators have modified the logistic model by including consideration of the effects of changing environmental factors, most often temperature but occasionally also humidity measures, leaf wetness, etc. These include barley powdery mildew (Hau 1990), pathogenic fungi (Analytis 1977), stripe rust in wheat (Zadoks 1971), *alternaria solani* (Waggoner and Parlange 1974), *Puccinia recondita* in wheat (Tomerlin *et al.* 1983), and late blight in potato (Fry *et al.* 1983). In other diseases, variable host size, when growth of new tissue outstrips the infection curve, needs to be brought into the basic model. These issues were addressed for rust of coffee by Kushalappa and Ludwig (1982), alfalfa by Thal and Campbell (1988), root invading fungi by Huisman (1982), vesicular-arbuscular mycorrhizal in onions by Tinker (1975), sweetcorn by Arnold (1974), foliar diseases in Waggoner (1986), and plant pathogens by Jeger (1987b), among others. In an entirely different direction, Madden *et al.* (1987) recognised the potential for competing diseases and infections in their study of the tobacco etch and tobacco vein mottling viruses.

Stochastic models, along the lines long being formulated for epidemic processes in human diseases (see e.g. Bailey 1975), have been much slower to emerge. Yet, these are arguably at least as important, some might say more important, than are deterministic formulations. One attempt to introduce a stochastic model is that by Marcus (1991) in a study of the zucchini yellow mosaic virus, in which, in effect, a Brownian model term is added to the original Van der Plank logistic model (though, technically, the Dennis (1988) generalization of the Van der Plank equation is proposed).

3   Stochastic Model for Leaf and Stem Lesions

3.1   The Model as a Bivariate Death Process

In this section, a specific generalization of the basic logistic process is taken with a view to presenting a more realistic biological model for some situations. More specifically, in addition to infection transmission being a function of the amount of susceptible and infected tissue, provision for additional infection from the surrounding environment is made. Suppose the susceptible and infected tissue under study are the leaves of a plant. Quite easily the basic logistic model can prevail. The rate of infection however can be higher if, for example, there are sources of infection elsewhere (such as on the ground, or, as is often the case from infected lesions on the plant's stem). For modelling purposes, this secondary source of infection will be referred to as the stem which itself may or not become infected. Furthermore, a stochastic rather than a deterministic process will be developed. In Section 3.3, the model will be fitted to *anthracnose* on *S. scabra*. Earlier, Pratt (1984) had recognized the leaf and stem as separate disease units in his investigation of disease in subterranean clover caused by *Cercospora*.

As before, let $Y(t)$ represent the number of uninfected leaves at time t; and let $Z(t) = 1 - Z_1(t)$ where $Z_1(t)$ represents the infectivity status of the stem, with $Z_1(t) = 0$ if the stem is uninfected and $Z_1(t) = 1$ if it is infected. Let the number of uninfected and infected leaves at time zero be N and K, respectively. Then, $\{Y(t), Z(t)\}$ can be represented as a stochastic bivariate death process. The infinitesimal transition probabilities in the interval $(t, t + h)$ are

$$P\{Y(t+h) = y - 1, Z(t+h) = z \mid Y(t) = y, Z(t) = z\}$$
$$= [\beta y(N + K - y) + \alpha y(1 - z)]h + o(h), \tag{3.1}$$
$$P\{Y(t+h) = y, Z(t+h) = 0 \mid Y(t) = y, Z(t) = 1\}$$
$$= \mu(N + K - y)h + o(h), \tag{3.2}$$

where $o(h)/h \to 0$ as $h \to 0$, and where in (3.1) the first term is the contribution to the infection rate from the infected leaves, and the second term is the influence of the stem if it is infected in which case there is a higher rate of infection. It is assumed in (3.2) that the stem itself becomes infected at a rate proportional to the number of infected leaves.

Let

$$p_{y,z}(t) = P\{Y(t) = y, Z(t) = z \mid Y(0) = N, Z(0) = 1\}.$$

Then, the differential-difference equations governing this process for $z \in \{0, 1\}$ become

$$\frac{d}{dt}p_{y,z}(t) = -[\beta y(N + K - y) + \alpha y(1 - z) + \mu(N + K - y)z]\, p_{y,z}(t)$$
$$+ [\beta + \mu(1 - z)](N + K - y - 1)(y + 1)p_{y+1,z}(t)$$
$$+ \mu(N + K - y)(1 - z)p_{y,1-z}(t)$$

for $y \in \{0, \ldots, N - 1\}$, and

$$\frac{d}{dt}p_{N,z}(t) = -[\beta N K + \alpha N(1 - z) + \mu(N + K - y)z]\, p_{N,z}(t)$$
$$+ \mu(N + K - y)(1 - z)p_{N,1-z}(t). \tag{3.3}$$

The boundary conditions are $p_{N,1}(0) = 1$ and $p_{y,z}(0) = 0$, otherwise. By using the method of integrating factors, these equations can be solved recursively. Thus, it can be shown that, for $y \in \{0, \ldots, N\}$,

$$p_{N-y,1}(t) = \sum_{j=0}^{y} A(N-y,j) \exp\{-tE_1(j)\} \qquad (3.4)$$

where

$$E_1(j) = (K+j)[\beta(N-j) + \mu],$$

and

$$A(N-y,j) = \frac{(-1)^j \beta^y (N-1)!(K+y-1)!(y-j-1)!}{(N-y)!(K-1)!j!y!} \times$$

$$\prod_{i=0, i \neq j}^{y} [\beta(N-K-i-j) + \mu]^{-1},$$

with $A(N,0) \equiv 1$; and, for $y \in \{0, \ldots, N\}$,

$$p_{N-y,0}(t) = \sum_{j=0}^{y} [B(N-y,j)\exp\{-tE_2(j)\} + C(N-y,j)\exp\{-tE_1(j)\}] \quad (3.5)$$

where

$$E_2(j) = (N-j)[\beta(K+j) + \alpha],$$

and

$$B(N-y,j) = B(N-y+1,j) \prod_{i=j}^{y-1} [D(i,j)]^{-1}, j \in \{0, \ldots, y-1\},$$

$$B(N-y,y) = -\sum_{j=0}^{y-1} B(N-y,j) - \sum_{j=0}^{y} C(N-y,j),$$

$$C(N-y,j) = \mu(K+j)A(N-j,j)[(N-j)\alpha - (K+j)\mu]^{-1} \prod_{i=j}^{y-1} D(i,j)$$

$$+\mu \sum_{l=j+1}^{y} (K+l)A(N-l,j)[E_2(l) - E_1(j)]^{-1} \prod_{i=l}^{y-1} D(i,j),$$

with

$$D(i,j) = E_2(i)[E_2(i+1) - E_2(j)]^{-1}.$$

3.2   Asymptotic Time to Stem Infection

The time T to first stem infection is important as this signifies another stage of plant deterioration, since stem infection will affect the productive use of the plant as pasture more than will the infection of leaves themselves.

Clearly, the distribution function of T is

$$P(T > t) = F(t) = 1 - \sum_{y=0}^{N} \sum_{j=0}^{y} A(N - y, j) \exp\{-tE_1(j)\}.$$

Then, the limiting distribution of T when the number of leaves N tends to infinity so that βN tends to a constant ν, is

$$\lim F(t) = 1 - \sum_{y=0}^{\infty} \binom{K + y - 1}{y} \exp\{-K(\mu + \nu)t\}[1 - \exp\{-(\mu + \nu)t\}]^y.$$

It therefore follows that the joint probability distribution of $\{Y(t), Z(t) = 1\}$ is a negative binomial distribution with parameter $[1 - \exp\{-(\mu+\nu)t\}]$. That is,

$$p_{y,1}(t) = \binom{K + y - 1}{y} exp\{-K(\mu + \nu)t\}[1 - \exp\{-(\mu+\nu)t\}]^y, \; y \in \{0, 1, \ldots\}.$$

3.3 Some Generalizations

In general, the infinitesimal infection rates for leaf and stem infection could be any arbitrary function of the variables (y, z). Thus, (3.1) and (3.20 become

$$\begin{aligned} P\{Y(t + h) &= y - 1, Z(t + h) = z \mid Y(t) = y, Z(t) = z\} \\ &= \gamma(y, z)h + o(h), \end{aligned} \tag{3.6}$$

$$\begin{aligned} P\{Y(t + h) &= y, Z(t + h) = z - 1 \mid Y(t) = y, Z(t) = 1\} \\ &= \mu(y, z)h + o(h), \end{aligned} \tag{3.7}$$

with corresponding differential-difference equations, for $y \in \{0, \ldots, N\}$ and $z \in \{0, \ldots, S\}$ where $S \equiv Z(0)$,

$$\begin{aligned} \frac{d}{dt} p_{y,z}(t) = &- [\gamma(y, z) + \mu(y, z)]p_{y,z}(t) + \gamma(y - 1, z)p_{y-1,z}(t) \\ &+ \mu(y, z - 1)p_{y,z-1}(t) \end{aligned} \tag{3.8}$$

where in (3.8), $p_{y,z}(t) \equiv 0$ if $y < 0$ and/or $z < 0$.

These can be solved along analogous lines to that used in subsection 3.2. In the following subsection, we consider three specific models, viz., (a) when $\mu(y, z) = \mu$ corresponding to the situation in which stem infection occurs at a Poisson rate (Model 1), (b) $\mu(y, z) = \mu_1$, or μ_0 depending on whether stem infection is absent or present (Model 2), and (c) $\mu(y, z) = \mu(N + K - y)$ where infection is proportional to the number of infected leaves (Model 3), as in Section 3.1 above, in each case using (3.1) as the basic leaf infection rate.

Stochastic Model 1	Stochastic Model 2	Stochastic Model 3	Reported data
0.3716345	0.3716548	0.3694241	0.411
0.3355214	0.3338983	0.3291592	0.411
0.3005241	0.3005415	0.2916268	0.353
0.2680315	0.2680476	0.2570901	0.294
0.2381203	0.2381350	0.2256191	0.176
0.2107939	0.2108073	0.1971910	0.176
0.1859993	0.1860115	0.1717107	0.118

$sse =$ 2.0368202×10^{-2} 2.0616006×10^{-2} 1.9351426×10^{-2}

Stochastic Model 1: $\mu = $ constant

Stochastic Model 2: $\mu = \mu_s$, (μ_0, μ_1)

Stochastic Model 3: $\mu(r) = \mu(N + K - r)$

Table 1: Expected uninfected proportions of three stochastic models with different stem infection rates vs. reported data.

3.4   Numerical Results

Table 1 gives the expected proportions of uninfected leaves for the three different stem infection rates described above, together with the actual data. The data consist of measures of *anthracnose* spread on *S. scabra* plants observed for eight weeks after initially healthy plants were inoculated with the disease. For a detailed description of the experiment, see Chakraborty *et al.* (1987). The unknown parameter values of the stochastic model (β, α, μ) were estimated by minimizing the error sum of squares (sse). The results are plotted in Figure 1.

It is clear that while all three models fit the downward trend in the data well, the third model in which the stem infection rate depends on the number of infected leaves, has the best fit $(sse = 1.935 \times 10^{-2})$. There is nothing to distinguish between the first two models in which stem infection is either constant or changes when stem infection occurs, with $sse = 2.037 \times 10^{-2}$ for Model 1 and $sse = 2.062 \times 10^{-2}$ for Model 2, respectively. Furthermore, the estimated parameters values for $\beta = 9.0 \times 10^{-3}$ and $\alpha = 8.08 \times 10^{-3}$ are the same for each of Models 1 and 2. The model of choice, Model 3, gives parameter estimates of $\beta = 9.9 \times 10^{-3}$, $\alpha = 7.68 \times 10^{-3}$ and $\mu = 0.81$.

In addition, from the plot of the data as observed in Figure 1, there is a question as to whether or not there is a cyclical component inherent to the true underlying model or whether this apparent cycle is an artifact of the particular data set at hand. Thus, while the three models fitted herein have identified the linear trend well, they are not capable of identifying any basic cyclical trend were one to exist.

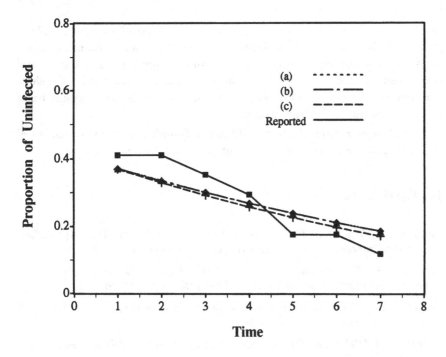

(a) Stochastic Model 1 : $\lambda = 9.0e - 3,\ \alpha = 8.08e - 3,\ \mu = 5.71$

(b) Stochastic Model 2: $\lambda = 9.0e - 3,\ \alpha = 8.08e - 3,\ \mu_1 = 0.01,\ \mu_0 = 5.51$

(c) Stochastic Model 3 : $\lambda = 9.9e - 3,\ \alpha = 7.68e - 3,\ \mu = 0.81$
$$\mu\ (r) = \mu\ (\ N + K - r\ )$$

Figure 1: Comparison of three stochastic models with different stem infection rates.

4   Conclusion and Extensions

It is clear that the stochastic model developed herein is one viable model at least for *anthracnose* in *S. scabra* in the case there is no essential cyclical component to the process. Though this particular model was based on the logistic model, it would be of interest to see how, or whether, some of the other types of models, such as monomolecular, Gompertz, Richards, Weibull, etc., fit as well or better. Of greater interest in general, however, would be the development of stochastic analogues of the numerous deterministic models fitted to the various plant epidemic disease data sets reviewed briefly in Section 2. These would constitute specific applications of the generalized model of equation (3.8). This system of equations can itself be further generalized by the use of transition rates which may be functions of entities outside of just the state space variables themselves. Finally, generalizations or extensions that allowed the identification of nonlinear trends such as the cyclical component alluded to in the *anthracnose* example, or extensions to include seasonal models developed over several years (or equivalent), would be of value and worthy of future consideration.

Partial support from the National Science Foundation, the Office of Naval Research and the Isaac Newton Institute is gratefully acknowledged.

References

Analytis, S. (1973) 'Methodik der Analys von Epidemien dargestellt am Appelschorf (*Venturia inaequalis* (Cooke) *Aderh*)', *Acta Phytomedica* 1, 5–75.

Analytis, S. (1977) 'Uber die Relation zwischen biologischer Entwicklung und Temperatur bei phytopathogenen Pilzen', *Phytopath. Z.* 90, 64–76.

Arnold, C.Y. (1974) 'Predicting stages of sweetcorn (*Zea mays L.*) development', *J. Am. Soc. Host. Sci.* 99, 501–505.

Bailey, N.T.J. (1975) *The Mathematical Theory of Infectious Diseases and its Applications*, Griffin, London.

Bronnimann, A. (1968) 'Zur Kenntnis von *Septoria nodorum* Berk., den Erreger der Spelzenbräune und einer Blattedürre des Weizens', *Phytopath. Z.* 61, 101–146.

Byrne, G.F. and Drummond, J.E. (1980) 'Fitting a growth curve equation to field data', *Agric. Meteorol.* 22,1–9.

Campbell, C.L. (1986) 'Interpretation and uses of disease progress curves for root diseases'. In *Plant Disease Epidemiology: Population Dynamics and Management*, Vol. 1, K.J. Leonard and W.E. Fry (eds.), MacMillan, 38–54.

Campbell, C.L., Jacobi, W.R., Powell, N.T. and Main, C.E. (1984) 'Analysis of disease progression and the randomness of occurrence of infected plants during tobacco black shank epidemics', *Phytopath.* 74, 230–235.

Campbell, C.L. and Madden, L.V. (1990) *Introduction to Plant Disease Epidemiology*, Wiley, New York.

Chakraborty, S. and Billard, L. (1994) 'Quantitative relationships between *Colletotrichum gloeosporioides* infection of *Stylosanthes scaba* and weather factors under field conditions', *Plant Pathology*, in press.

Chakraborty, S., Cameron, D.F., Irwin, J.A.G. and Ratcliff, D. (1987) 'Epidemiology of anthracnose in stylosanthes: Disease assessment and sampling unit', *Proc. Austral. Plant Path. Confc.*

Dayananda, P.W.A., Billard, L. and Chakraborty, S. (1995) 'Estimation of rate parameter and its relationship with latent and infectious periods periods in plant disease epidemics', *Biometrics*, in press.

Delp, C. J. (1953) *Some environmental factors which influence the development of the grape powdery mildew fungus*, Uncinula necator *(Schw.) Burr.* Unpublished PhD dissertation, University of California, Davis.

Dennis, B. (1988) 'Stochastic differential equations as insect population models'. In *Estimation and Analysis of Insect Populations*, L. MacDonald, B.G. Manly, J. Lockwood and J. Logan (eds.), Lecture Notes in Statistics, Springer-Verlag, 219–238.

Fenton, C.A.L., Kester, D.E. and Kuniyuski, A.H. (1988) 'Models for noninfectious bud failure in almond', *Phytopath.* **78**, 139–143.

Fleming, R.A. (1983) 'Development of a simple mechanistic model of cereal rust progress', *Phytopath.* **73**, 308–312.

Fracker, S.B. (1936) 'Progressing intensification of uncontrolled plant-disease outbreaks', *J. Econ. Entomol.* **29**, 923–940.

Fry, W.E., Apple, A.E. and Bruhn, J.A. (1983) 'Evaluation of potato late blight forecaster modified to incorporate host resistance and fungicide weathering', *Phytopath.* **73**, 1054–1059.

Gessler, C. and Blaise, P. (1992) 'An extended progeny/parent ratio model II. Application to experimental data', *J. Phytopath.* **134**, 53–62.

Goidanich, G. (1982) *Manuale di patologia vegetale. Vol. II.* Ed. Agricole Bologna.

Hau, B. (1990) 'Analytic models of plant disease in a changing environment', *Ann. Rev. Phytopathol.* **28**, 221–245.

Huisman, O.C. (1982) 'Interrelations of root growth dynamics to epidemiology of root-invading fungi', *Ann. Rev. Phytopath.* **20**, 303–327.

Jeger, M.J. (1982) 'Using growth curve relative rates to model disease progress of apple powdery mildew', *Prot. Ecol.* **4**, 49–58.

Jeger, M.J. (1984) 'Relating disease progress to cumulative numbers of trapped spores: apple powdery mildew and scab epidemics in sprayed and unsprayed orchard plots', *Plant Pathol.* **33**, 517–523.

Jeger, M.J. (1987a) 'The influence of root growth and inocular density on the dynamics of root disease epidemics: Theoretical analysis', *New Phytol.* **107**, 459–478.

Jeger, M.J. (1987b) 'Modelling the dynamics of plant pathogens'. In *Populations of Plant Pathogens: Their Dynamics and Genetics*, M.S. Wolfe and C.E. Caten (eds.), Blackwell, Oxford, 91–107.

Kushalappa, A.C. and Ludwig, A. (1982) 'Calculation of apparent infection rate in plant diseases: Development of a method to correct for host growth', *Phytopath.* **72**, 1373–1377.

Large, E.C. (1952) 'The interpretation of progress curves for potato late blight and other plant diseases', *Plant Pathol.* **1**, 109–117.

Madden, L.V., Pirone, T.P. and Raccah, B. (1987) 'Temporal analysis of two viruses increasing in the same tobacco fields', *Phytopath.* **77**, 974–980.

Madden, L.V. and Campbell, C.L. (1990) 'Nonlinear disease progress curves'. In
  Epidemics of Plant Diseases: Mathematical Analysis and Modelling, J. Kranz
  (ed.), Springer-Verlag, 181–229.

Marcus, R. (1991) 'Deterministic and stochastic logistic models for describing increase of plant disease', *Crop Protection* 10, 155–159.

Pegelow, E.J., Taylor, B.B., Horrocks, R.D, Buxton, D.R., Marx, D.B. and Wan-
  jura, D.F. (1977) 'The Gompertz function as a model for cotton hypocotyl
  elongation', *Agron. J.* 69, 875–878.

Pratt, R.G. (1984) 'A new *Cercospora* leaf and stem disease of subterranean cloven',
  Phytopath. 74, 1152–1156.

Rapilly, F. (1979) 'Yellow rust epidemiology', *Ann. Rev. Phytopathol.* 17, 59–73.

Richards, F.J. (1959) 'A flexible growth function for empirical use', *J. Exp. Bot.*
  10, 290–300.

Thal, W.M. and Campbell, C.L. (1988) 'Analysis of progress of alfalfa leafspot
  epidemics', *Phytopath.* 78, 389–395.

Tinker, P.B. (1975) 'Effects of vesicular-arbuscular mycorrhizas on higher plants',
  Symp. Soc. Exp. Biol. 29, 325–349.

Tomerlin, J.R., Eversmeyer, M.G., Kramer, C.L. and Browder, L.E. (1983) 'Temperature and host effects on latent and infectious periods and on urediniospore
  production of *Puccinia recondita f. sp. tritici*', *Phytopath.* 73, 414–419.

Van der Plank, J.E. (1963) *Plant Diseases: Epidemics and Control*, Academic
  Press, new York.

Van der Plank, J.E. (1982) *Host-Pathogen Interactions in Plant Disease*, Academic
  Press, New York.

Waggoner, P.E. (1986) 'Progress curves of foliar diseases: their interpretation and
  use'. In *Plant Disease Epidemiology: Population Dynamics and Management*,
  Vol. I K.J. Leonard and W.E. Fry (eds.), MacMillan, 3–37.

Waggoner, P.E. and Parlange, J.Y. (1974) 'Verification of a model of spore germination at variable, moderate temperatures', *Phytopath.* 64, 1192–1196.

Zadoks, J.C. (1961) 'Yellow rust on wheat studies in epidemiology and physiologic
  specialization', *T. Pl. Ziekten* 67, 69–256.

Zadoks, J.C. (1971) 'Systems analysis and the dynamics of epidemics', *Phytopath.*
  61, 600–610.

Part 3
Space-time Dynamics

Detecting Nonlinearity and Chaos in Epidemic Data

Stephen Ellner

A. Ronald Gallant

James Theiler

1 Summary

Historical data on recurrent epidemics have been central to the debate about the prevalence of chaos in biological population dynamics. Credit for this interest in epidemics goes to Schaffer and Kot (1985, 1986), who first recognized that the abundance and accuracy of disease incidence data opened the door to applying a range of methods for detecting chaos that had been devised in the early 1980's. Using attractor reconstruction, estimates of dynamical invariants, and comparisons between data and simulation of SEIR models, the 'case for chaos in childhood epidemics' was made through a series of influential papers beginning in the mid 1980's (reviewed by Schaffer *et al.* 1990). The proposition that the precise timing and magnitude of epidemic outbreaks are deterministic but chaotic is appealing, since it raises the hope of finding determinism and simplicity beneath the apparently stochastic and complicated surface of the data.

However the initial enthusiasm for methods of detecting chaos in data has been followed by critical re-evaluations of their limitations. Early hopes of a 'one size fits all' algorithm to diagnose chaos *vs.* noise in any data set have given way to a recognition that a variety of methods must be used, and interpretation of results must take into account the limitations of each method and the imperfections of the data (e.g., Theiler 1990).

Our goals here are twofold. First, we present an overview of methods for detecting nonlinearity and chaos in epidemic data. We identify features of epidemic data that create problems for the older, better known methods of detecting chaos (Section 2), and we then review some newer methods for detecting nonlinearity and chaos that are suited to epidemic data, and have a more solid statistical basis (Sections 3-5). Our emphasis is on the essential ideas of each method, referring the reader to the relevant literature for the technical details which we omit. Second, we begin a re-evaluation of the claims for nonlinear dynamics and chaos in epidemics, by applying each of the newer methods to a collection of data sets on measles, mumps, rubella, and chicken pox. These results are new, and publication elsewhere is not planned, so a fairly complete description is given.

When we ask 'are epidemics nonlinear?', we are not questioning the existence of global nonlinearities in epidemic dynamics, such as nonlinear transmission rates. Our question is whether the data's deviations from an annual cycle (for example, the biennial or triennial cycles that are often observed) are adequately described by a linear, noise-driven stochastic process, or whether a nonlinear description is mandated by the data.

Our conclusion is that evidence for chaos is generally lacking, but at least for measles we can reject the hypothesis of linear noise superimposed on an annual cycle. Thus nonlinearity in the dynamics, and its interactions with stochastic perturbations, are manifested in the data and should be taken into account when interpreting or attempting to predict fluctuations in the number of cases. In particular, our results suggest that short-term noise amplification (Deissler and Farmer 1992) and 'transient chaos' are likely to be common.

2   Noise, seasonality, and the hunt for chaos

The task of detecting nonlinearity or chaos in epidemics is complicated by two unavoidable features of the data: dynamic noise and seasonality. The literature on detecting chaos mostly ignores these features (apart from lip service), so many 'consumers' of the literature are unaware of their immense effects on methods for detecting chaos. Those effects are the subject of this section.

2.1   Dynamic noise

The prevalent attitude in the chaos literature is that any stochasticity is an undesirable corruption of the data. This attitude is reasonable for random measurement errors – accurate data are indeed better than inaccurate data – and physicists have devoted considerable effort to methods for reducing measurement errors. However epidemic dynamics also are affected by 'dynamic noise' – external, unpredictable perturbations (e.g., fluctuations in weather, teacher strikes, etc.) that affect disease transmission and consequently are an intrinsic part of the dynamics.

Here we take the view, following Eckmann and Ruelle (1985), that the defining feature of chaos is bounded fluctuations with sensitive dependence on initial conditions. This definition of chaos applies equally to completely deterministic systems and to systems with dynamic noise. Formally, suppose that the data are generated by a stationary ergodic process of the form

$$X_{t+1} = F(X_t, E_t)$$

where $X_t \in \mathcal{R}^d$ and E_t is a sequence of i.i.d. random variables. The system's sensitivity to small changes in initial conditions is quantified by the dominant Lyapunov exponent λ, given by

$$\lambda = \lim_{m \to \infty} \frac{1}{m} \log \|DF(X_m, E_m)DF(X_{m-1}, E_{m-1}) \cdots DF(X_1, E_1)\|, \quad (2.1)$$

where $DF(\bullet, E)$ is the Jacobian matrix of $F(\bullet, E)$. λ is well-defined and constant with probability 1 under some mild regularity conditions (Kifer 1986). Thus λ is a specific number, rather than a random variable, even for systems with dynamic noise. Note that the Jacobians in (2.1) only involve derivatives with respect to the state (X). Thus for noisy systems the Lyapunov exponent characterizes the exponential divergence of two trajectories with slightly perturbed initial conditions, but subject to the same random shocks (E).

Dynamic noise can move systems into or out of chaos (Crutchfield *et al.* 1982); in particular, the stability of seasonally forced SEIR models is very sensitive to small random fluctuations in the contact rate (Rand and Wilson 1991). Removing dynamic noise by 'noise reduction' techniques is not desirable: we want to characterize the real dynamics, which are noisy due to random forcing. Most methods for detecting chaos or nonlinearity in data, even methods that are robust against (or explicitly designed to handle) measurement errors, have serious problems with dynamic noise. Methods in this category include:

Fractal dimension. Estimates of fractal dimension (see Theiler (1990) for a review) are seriously degraded by dynamic noise much smaller than the system's range of fluctuations, even though much higher levels of measurement error can be dealt with (R. Smith, 1992a,b). This reflects a fundamental difference between the effects of measurement errors and dynamic noise. With measurement errors, we are viewing a low-dimensional attractor through fogged-up glasses; with dynamic noise the attractor is infinite dimensional.

Lyapunov exponents by the Wolf *et al.* (1985) method. This method quantifies the sensitive dependence on initial conditions by finding segments of the time series that come close together in phase space, and monitoring their subsequent divergence. Because divergence due to dynamic noise is confounded with divergence due to sensitive dependence on initial conditions, dynamic noise generates 'false positives' in the hunt for chaos (Sayers 1990).

Nonlinear prediction (Sugihara and May 1990). The method of Sugihara and May (1990) distinguishes between measurement error and deterministic chaos by comparing the accuracy of short-term and long-term out of sample forecasts. In a chaotic system, long-term forecasts are less accurate due to sensitive dependence on initial conditions. However dynamic noise also decreases long-term forecast accuracy, so distinguishing between chaos and dynamic noise by this method is generally not possible (Ellner 1991, Stone 1992).

2.2 Seasonality

Seasonality should not create any problems for methods of detecting chaos in data, because any periodically forced system can be re-expressed as an equivalent autonomous system by adding a state variable to serve as a clock. This frees us (in theory) to behave as if our data come from an autonomous system. In practice, however, data analyses can be confounded by strong seasonal forcing:

Attractor reconstruction. The early claims of evidence for chaos in epidemics was based on the now-classic method of attractor reconstruction in time delay co-ordinates (Packard *et al.* 1980, Takens1981, Sauer *et al.* 1991). However, Ellner (1991) showed that the fieldmarks of low-dimensional chaos which had been observed in measles data – graphically reconstructed attractors, Poincare sections, and Poincare maps – were also observed in a seasonally forced nonchaotic stochastic model which is really infinite-dimensional.

Lyapunov exponents. In the Wolf *et al.* (1985) method, and the modified Wolf method proposed by Rand and Taylor (D. Rand, *pers. comm.*), data segments nearby in phase space can correspond to different times of year. Subsequent trajectories will diverge simply because they are following different 'clocks', creating a positive bias in estimates of λ. The spurious neighbors also affect our method based on time series modeling (Nychka *et al.* 1992, McCaffrey *et al.* 1992); this invalidates Ellner's (1991) conclusion that measles exhibits weak chaos. A fix-up for the method and updated conclusions are described below.

Some influential figures are now arguing, based on the problems with the older methods, that the program of 'detecting chaos' is doomed to failure by the need for massive amounts of very accurate data. We disagree, so long as the standards of 'success' are those of field biology, where imperfect and limited data are the norm, rather than those of laboratory physics. A limited data set may not allow us to reject a null hypothesis that could be rejected with additional data, but with methods grounded in experimental statistics we can still say that a given data set does or does not provide evidence for a given hypothesis, and attach statistical measures of confidence to our conclusions. A chance of error is unavoidable, so overall conclusions often must emerge from a series of studies with different limitations, rather than from a single decisive experiment (Hastings *et al.* 1993).

3 Surrogate data

We now turn to some more promising methods for epidemic data. Surrogate data methods provide a Monte-Carlo approach for testing whether data are consistent with a (possibly transformed) linear autoregressive model with

Gaussian dynamic noise (Theiler *et al.* 1992, and references therein). The basic procedure is to simulate 'surrogate' data sets which have the same power spectrum as the real data, and compare the values of a test statistic on the real and simulated data. One method for generating surrogates is to Fourier transform the data, randomize the phases in the complex Fourier coefficients while preserving the amplitudes, and inverse Fourier transform to obtain a surrogate data set. The surrogate data have the same discrete power spectrum and therefore the same (circular) linear autocorrelations as the real data, but any couplings between modes due to nonlinear structure in the data have been obliterated. Repeat as often as desired, using an apt test statistic, and you have a statistical hypothesis test of

H_0 : the data arise from a static transform of a Gaussian

linear autogressive process. (3.1)

An important strength of the surrogate data method is that any computable measure of nonlinearity can be used as the test statistic. Even if the numerical value of the measure on any single data set may be inaccurate (e.g., biased due to dynamic noise), differences between the real and surrogate data still can provide evidence of nonlinearity which is no less reliable than any other statistical test of a null hypothesis.

Of course it is not quite that simple. If the real data aren't Gaussian they should be made Gaussian by a transformation; care is needed when computing the power spectrum; and it is not clear how to generate good surrogates for data with strong spectral peaks. See Theiler *et al.* (1992, 1994) for the details. To avoid false negatives, the test statistic must key into some difference between linear and nonlinear dynamics: a statistic that can be computed from the linear autocorrelations is useless because it will have exactly the same value on the real and surrogate data. It is also helpful if the test statistic measures a physical or intuitively identifiable quantity. Detecting nonlinearity is just the first step; ultimately, one wants to be able to characterize it.

For epidemic data the null hypothesis given above is clearly false due to seasonality. We therefore examined the more interesting null hypothesis

H_0 : data = seasonal trend + transform of a Gaussian linear AR process.

(3.2)

In many cases the data appear to have a biennial or triennial cycle. This is clearly a departure from an annual cycle, but it is not necessarily a *nonlinear* departure, because a linear filter acting on white noise can produce spectral peaks at biennial or triennial periods. If the data exhibit a biennial or triennial cycle, failure to reject (3.2) would indicate that the multi-year cycle can be described as a linear response by the system to external forcing; while rejection of (3.2) would imply that the system's response is nonlinear.

To test (3.2) we subtracted off the seasonal trend (estimated by averaging over years in the data), normalized the deviations from the trend to have seasonally constant variance, and generated surrogates for the normalized deviations. We used several test statistics:

1. The Ramsay and Rothman 'time-reversal' statistic

$$\rho_{i,j}(m) = \text{Sample average of}(x_t^i \, x_{t+m}^j - x_t^i \, x_{t-m}^j),$$

for $i \neq j$ (Rothman 1990, Ramsay and Rothman 1991). The distribution of a linear process with independent Gaussian innovations is unchanged by time reversal, so excessively large values of $|\rho_{i,j}|$ signal a departure from H_0. We calculated $|\rho_{1,2}(m)|$ for $m =1$ through 16 quarters and used the maximum and median of the 16 values as our test statistics.

2. Statistics related to the correlation integral $C(r)$, which is the fraction of reconstructed data vectors whose distance apart is less than or equal to r. The statistics we used were two percentiles of the distance distribution, $r_{.01}$ and $r_{.001}$, defined by $C(r_p) = p$, and a crude estimate of the correlation dimension D_2 (Grassberger and Procaccia 1983):

$$\hat{D}_2 = \frac{\log C(r_1) - \log C(r_2)}{\log(r_1) - \log(r_2)},$$

using $r_{.01}$ and $r_{.001}$ as r_1 and r_2. This formula for $\hat{D}_2$ does not give a very accurate estimate of fractal dimension. However, as noted above, such inaccuracies do not affect the validity of surrogate data methods because the conclusions are based on differences between real and surrogate data sets. We used reconstruced state vectors of dimension 8 (i.e, each state vector consisted of 8 consecutive quarterly case counts), so that these statistics would be looking for 'long-range' structures not captured by the linear autocorrelations.

3. 'Prediction' accuracy backwards in time (suggested by Robert May following our talk). For nonlinear maps with stretching and folding, the folds make it hard to tell where you came from even if you can predict where you're going. For example in the logistic map, given x_t you can predict x_{t+1} exactly but there are two possibilities for x_{t-1} and no way to identify the correct choice. Our test statistics were the 'prediction' accuracy 1 year into the past for kernel time series models using 2, 3, and 4 future values, with the kernel bandwidth chosen by ordinary cross validation. For these statistics only the seasonal trend was not removed from the data, because trend removal could obscure a simple nonlinear relationship.

The results (Table 1) give consistent, and occasionally very strong, evidence for nonlinearity in measles. Of the 12 measles series analyzed, 10 were significantly nonlinear at the .05 level for at least one of the test statistics.

	Time reversal		C(r)			Back-prediction		
	Max	Median	$\widehat{D}_2$	$r_{.001}$	$r_{.01}$	d= 2	d= 3	d= 4
MEASLES								
NYC	*	-	**	*	-	+	-	-
Baltimore	-	*	*	*	-	-	-	-
Detroit	-	-	-	-	-	+	+	+
Milwaukee	-	+	-	-	-	-	-	-
Copenhagen	-	-	-	*	**	**	**	**
London	**	**	-	+	*	-	-	-
Bristol	-	-	-	-	-	-	-	+
Liverpool	-	-	-	-	-	**	**	**
Manchester	**	+	-	-	*	+	*	*
Newcastle	-	-	-	+	**	-	-	-
Birmingham	**	**	-	-	-	-	-	-
Sheffield	-	-	+	*	+	-	-	-
MUMPS								
NYC	-	-	-	-	-	-	-	-
Milwaukee	-	-	-	-	-	-	-	-
Copenhagen	-	-	-	**	**	-	-	-
RUBELLA								
St.Louis	-	-	-	-	-	-	-	-
Copenhagen	-	-	-	-	-	-	-	-
CHICKENPOX								
NYC	-	-	-	-	-	-	-	-
Detroit	-	-	*	**	*	-	-	-
St.Louis	-	-	-	-	+	-	-	-
Milwaukee	-	*	-	+	+	-	-	-
Copenhagen	-	-	-	-	-	-	-	-

Table 1. Surrogate data tests for nonlinearity based on quarterly case reports, using test statistics based on time reversal, the correlation integral C(r), and 'prediction' accuracy 1 year backwards in time. The test statistics are described in the text. Reported significance levels are based on $n = 500$ surrogates for each data set for time-reversal and C(r) statistics, $n = 250$ for back-prediction. Symbols indicate significance levels $P > .1(-)$, $P < .1(+)$, $P < .05(*)$ and $P < .01(**)$.

This conclusion is modest relative to other claims which have been made about measles, but it rests on solid statistical foundations and should be difficult to dispute. The pattern is reversed in the other diseases: only 3 of the 10 data sets had a significant nonlinearity at the .05 level.

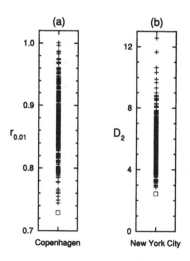

Figure 1. (a) The statistic $r_{.01}$ is shown for the Copenhagen measles data ($\square$), and for 500 surrogate time series (+). The value is significantly smaller for the actual data than for the surrogates. (b) The estimated correlation dimension D_2 is shown for New York City measles data ($\square$), and for 500 surrogate time series (+). Again, the actual data exhibit a much smaller dimension than is seen in the surrogate time series.

We chose two of the cases where nonlinearity was detected with $P < 0.01$, and plotted the value of the summary statistic for both the original and the surrogate data sets. As Figure 1 shows, the differences are not only statistically significant, but are numerically substantial as well. The value of $r_{0.01}$ for detrended Copenhagen measles is roughly 20% smaller than the average value for the surrogate time series; and the crudely estimated dimension D_2 for detrended New York City measles is less than half of the average value for the surrogates.

On the other hand, we remark that no one statistic consistently identifies nonlinearity in all of the measles time series. So we cannot say that measles epidemics in general exhibit low dimension, or high backward predictability. The data provide convincing evidence that nonlinearities are present in the underlying process, and also are manifested in the observed dynamics. However, the tests in this section do little to characterize the nature of that nonlinearity.

Our findings are in line with Casdagli's (1992) results for NYC measles, based on his exploratory method for detecting nonlinear dynamics. Casdagli's (1992) method involves comparing the short term prediction accuracy of a series of models that range from linear to strongly nonlinear (specifically, locally affine models based on different numbers of nearest neighbors). A substantial improvement in forecasting accuracy by nonlinear vs. linear models is taken as indicating nonlinear dynamics. For NYC measles, Casdagli (1992) found that nonlinear models could achieve a 25% reduction in RMS forecasting error compared with the linear model, which was interpreted as evidence for nonlinear (though not necessarily chaotic) dynamics.

4 Lyapunov exponents via time series modeling

One rough characterization of nonlinear dynamics is whether the dynamics are chaotic or stable, as indicated by the value of the Lyapunov exponent λ (defined above). In this section we describe methods for estimating λ from time series data, and present estimates of λ for epidemic data.

Our approach is to estimate λ by first estimating the nonlinear map generating the data. This allows us to account explicitly for dynamic noise and to estimate its magnitude, and to estimate λ in a way that is not positively biased by dynamic noise. The first step is reconstruction in time delay coordinates (Sauer *et al.* 1991, Casdagli 1992b), so in practice the procedure amounts to fitting a nonlinear autoregressive model

$$x_{t+T} = f(x_{t-L}, x_{t-2L}, \cdots x_{t-dL}) + e_t. \tag{4.1}$$

and using derivatives of the estimated map to compute an estimate of λ. In equation (4.1), L is called the 'time delay' and T is the prediction time.

Equation (2.1) is positively biased for finite m, and our simulation results suggest that a better estimate is

$$\hat{\lambda} = \frac{1}{m} \log \|DF(X_m, E_m)DF(X_{m-1}, E_{m-1}) \cdots DF(X_1, E_1)\vec{v}\|, \tag{4.2}$$

where $\vec{v} = (1, 0, 0, ..., 0)'$. McCaffrey *et al.* (1992) give supporting statistical theory, Nychka *et al.* (1992) discuss practical implementation on short, noisy data series, and Ellner *et al.* (1991) discuss convergence rates.

Once again, it is not *quite* that simple. Some families of prediction models work much better than others. With short, possibly noisy data sets we have achieved the best overall performance from the 'feedforward neural net' (FNN) model. The FNN model decomposes an arbitrary function into a sum of sigmoids,

$$f(x_1, x_2, \cdots x_d) = \beta_0 + \sum_{i=1}^{k} \beta_i G(\mu_i + \sum_{j=1}^{d} \gamma_{ij} x_j), \tag{4.3}$$

where G is a univariate sigmoid function such as the logistic $e^u/(1+e^u)$. FORTRAN source code and a user's manual for our implementation are available by anonymous ftp at lyapunov.ucsd.edu in /pub/ncsu. Thin-plate splines and similar extensions of polynomial models are also effective for low-dimensional fitting and are much faster to compute, but the number of parameters increases too rapidly for use in higher dimensions (Ellner and Turchin 1995).

Also, precautions must be taken both against overfitting and against underfitting. To guard against overfitting, Nychka *et al.* (1992) recommend that the model complexity (e.g., the value of k the FNN model) be chosen by the GCV (generalized cross validation) criterion with the number of model parameters inflated by a factor of 2; this tactic appeared to drastically reduce the chance of overfitting without introducing much bias. If the data are highly autocorrelated, it is likely that GCV will select a linear model that makes accurate short-term predictions but ignores the long-term dynamics. To guard against this, Ellner and Turchin (1995) recommend choosing L to be the smallest lag such that the autocorrelation between x_t and x_{t-L} is below 0.5, and using T$= L$. Here we simply used quarterly total case reports, which did not have a tight autocorrelation between successive values.

Seasonality also requires special treatment. When model (4.1) is fitted to data with a strong seasonal trend, one of the lagged variables usually winds up serving as a surrogate 'clock'. The estimate of λ then includes derivatives with respect to time, but it shouldn't: resetting the clock is not a perturbation of the system's state. To remove the need for a surrogate clock, we explicitly added a real clock to the model:

$$x_t = f(x_{t-1}, x_{t-2}, \cdots x_{t-d}, \sin(2\pi t/K), \cos(2\pi t/K)) + e_t$$

where K is the number of data points per year. The effect of including the clock is as expected (Table 2): the estimated λ drops, and fewer past values are needed to make predictions.

The results on epidemic data (Table 3) are again quite consistent: the dynamics are identified as stable rather than chaotic. In fact there appears to be a mode at or just below the transition to chaos ($\lambda = 0$) in the distribution of Lyapunov exponents (Figure 2). The location of the mode is probably influenced by the weak bias towards underfitting in the procedures used here (Nychka *et al.* 1992). In simulation trials on low-dimensional models (Ellner and Turchin 1995), the bias towards underfitting was too small to alter the qualitative conclusion from Table 3, that epidemics tend to be neither strongly stable nor strongly chaotic.

Contrary to our urgings that the hunt for chaos should be pursued in a statistical framework, we have not provided standard errors for the estimates in Table 3. Our feeling is that given the current state of the art, it would be easy to compute a standard error but hard to say exactly what that number means, and we wish to avoid overstating the (statistical) significance of our conclusions. The reliability of our conclusions is best indicated by the consistency across multiple data sets, which we leave for the reader to evaluate.

	SEASONAL			NON-SEASONAL		
	#lags	#units	λ	#lags	#units	λ
Baltimore	5	4	−0.11	8	7	+0.09
NYC	5	3	−0.08	6	6	+0.02
Detroit	6	5	−0.05	6	6	+0.025
Copenhagen	5	6	−0.01	8	6	+0.06

Table 2. Estimated Lyapunov exponents by neural net time series models for measles monthly data. All models used $L = 3$, with the numbers of lags d and units k in the model chosen by the GCV criterion as described in the text. Non-seasonal models only use lagged values of the time series; seasonal models include $\sin(2\pi j/12)$ and $\cos(2\pi j/12)$ as covariates (j = time in months).

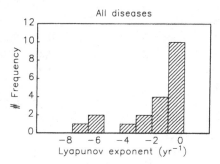

Figure 2. Histogram of estimated Lyapunov exponents for quarterly disease case reports. Values in Table 3 were multiplied by 4 to express exponents in units year^{-1}.

5   Efficient generalized method of moments

If enough is known about the system of interest, we may prefer to fit a mechanistic model rather than a purely descriptive time series model. A mechanistic model may be overly (or incorrectly) constrained and therefore unable to really match the dynamics, but mechanistic models have the advantage that time series data can be supplemented with information from other sources. For example, the duration of the infectious period can be hard-wired into an SEIR epidemic model.

Fitting of mechanistic models is frequently complicated by the unavailability of the likelihood in a closed or easily computed form. A popular alternative is to use a 'method of moments': choose parameters so that model output matches some features of the data. The features may be genuine moments (mean, variance, autocorrelations, etc.), or any other functions of a simu-

	#lags	#units	λ	r^2	df
MEASLES					
NYC	3	2	-0.67	0.93	123
Baltimore	4	2	-0.07	0.83	109
Detroit	6	2	-0.08	0.85	145
Milwaukee	2	2	-7.78	0.77	103
Copenhagen	2	3	-0.06	0.87	135
London	2	1	-0.23	0.67	51
Bristol	3	1	-0.13	0.77	50
Liverpool	2	1	-1.56	0.72	51
Manchester	2	2	-0.24	0.90	45
Newcastle	2	1	-3.61	0.71	51
Birmingham	2	2	-0.16	0.92	45
Sheffield	5	1	-1.93	0.84	48
MUMPS					
NYC	5	2	$+0.01$	0.94	119
Milwaukee	2	2	-0.39	0.74	153
Copenhagen	2	3	-0.24	0.86	135
RUBELLA					
St.Louis	2	2	-0.27	0.76	61
Copenhagen	2	1	-0.87	0.71	99
CHICKENPOX					
NYC	6	2	-0.14	0.95	117
Detroit	2	1	-0.33	0.78	61
St.Louis	1	1	-1.46	0.86	68
Copenhagen	1	1	-0.61	0.81	107
Milwaukee	2	2	-0.37	0.86	129

Table 3. Estimated Lyapunov exponent λ for quarterly case reports using seasonal neural net model. All models used $L = 1$, with the number of lags d and units k chosen by the GCV criterion as described in the text.

lated trajectory (period of a limit cycle, fractal dimension,etc.). This leads to fitting criteria such as

$$\text{Minimize} \quad \sum_i C_i (M_i(\rho) - M_i(\text{data}))^2$$

where M_i are the features, ρ is the parameter vector of the mechanistic model, and C_i are positive weights. However it is not clear which 'moments' M_i to use, and how they should be weighted, to get the most accurate estimates of ρ.

Gallant and Tauchen (1992) have proved that with appropriate M_i and weighting, and some smoothness and identifiability conditions, GMM is asymptotically equivalent to maximum likelihood estimation of the mechanistic model's parameters. The M_i are obtained by choosing a statistical model $f(x_{t+1} \mid x_t, \theta)$ for the transition probabilities governing the time series, such that the parameter vector θ of the statistical model is easy to estimate by maximum likelihood. For example, f may be a nonparametric regression model with appropriate error structure. The generalized moments to be matched as well as possible are then

$$M_i(\rho) = E_\rho[\frac{\partial}{\partial \theta_i} \ln f(x_{t+1} \mid x_t, \tilde{\theta})], \qquad (5.1)$$

where $\tilde{\theta}$ is the maximum likelihood estimate of θ from the empirical data, and $E_\rho(\ )$ is expectation with respect to the distribution of (x_{t+1}, x_t) in the mechanistic model with parameter vector ρ.

$E_\rho(\ )$ in (5.1) is computed by simulating the model (i.e., by Monte Carlo integration). If E_ρ is replaced by the empirical distribution of (x_{t+1}, x_t), then the expression in (5.1) is exactly 0 by the first order condition for maximizing the likelihood. Thus a good mechanistic model should give small values of $M_i(\rho)$. The right weighting is a quadratic form $M^T \tilde{I}^{-1} M$ where $\tilde{I}$ is an estimated information matrix; see Gallant and Tauchen (1992) for precise statement of the results, extension to more general settings, and proofs.

The advantage of GMM is that the statistical model f doesn't have to be 'right', i.e. it doesn't need to duplicate exactly the transition probability of the process generating the data. It just needs to be sufficiently general, or well enough adapted to the application, so that it discriminates parameters of the mechanistic model, i.e., $M_i(\rho) = 0$ for all i if and only if $\rho = \rho_0$, where ρ_0 is the true value of ρ.

For an epidemiological application of this method, we estimated contact rate parameters for a deterministic SEIR model, using the monthly measles case reports series from New York City 1928-1963. To mitigate excessive fadeouts in the model we added a small exchange of individuals (at rate δ) with an 'outside world' having fixed levels of the disease:

$$\frac{dS}{dt} = m(1 - S) - \beta(t)SI + \delta(S_0 - S) \qquad (5.2)$$

$$\frac{dE}{dt} = \beta(t)SI - (m + a)E + \delta(E_0 - E) \qquad (5.3)$$

$$\frac{dI}{dt} = aE - (m + g)I + \delta(I_0 - I) \qquad (5.4)$$

This model is a bit simplistic for measles (see Grenfell, Kleczkowski and Bolker, this volume), and the migration terms are admittedly an *ad hoc* way of bringing the model more closely in line with the data. Our justification is simply that this is our first exploratory attempt at using GMM for fitting a mechanistic epidemic model. As we gain experience and hone the implementation, it should become possible to deal with more realistic models.

We assumed that the contact rate $\beta(t)$ has the form

$$\beta(t) = b_0 \left(1 + \sigma e_t\right) + b_1 \phi(t)$$

where $\phi(t)$ is the seasonal forcing function proposed by Kot *et al.* (1988),

$$\phi(t) = 1.5 \left(\frac{0.68 + \cos(2\pi t)}{1.5 + \cos(2\pi t)}\right) - .4$$

(we added the '$-.4$' so that the average of ϕ over the year would be zero), and σe_t are autocorrelated random fluctuations with mean 0, variance σ^2, and autocorrelation 0.95 between values 1 month apart. We estimated the values of b_0 and b_1, assuming that all other parameters of the model were known. We took $\sigma = .05$ to represent small year-to-year fluctuations in contact intensity; results for $\sigma = .01$ (not presented) were essentially the same. The statistical model was a neural net with 5 lags and 3 units, as in the best-fit neural net model for monthly NYC measles data (Table 2).

Simulated measurement errors were added to the output from the SEIR model; this was necessary to produce a reasonable match between the power spectra of the simulated and real data at higher frequencies (1-2 months). The simulated errors were lognormal with coefficient of variation based on the estimate that 1/8 of all cases are reported (B. Grenfell, *pers. comm*), and assuming that cases are reported or not in independent clusters of size 2 representing a pair of cases in a family. The clustering assumption increases the variance of the simulated measurement errors, and a cluster size of 2 or 3 was necessary to produce the observed amount of power at high frequencies in the data.

The results are encouraging for the method, but somewhat discouraging for fitting SEIR models from time series data alone. The encouraging result is that our automatic procedure produced a value of the relative forcing intensity b_1/b_0, that is in line with generally accepted estimates. A contour plot of the GMM fitting criterion (Figure 3a) has a steep 'valley' of better fits (smaller values of the criterion) roughly along the line $b_1 = 0.2b_0$, and a univariate plot of optimal GMM vs. b_1/b_0 has a well-defined minimum (Figure 3b). The discouraging results are first that, as can be seen in Figure 3a, the terrain along the valley floor is rather flat, so the absolute values of b_0 and b_1 are less well identified. Second, the entire terrain is rough (Figure 4). It is not clear how much of the roughness is due to Monte Carlo error (finite sample size in computing E_ρ), vs. intrinsic roughness of the exact surface. If the latter is dominant, then standard asymptotic methods based on Taylor series approximations will not be available for setting confidence regions or for hypothesis testing based on GMM.

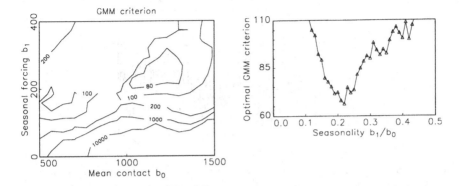

Figure 3. (a) Contour plot of the GMM objective function; smaller values correspond to better fits between model and data. Contours based on values computed at a regular 31×31 grid over the range of values shown for b_0 and b_1, with a simulation of 5000 months duration for each parameter combination. (b) Plot of minimum GMM objective function as a function of the relative intensity of seasonal forcing b_1/b_0. For both (a) and (b) the following parameter values were used in the SEIR model: m= 0.02, a= 55, g= 60, $S_0 = 0.05$, $E_0 = I_0 = 0.001$, $\delta = .01$.

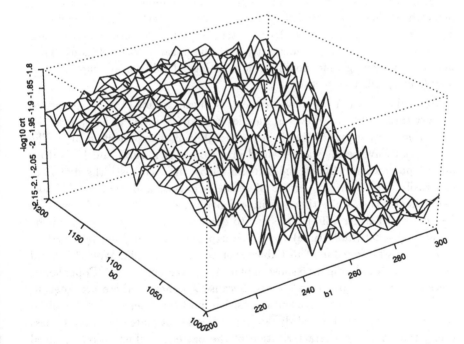

Figure 4. Plot of GMM objective function (computed as in Figure 3) at a grid of values near the best-fit parameter values.

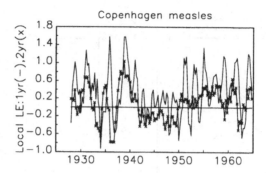

Figure 5. Finite-time 'local' Lyapunov exponents for Copenhagen measles data based on the best-fit seasonal neural net model for quarterly data.

6   Conclusions

We would like to close by speculating on the implications of our findings. Our 'surrogate data' results indicate that nonlinear departures from annual periodicity are a consistent feature of the measles data, but less common in the other diseases examined. The statistics $r_{.01}$ and $r_{.001}$, based on the correlation integral, were especially powerful at picking out nonlinearity. The property detected by these statistics (as used here, with state vectors corresponding to 2 years of data), is that 2-year-long stretches of data are more similar to each other than would be expected strictly from the linear autocorrelations. Thus nonlinear modeling, and nonlinear forecasting, should be an improvement over linear prediction methods.

According to our Lyapunov exponent estimates, chaos ($\lambda > 0$) appears to be very rare or absent. However, measles is often identified as being near the transition to chaos, with a mode in the distribution of exponents near 0. The same qualitative result was obtained in a survey of natural and laboratory animal populations (Ellner and Turchin 1995). In such cases the dynamics can easily vary between periods of stable behavior, and periods of chaos-like behavior (i.e., finite-time sensitive dependence on initial conditions: see Deissler and Farmer 1992). One way to quantify this type of behavior is by computing local (finite-time) Lyapunov exponents λ_m, defined by equation (2.1) with a finite value of m (Abarbanel *et al.* 1991, 1992, Wolff 1992 and references therein). Figure 5 shows a plot of λ_m over time for the Copenhagen measles series, for m= 1 or 2 years; because λ is near 0 there are frequent transitions between sensitive and insensitive short-term dependence on initial conditions. For this type of dynamics, a precise estimate of λ may be less useful than a rough characterization of the pattern of fluctuations in local exponents (e.g., their variance, autocorrelation, frequency of sign changes).

Methods are still evolving rapidly, so our results and conclusions are hardly the last word on nonlinearity and chaos in epidemics. One promising direction, encouraged by the feasibility of GMM model fitting, is to hybridize between mechanistic and statistical modeling. We expect that models that are mechanistic insofar as possible, but rely on state-space reconstruction and nonparametrics where ignorance forces that upon us, have the potential to provide more reliable characterizations of the dynamics, and more reliable prediction methods.

References

Abarbanel, H.D.I., Brown, R. and Kennel, M.B. (1991) 'Variation of Lyapunov exponents on a strange attractor', *J. Nonlin. Sci.* **1**, 175–199.

Abarbanel, H.D.I., Brown, R. and Kennel, M.B. (1992) 'Local Lyapunov exponents computed from observed data', *J. Nonlin. Sci.* **2**, 343–365.

Casdagli, M. (1992a) 'Chaos and deterministic versus stochastic and non-linear modelling', *J. R. Statist. Soc. B* **54**, 303–328.

Casdagli, M. (1992b) 'A dynamical systems approach to modeling input-output systems'. In *Nonlinear Modeling and Forecasting*, M. Casdagli and S. Eubank (eds.), SFI Studies in the Sciences of Complexity Proc. Vol. XII. Addison-Wesley, New York, 265–281.

Crutchfield, J.P., Farmer, J.D. and Huberman, B.A. (1982) 'Fluctuations and simple chaotic dynamics', *Phys. Rep.* **92**, 45–82.

Deissler, R.J. and Farmer, J.D. (1992) 'Deterministic noise amplifiers', *Physica D* **55**, 155–165.

Eckmann, J.-P. and Ruelle, D. (1985) 'Ergodic theory of chaos and strange attractors', *Rev. of Mod. Phys.* **57**, 617–656.

Ellner S. (1991) 'Detecting low-dimensional chaos in population dynamics data: a critical review'. In *Chaos and Insect Ecology* J.A. Logan and F.P. Hain (eds.) VPI and SU, Blacksburg VA, 63–90.

Ellner, S., Gallant, A.R., McCaffrey, D. and Nychka, D. (1991) 'Convergence rates and data requirements for Jacobian-based estimates of Lyapunov exponents from data', *Phys. Lett. A* **153**, 357–363.

Ellner, S., Nychka, D.W. and Gallant, A.R. (1992) 'LENNS, a program to estimate the dominant Lyapunov exponent of noisy nonlinear systems from time series data'. Institute of Statistics Mimeo Series **2235**, Statistics Department, North Carolina State University, Raleigh NC 27695-8203.

Ellner, S. and Turchin, P. (1995) 'Chaos in a noisy world: new methods and evidence from time series analysis', *Amer. Naturalist*, in press.

Gallant, A.R. and Tauchen, G. (1992) 'Which moments to match?' Working Paper, Department of Economics, Duke University, Durham NC.

Grassberger, P. and Procaccia, I. (1983) 'Measuring the strangeness of strange attractors', *Physica D* **9**, 189–208.

Hastings, A., Hom, C.L., Ellner, S., Turchin, P. and Godfray, H.J.C. (1993) 'Chaos in ecology: is mother nature a strange attractor?' *Ann. Rev. of Ecol. and Systematics* **24**, 1-33.

Kifer, Y. (1986) *Ergodic Theory of Random Transformations.* Birkhäuser, Boston, MA.

Kot, M., Schaffer, W.M., Truty, G.L., Graser, D.J. and Olsen, L.F. (1988) 'Changing criteria for imposing order', *Ecol. Modell.* **43**, 75–110.

McCaffrey, D., Ellner, S., Nychka, D.W. and Gallant, A.R. (1992) 'Estimating the Lyapunov exponent of a chaotic system with nonlinear regression', *J. Amer. Statist. Assoc.* **87**, 682–695.

Nychka, D.W., Ellner, S., McCaffrey, D. and Gallant, A.R. (1992) 'Finding chaos in noisy systems', *J. R. Statist. Soc. B* **54**, 399–426.

Packard, N.H., Crutchfield, J.P., Farmer, J.D. and Shaw, R.S. (1980) 'Geometry from a time series', *Phys. Rev. Lett.* **45**, 712–716.

Ramsay, J.B. and Rothman, P. (1992) 'Time irreversibility and stationary time series: estimators and test statistics'. Preprint.

Rand, D.A. and Wilson, H.B. (1991) 'Chaotic stochasticity: a ubiquitous source of unpredictability in epidemics', *Proc. R. Soc. Lond. B* **246**, 179–184.

Rothman, P. (1990) *Characterization of the Time Irreversibility of Economic Time Series.* PhD Dissertation, Department of Economics, New York University.

Sauer, T., Yorke, J.A. and Casdagli, M. (1991) 'Embedology', *J. Stat. Phys.* **65**, 579–616.

Sayers, C. (1990) 'Chaos and the business cycle'. In *The Ubiquity of Chaos*, S. Krasner (ed.), AAAS, Washington DC, 115–125.

Schaffer W.M. and Kot, M. (1985) 'Nearly one-dimensional dynamics in an epidemic', *J. Theor. Biol.* **112**, 403–427.

Schaffer W.M. and Kot, M. (1986) 'Chaos in ecological systems: the coals that Newcastle forgot', *Trends Ecol. Evol.* **1**, 58–63.

Schaffer W.M., Olsen L.F., Truty G.L. and Fulmer S.L. (1990) 'The case for chaos in childhood epidemics'. In *The Ubiquity of Chaos*, S. Krasner (ed.) AAAS, Washington DC, 138–166.

Smith, R.L. (1992a) 'Estimating dimension in noisy chaotic time series', *J. R. Statist. Soc. B* **54**, 329–351.

Smith, R.L. (1992b) ' Relation between statistics and chaos', *Statist. Sci.* **7**, 109–113.

Stone, L. (1992) 'Coloured noise or low-dimensional chaos?', *Proc. R. Soc. Lond. B* **250**, 77–81.

Sugihara, G. and May, R.M. (1990) 'Nonlinear forecasting as a way of distinguishing chaos from measurement error in time series', *Nature* **344**, 734–741.

Takens, F. (1981) 'Detecting strange attractors in turbulence' In *Dynamical Systems and Turbulence, Warwick 1980*, D. Rand and L-S. Young, (eds.) Lecture Notes in Mathematics **898**, Springer-Verlag, Berlin, 366–381.

Theiler, J. (1990) 'Estimating fractal dimension', *J. Opt. Soc. Am. A* **7**, 1055–1073.

Theiler, J., Eubank, S., Longtin, A., Galdrikian, B. and Farmer, J.D. (1992) 'Testing for nonlinearity in time series data: the method of surrogate data', *Physica D* **58**, 77–94.

Theiler, J., Linsay, P.S. and Rubin, D.M. (1994) 'Detecting nonlinearity in data with long coherence times'. In *Times Series Prediction. Forecasting the Future and Understanding the Past*, A.S. Weigend and N.A. Gershenfeld (eds.) SFI Studies in the Sciences of Complexity Proc. Vol XV. Addison-Wesley, New York, 429–455.

Wolf, A., Swift, J.B., Swinney, H.L. and Vastano, J.A. (1985) 'Determining Lyapunov exponents from a time series', *Physica D* **16**, 285–315.

Wolff, R.C.W. (1992) 'Local Lyapunov exponents: looking closely at chaos', *J. R. Statist. Soc. B* **54**, 353–371.

Seasonality, Demography and the Dynamics of Measles in Developed Countries

Bryan Grenfell
Ben Bolker
Adam Kleczkowski

1 Introduction

Measles is among the best documented of human diseases in terms of epidemiology and population dynamics. This special status arises partly from the historical and current public health importance of the disease (Black 1984, Anderson and May 1991), which has led to relatively efficient case notification schemes in many developed countries. These reports document the dynamics of measles, which occurs in recurrent (and often remarkably regular) epidemics in large urban populations (Brownlee 1919, Anderson *et al.* 1984, Cliff and Haggett 1988). Analysing the structure and persistence of these epidemics has been a major preoccupation amongst epidemiological and ecological dynamicists, particularly given the comparatively simple natural history of transmission of measles virus (Black 1984), which lends itself readily to modelling (Hamer 1906, Soper 1929, Bartlett 1957, Bartlett 1960, Black 1966, Schenzle 1984, Anderson and May 1991).

In terms of quantitative epidemiological research on measles, the public health importance and dynamically interesting epidemic behaviour of the disease have generated two distinct bodies of work.

Epidemiological analyses There is an extensive literature examining the dynamics of measles infection, its persistence in communities and the effects of heterogeneities in transmission with respect to age, season and spatial organization of the host population (Hamer 1906, Soper 1929, Bartlett 1957, Bartlett 1960, London and Yorke 1973, Anderson and May 1985, Dietz and Schenzle 1985, May 1986, Anderson and May 1991). The onset of mass vaccination during the last three decades (Black 1984) has also prompted a major area of development of this theory, which aims to estimate the critical level of vaccination required to eradicate the infection from a community (Dietz 1976, Anderson and May 1982). In addition to these theoretical developments, the

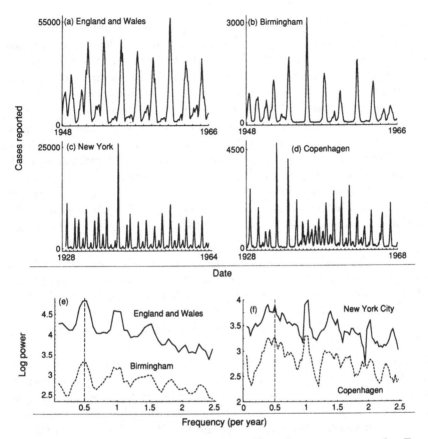

Figure 1: Measles time series (cases notified) and power spectra for England and Wales, Birmingham, Copenhagen and New York. (a),(b) Weekly case reports for England and Wales and Birmingham respectively, 1948–1968. (c) Monthly case reports for New York City, 1928–1964. (d) Monthly case reports for Copenhagen, 1928–1968. (e) Power spectra for England and Wales and Birmingham data; spectra smoothed with a 3-point running mean (Chatfield 1975, Priestley 1982). (f) Power spectra for New York City and Copenhagen data, method as above.

relatively long time series of measles case notifications, which are available for a number of countries, have been analyzed statistically by a number of workers (Brownlee 1919, Fine and Clarkson 1982, Anderson *et al.* 1984, Cliff and Haggett 1988), in order to assess the relative importance of annual and longer-term periodicities in the pattern of epidemics (Fig. 1).

Ecological analyses: non-linear dynamics The combination of relatively long time series of measles incidence, and the availability of simple population models to analyze them, have also recently drawn the attention

of population ecologists (May 1986). In particular, a number of workers –
notably W.M. Schaffer and his collaborators (Schaffer (1985a), Schaffer and
Kot (1985), Olsen *et al.*(1988), Kot *et al.* (1988), Olsen and Schaffer (1990)) –
have sought to identify fluctuations in measles incidence as candidates for low-
dimensional chaotic dynamics. There have been attempts to identify chaotic
attractors for measles, both from observed incidence data (Olsen *et al.* 1988,
Sugihara and May 1990) and based on the simplest homogeneous epidemiological model, the SEIR model (Schaffer and Kot 1985, Rand and Wilson
1991). However, there are problems with this approach. First, the available
measles time series may simply be too short for the statistical methods used
to detect chaos (Nychka *et al.* 1992). Second, the modelling approaches to
this problem have tended to omit much biological detail, ignoring more realistic formulations of measles dynamics developed for epidemiological purposes
(Bolker and Grenfell 1993).

A crucially important process in the dynamics of measles in developed
countries is the *seasonal variation* in infection rate, induced by the annual
pattern of aggregation of children in schools (London and Yorke 1973, Fine
and Clarkson 1982). The epidemiological effects of seasonality in measles
transmission have been extensively studied (London and Yorke 1973, Dietz
1976, Grossman 1980, Aron and Schwartz 1984, Schenzle 1984, Schaffer and
Kot 1985, Aron 1990), particularly in terms of overall patterns of incidence,
the maintenance of recurrent epidemics and the persistence of infection in
communities (Yorke *et al.* 1979). As discussed below, this seasonal forcing of
the system is also intimately bound up with the generation of chaos in simple
deterministic measles models (Schaffer and Kot 1985), Olsen *et al.*1988).

This paper describes recent attempts to bring together epidemiological and
nonlinear approaches to measles dynamics. We begin by comparing the nonlinear chaotic behaviour of the forced SEIR model with an epidemiological
formulation, based on a more mechanistic model for the origins of seasonality. Seasonal variation in infection rate is an example of non-autonomous
(time-dependent) oscillations in a system parameter on an annual timescale.
However, there are also likely to be significant variations at longer timescales,
particularly in response to secular trends in birth rate (Grenfell and Anderson
1985), which controls the recruitment of infants to the susceptible population.
We explore the effects of such long term demographic variations, using analyses of measles data sets from Europe and the USA. Like much else in measles
dynamics, these effects are shown to be intimately bound up with spatial heterogeneity in transmission; we therefore conclude with a discussion of possible
directions for future work in this area.

2 Seasonality and Measles Dynamics

2.1 The forced SEIR model

Fig. 1 shows observed incidence and basic time series analyses for a selection of measles data sets from Europe and the USA. For simplicity, we restrict ourselves to the situation before the onset of mass vaccination — the widespread use of vaccines introduces extra complexities to the dynamics (Bolker and Grenfell, in preparation). As shown in the time series analysis of Fig. 1, the series all show an annual periodicity, superimposed on longer term (biennial or triennial) epidemic patterns. The annual variation in incidence is mainly caused by changes in the contact rate of children, associated with the seasonal pattern of school terms (Kharat *et al.* 1989, Campanella and Tarantini 1989, Fine and Clarkson 1982). A number of workers have modelled the effects of seasonal variations in infection rate (London and Yorke 1973, Dietz 1976, Grossman 1980, Aron and Schwartz 1984, Schenzle 1984, Schaffer and Kot 1985, Aron 1990). The simplest approach is to start with the standard homogeneous SEIR (Susceptible/ Exposed/ Infectious/ Recovered) model:

$$\frac{dS}{dt} = \mu N - (\mu + \beta I)S \qquad (2.1)$$

$$\frac{dE}{dt} = \beta I S - (\mu + \sigma)E \qquad (2.2)$$

$$\frac{dI}{dt} = \sigma E - (\mu + \gamma)I. \qquad (2.3)$$

S, E, I and R respectively represent the densities of Susceptible, Exposed, Infectious and Recovered individuals, in a constant total population of size $N = S + E + I + R$ (given this identity, only the 3 equations for S, E and I are necessary to specify the system). Average per capita mortality rate due to all causes is μ years^{-1}, indicating an average life expectancy of $1/\mu$ years; given that infection is assumed not to cause extra mortality, the net birth and death rates (μN and $\mu[S + E + I + R]$ respectively) are equal. In this simplest version of the model (which ignores the effect of passive maternally-derived immunity in infants), individuals are assumed to be born susceptible. The net infection rate, $\beta I S$, is controlled by the infection parameter β (year^{-1}, infective^{-1}) which is assumed to be constant. Finally, σ and γ (year^{-1}) are rate parameters controlling the onset of infectivity and recovery respectively, such that $1/\sigma$ and $1/\gamma$ are the average incubation and infectious periods.

Seasonal forcing of the infection process can be modelled by replacing the constant infection parameter, β, of equations (2.3) with a time-varying periodic function, such as

$$\beta(t) = b_0[1 + b_1 \cos(2\pi t)]. \qquad (2.4)$$

Here, b_0 is the average infection rate and b_1 controls the amplitude of variation around it. The behaviour of this model has been analyzed both in the epidemiological literature (London and Yorke 1973, Dietz 1976) and in the exploration of nonlinear dynamics in measles incidence (Aron and Schwartz 1984, Schaffer 1985b, Schaffer and Kot 1985, Olsen and Schaffer 1990, Rand and Wilson 1991). Fig. 2 illustrates the dynamic properties of the seasonally forced SEIR model with a series of numerical simulations for a range of values of the amplitude of sinusoidal forcing, controlled by the parameter b_1 in Equation (2.4). There is a progression with increasing b_1, from a simple annual cycle ($b_1 = 0.01$) through a sequence of period doublings as b_1 increases, to irregular chaotic fluctuations at $b_1 = 0.28$, the value proposed by Schaffer and his collaborators (Olsen *et al.* 1988). Although it has been suggested that this degree of seasonal forcing may be unrealistically high (Pool 1989, Grenfell 1992), recent work on the impact of demographic and environmental noise indicates that chaos-like behaviour can be produced in noisy systems for lower degrees of forcing, via the operation of long transients, known as 'chaotic repellors' (Rand and Wilson 1991).

Fig. 3 displays a more synoptic view of the model's dynamics, via a bifurcation diagram for infectives, over a range of values of the amplitude of seasonal forcing (b_1). Simulated data are annually sampled (near the minimum incidence), so that a single point at a particular value of b_1 corresponds to an annual cycle. This picture clearly illustrates the transition to chaos with increasing seasonal forcing of the infection rate. The points in Fig. 3 represent the 'main sequence' of bifurcations (Rand and Wilson 1991). However, depending on the initial conditions, the system can fall onto other attractors (Engbert and Drepper 1994), sometimes with bifurcations to chaos below $b_1 = 0.28$. These multiple domains are illustrated in Fig. 3 (as pluses) and illustrate the dynamic complexities possible in even such a simple model as the SEIR.

Fig. 3 also shows that the 'large scale' chaos for $b_1 > 0.28$ is characterized by high amplitude fluctuations with very low infective minima (down to $10^{-14} \times$ population size in Fig. 3). This unrealistically low figure is the basis of a number of criticisms of the SEIR/chaos result (Pool 1989, Grenfell 1992). In particular, the associated degree of 'fadeout' of infection appears to be significantly larger than that observed, even in model 'cities' of a million people (i.e., over twice the population threshold empirically derived by Bartlett (1960) and Black (1966)). Although spatial heterogeneity appears to reduce the degree of fadeout slightly, fadeout remains a significant problem, in terms of modelling the nonlinear dynamics of measles with the SEIR model (Bolker and Grenfell 1993). We explore this situation, in terms of the dynamics of more realistic epidemiological models for measles, in the next section.

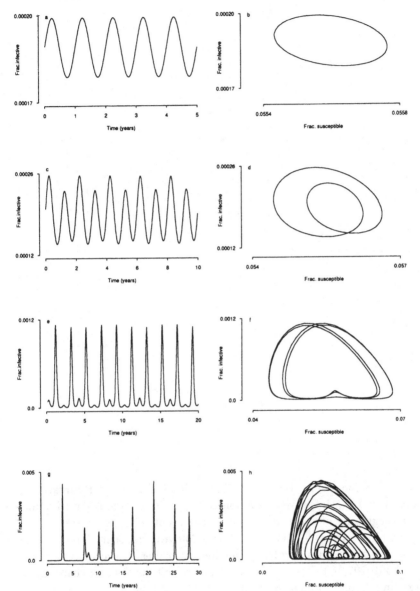

Figure 2: Dynamics of the seasonally forced SEIR model, time (I vs. t) and phase (S vs. I) plots, for different seasonal amplitudes b_1. Vertical axis shows proportion of population infective, horizontal axis shows time in years. (a) Annual cycle ($b_1 = 0.01$); (b) Biennial cycle ($b_1 = 0.05$); (c) Eight-year cycle ($b_1 = 0.267$); (d) Large amplitude chaos ($b_1 = 0.28$). Other model parameters: $\mu = 0.02$, $\gamma = 73.0$, $\sigma = 45.6$, $b_0 = 1010.7$; all units year^{-1} except contact rate (year^{-1} infective^{-1}). Population size, N, is scaled to unity.

SEIR

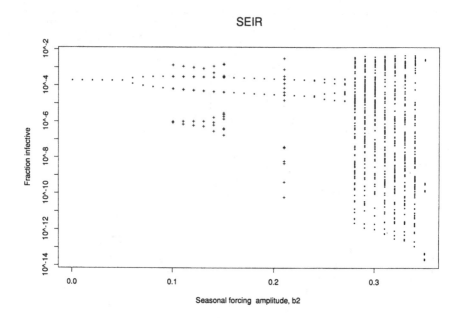

Figure 3: A more synoptic view of forced SEIR dynamics. Bifurcation diagrams show $\log_{10}$(infectives) in a population of 50 million, sampled annually at the beginning of the epidemiologic year (September, near the minimum number of infectives) for 100 years after a 200-year transient, for given values of seasonal forcing amplitude. Parameters as in Fig. 4, except $N = 5 \times 10^7$, $b_1 = 0.0010107$. (·) show the 'main sequence' bifurcations to chaos and (+) coexisting domains found from some initial conditions.

2.2   Seasonality and age-structure in transmission dynamics

Since these seasonal variations in transmission arise from the pattern of schooling, they are also intimately related to heterogeneities in measles transmission with age. In an important paper, Fine and Clarkson (1982) used measles data for England and Wales to explore this issue. In particular, they document the seasonal increase in infection rate, particularly of primary school children, associated with the pattern of school terms.

Although introducing age-structure alone into the SEIR model does not affect its behaviour qualitatively, the combination of age-structure and seasonality in transmission has a profound impact. In particular, Schenzle (1984) implemented Fine and Clarkson's qualitative model in a continuous time age-cohort formulation which mimics the average pre-vaccination pattern of measles epidemics in England and Wales very closely (Fig. 4), as well as the qualitative behaviour of the infection after the onset of vaccination. This model (which we shall call the RAS — Realistic Age-Structured — model) therefore serves as a useful epidemiological yardstick against which to judge the biological accuracy of the nonlinear dynamic approach to measles modelling.

Fig. 4 shows a bifurcation diagram for the RAS model, equivalent to the SEIR bifurcation diagram of Fig. 3. Although the RAS model does undergo some period doubling as seasonal forcing increases, there is no evidence of the irregular chaotic fluctuations in the density of susceptibles generated by the SEIR model. The important biological point to emerge from Fig. 4 is that the (interepidemic) infective minima for the RAS model are much higher (and therefore more biologically realistic) than for the SEIR model. Bolker and Grenfell (1993) show that this, in turn, leads to a lower propensity for chaos, which is associated, in this class of models, with divergence of model trajectories at low infective densities.

The fundamental difference between SEIR and RAS model dynamics arises from the additional **population heterogeneity** introduced in the latter, more realistic, model. In particular, the comparatively small force of infection in the preschool age group allows this segment of the population to act as a 'reservoir' of infection, preventing the violent swings in infective density generated in the highly forced SEIR model (and its age structured analogues which assume a homogeneous infection rate with respect to age).

Adding more realism in terms of demographic noise leaves this picture essentially intact although, as discussed by Bolker and Grenfell (1993), further dynamic complexities emerge as human population size in the models is decreased. Specifically, whereas stochastic models for 'large' populations (for example, 50 million) exhibit regular biennial epidemics, these can break down into more complex behaviour, with mixtures of 1, 2 and 3 year cycles, in populations of 1 million. It seems likely that the biological relevance of these patterns can only be clarified by including explicit **spatial dynamics** into the models. We shall return to a discussion of this issue after considering the impact of (non-seasonal) demographic variations on measles dynamics.

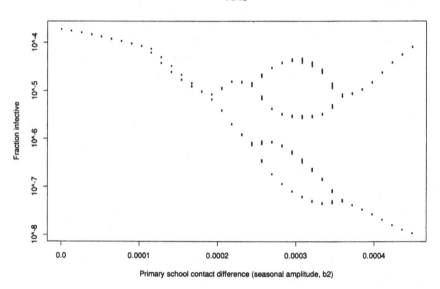

Figure 4: Bifurcation diagram for the RAS model, equivalent to Fig. 3 (parameters as given by Schenzle 1984): $N = 5 \times 10^7$, $\mu = 0.018$, birth rate = 666666 (death does not start until age 20), $\gamma = 73.0$, $\sigma = 45.6$ contact rates are from a least squares fit of the model to per-vaccination measles time series for England and Wales (Bolker and Grenfell 1993). Seasonal amplitude, the additional contact rate among primary-school children (effective only during school terms), is scaled so that the x-axes in Figs 3 and 4 are equivalent.

3   Demographic Variations and Measles Dynamics

Since birth rate is essentially the 'engine' which controls the recruitment of new susceptibles, its average level and temporal dynamics are likely to have significant impact on patterns of measles incidence. The most extensive quantitative studies in this area have concerned the influence of high birth rate and growing populations on measles dynamics in developing countries (McLean and Anderson 1988a, 1988b). In terms of prevaccination dynamics, both models and epidemiological data analysis indicate that high birth rates tend to move measles into a regime of annual cycles.

The effect of demographic variations on endemic measles dynamics in **developed** countries has been much less analyzed. The most detailed examination of demographic effects on a large scale in this context is Stocks' (1942) analysis of the impact on measles and whooping cough incidence of the dispersal of children from London and other major southern English cities during 1939 and 1940. Unlike birth rate, this population movement does not exert a direct effect on the recruitment of susceptibles; however, it might be expected to have a significant effect on measles dynamics, due to the reduction in contact between children in schools. Stocks found that the immediate effect of the dispersal was to reduce measles incidence in these major centres during 1940. Though he went on to speculate about the possible longer term epidemiological effects of this demographic perturbation, these have not been explored. The possible consequences of this perturbation for spatial dynamics of measles will be discussed below.

In the following section, we present a preliminary analysis of the effects of long term variations in the recruitment of susceptibles on measles dynamics in developed countries. In particular, we use simple models and descriptive analyses of notification time series to examine the possible effects on measles dynamics of the 'baby boom' observed during the 1940s in developed countries.

3.1   Measles incidence and birth rate variations

3.1.1   Models

In order to focus the data analysis, we begin with some simple models of the influence of demography on measles incidence. From the equilibrium of the standard SEIR model (equation (2.3)), the steady state incidence of measles obeys:

$$I^* = \frac{\mu}{\beta}\left[\frac{\beta\sigma N - (\mu+\sigma)(\mu+\gamma)}{(\mu+\sigma)(\mu+\gamma)}\right], \tag{3.1}$$

$$\approx \frac{\mu}{\beta}\left[\frac{\beta N - \gamma}{\gamma}\right] \tag{3.2}$$

since, on biological grounds, $\sigma, \gamma \gg \mu$ (May 1986, Anderson and May 1991).

Average measles incidence is therefore predicted to increase linearly with the population 'turnover rate', μ, which effectively represents the birth rate

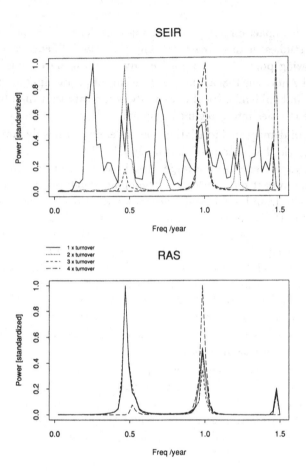

Figure 5: Effect of increasing population turnover (μ, i.e., effectively the birth rate) on the dynamics of forced SEIR and RAS models. The figures show spectra (peaks standardized to unity) for: (a) the SEIR model, with parameters as in Fig. 3, and seasonal forcing parameter, $b_1 = 0.28$, placing the model in the chaotic region; (b) the RAS model, with parameters as in Fig. 4 and seasonal forcing corresponding to the least squares fit to the observed biennial pattern observed in England and Wales before vaccination.

of susceptibles. This is a standard result in the literature on measles in high birth rate countries (McLean and Anderson 1988a), where another major preoccupation is the effect of high birth rates on measles *dynamics*. The basic result here is that high birth rates decrease the interepidemic interval, generating basically annual cycles of infection. However, these findings are based on models which ignore seasonality so that, for our purposes, we need to reevaluate them in the presence of seasonal forcing. Fig. 5 presents preliminary results for this analysis, comparing the effects of increasing birth rate on the dynamics of simulated epidemics (expressed as frequency spectra) for the forced SEIR and RAS models. As shown in Fig. 5, the minimum 'developed country' birth rates for the SEIR and RAS models generate irregular chaotic dynamics and biennial patterns respectively, superimposed on the annual driving frequency. In essence, increasing birth rate by a factor of 2–3 shifts the dynamics towards annual cycles in both models. For the SEIR model, biennial cycles come to dominate the low (longer than annual) frequency component at a relative birth rate of 1.5, with a transition to annual cycles at 3× the basic birth rate. By contrast, the RAS model retains a basically biennial pattern until a relative birth rate of 2.5. These results are based on simulations of the deterministic equations – qualitatively similar results are obtained from equivalent Monte Carlo simulations of the stochastic systems.

This analysis is preliminary and will be extended elsewhere, in particular to examine the impact of *dynamic* changes in birth rate. The results do, however, indicate the following hypotheses for evaluation by data analysis:

1. Average measles incidence increases with birth rate.

2. As birth rate increases, annual epidemics will tend to increase in importance.

3.1.2   Data analysis

We base our analysis on pre-vaccination measles notification and demographic data from Copenhagen, New York and several English cities. In terms of measles dynamics, measles cases in a given year are likely to be influenced by some weighted average of births over past years. Fig. 6 superimposes the raw measles and birth rate data. Though there is some indication of a positive association between births and subsequent cases for Copenhagen, the results are inconclusive overall. Part of the problem lies in the variability of raw measles incidence data. Fig. 7 therefore recasts the comparison in terms of a running average of measles data. Given this smoothing, more patterns emerge. First, (as suggested in the previous section) all the data sets for English cities show a positive association between measles incidence and birth rates over around the previous 5 years. Fig. 8 shows the equivalent cross correlations, which in most cases indicate a strong correlation between average measles cases and birth rates at a lag of 4 to 6 years. In reality, these patterns are likely to reflect a relationship between measles incidence and some *integral* over past birth rates. The data for Copenhagen also shows some evidence of a lagged relationship, though this may be obscured by a lack of data – the analysis is currently based only on birth rates up to 1950.

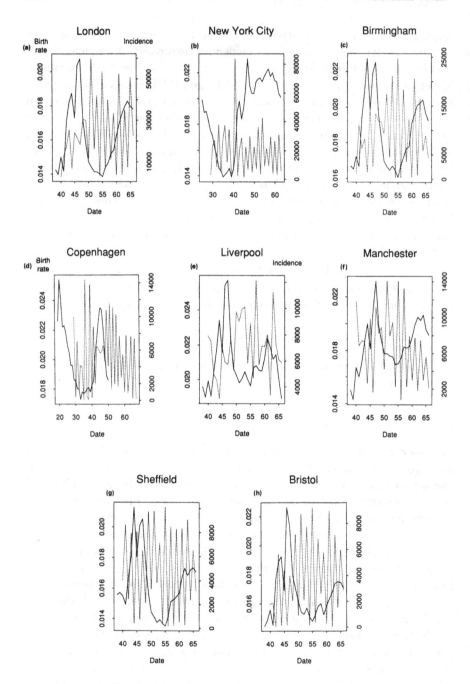

Figure 6: Raw measles notifications (dotted lines) and crude birth rates (solid lines) for English cities, New York and Copenhagen.

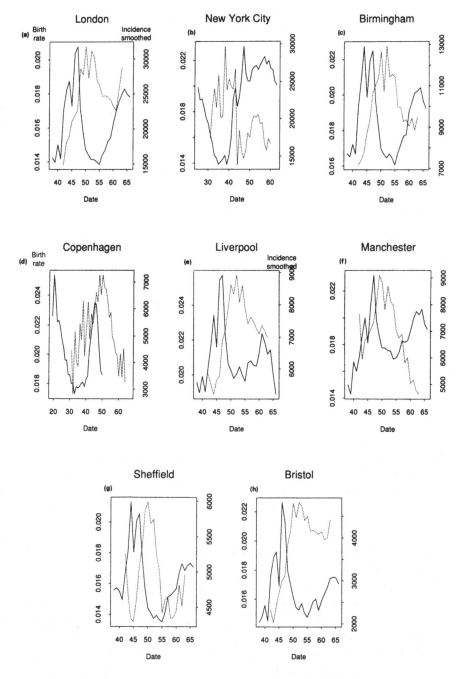

Figure 7: As Fig. 6, except the measles notifications are smoothed with a 6 year running average.

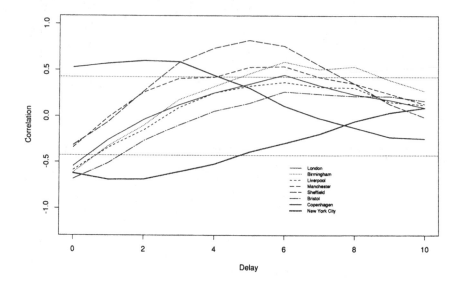

Figure 8: Cross correlations between birth rate and smoothed measles notifications, corresponding to Fig. 7. The dotted lines are 95% confidence bands for zero correlation.

The pattern for New York, is much more irregular and we discuss possible causes for this phenomenon below.

The overall patterns for English cities shown in Figs 7 and 8 indicate that average measles incidence appears to track the rise and fall in birth rates during the baby boom of the 1940s. The predicted effect on measles *dynamics* is much more difficult to discern. Though the baby boom in Copenhagen is followed by a period of annual cycles during 1940 to 45 (Fig. 6), there are no such obvious associations between epidemic cycle period and birth rate for the other cities. Nevertheless, this preliminary analysis does point to the need for future work on the relationship between long term demographic trends and the dynamics of measles.

4 Discussion

This paper presents a brief synoptic summary of the impact of seasonal and longer term temporal variation in epidemiological and demographic parameters on the population dynamics of measles. Although the focus has been on measles in developed countries, the simulation results of Fig. 5 indicate that the high birth rates of developing countries (typically 2 to 3 times those in developed countries; (McLean and Anderson 1988a, 1988b) may generate annual epidemics, swamping any tendency for seasonality to produce complex dynamics. This preliminary result is consistent with the predictions of unforced models (McLean and Anderson 1988a, 1988b). Nevertheless, we suggest that there is considerable scope for further work in this area, especially given the long term temporal variability of birth rates in developing countries.

For developed country measles parameters, the simple SEIR model indicates that relatively strong and predictable seasonality could interact with the propensity for longer-term cycles to produce complex chaotic dynamic behaviour. Our initial evaluation of this result using more realistic epidemiological models indicates that population heterogeneity, in terms of the age-distribution of infection, has the potential to simplify this picture. However, these results interact with the population size (and therefore spatial arrangement) of the host population, (Bolker and Grenfell, in preparation).

Whatever the rights and wrongs of the chaos debate, it is clear that measles dynamics in developed countries are markedly nonlinear and that seasonal forcing is a crucial influence in this context. Our preliminary analysis of measles and demography indicates that longer term temporal variations (in this case of birth rate) can also have a significant effect, particularly on the average level of measles incidence. Given that recruitment of new susceptibles provides the raw material for epidemics, some relationship between measles incidence and some integral over lagged birth rates is to be expected. However, this relationship again interacts with spatial heterogeneity. This is reflected both in local variations in the birth rate-measles incidence relationship for English cities (Grenfell 1992) and also in the fact that New York appears to show no simple relationship between average measles incidence and birth rate. More work is required here to clarify the relative effects of stochasticity and secular changes in demographic variables. In particular, it would be important to establish whether immigration into New York in the pre-vaccination era may complicate any simple relationship between measles incidence and demography. It is also worth noting that the proportion of total cases notified for New York (assuming that effectively all individuals before the vaccination era acquired the infection) is only around 12%, compared with 60% for England and Wales (Clarkson and Fine 1985).

4.1   Spatial heterogeneity and measles dynamics

In an interesting discussion of measles dynamics, Olsen *et al.* (1988) under-line the importance of spatial heterogeneity and, in particular partial spatial coupling between cities, in perpetuating the infection. This nonlinear per-spective echoes a large and sophisticated body of work on the spatial geog-raphy of measles epidemics (Murray and Cliff 1975, Cliff and Ord 1978, Cliff and Haggett 1988). Although the degree of coupling does not appear to be able to explain completely measles persistence in seasonally-forced systems, without an appeal to the age effects noted above (Bolker and Grenfell 1993), the question of spatial heterogeneity is clearly very important. In particular, more theoretical work is needed to examine the impact of seasonality and age-structure on the balance between measles fadeout and coupling in spatial grids with relatively small individual population sizes, corresponding to the spatial arrangement of hosts within and between cities.

These questions can also be explored in terms of the available empirical data. For example, Fig. 9 shows observed annual measles notifications for seven cities in England and Wales, before and after the onset of vaccination in 1968. In the pre-vaccination era (Fig. 9a), epidemics in the cities are relatively in phase, although there are significant heterogeneities (Bartlett 1957), particularly with respect to the Liverpool notifications (which show much higher epidemic minima). The task for theory here is to establish whether England and Wales was sufficiently coupled to be an epidemiological unit before vaccination and the origins (possibly arising from local differences in demography) of systematic departures from the overall pattern. After the onset of vaccination (Fig. 9b), the epidemics in cities are much more irregular in timing and apparently less in phase with each other. Again the basis of this irregularity (whether associated with spatial dynamics *per se*, or for example regional variations in vaccine uptake) goes to the heart of the problem of measles spread and persistence. This issue is also of considerable applied importance as vaccine uptake continues to rise to different extents in different areas.

Finally, though measles epidemics in the English cities were in phase dur-ing the 1950s and 60s, this was not always the case. For example, biennial epidemics in London and Birmingham were completely out of phase during the 1930s, then came into phase early in the 1940s (Stocks 1942, Grenfell *et al.*, in preparation). Whether this reflects the demographic perturbations of the War discussed above (Stocks 1942), or simply some increase in epidemio-logical coupling between the centres, is unclear. In does, however, underline the general point that we have much to learn about the spatial dynamics of even such a simple and well documented infection as measles.

Overall, recent developments suggest that measles dynamics will continue to present a fascinating challenge for epidemiologists, ecologists and applied

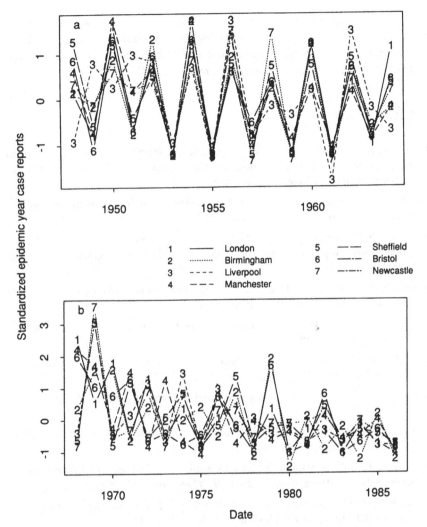

Figure 9: Standardized total measles incidence in epidemiologic years (1 Oct.–30 Sept.), for seven cities in England and Wales. Annual totals for each city were standardized by subtracting the city mean annual incidence, then dividing by the city standard deviation of annual incidence. (a) 1948–1966. (b) 1968–1988.

mathematicians. The whole question of the interaction between spatial dynamics and the possibility of chaotic dynamics at some populations scales is, in our opinion, likely to be particularly fruitful.

We thank Klaus Dietz, Steve Ellner and Robert May for helpful discussions. Financial support was provided by the Mellon Foundation (BMB), the Royal Society, Polish Academy of Sciences and AFRC (AK) and The Isaac Newton Institute for Mathematical Sciences, Cambridge (BG).

References

Anderson, R.M., Grenfell, B.T. and May, R.M. (1984) 'Oscillatory fluctuations in the incidence of infectious disease and the impact of vaccination: time series analysis', *J. Hyg. (Camb.)* **93**, 587–608.

Anderson, R.M. and May, R.M. (1982) 'Directly transmitted infectious diseases: control by vaccination', *Science* **215**, 1053–1060.

Anderson, R.M. and May, R.M. (1985) 'Age-related changes in the rate of disease transmission: implications for the design of vaccination programmes', *J. Hyg. (Camb.)* **94**, 365–436.

Anderson, R.M. and May, R.M. (1991) *Infectious diseases of humans: dynamics and control*, Oxford University Press, Oxford.

Aron, J.L. (1990) 'Multiple attractors in the response to a vaccination program', *Theor. Popul. Biol.* **38**, 58–67.

Aron, J.L. and Schwartz, I.B. (1984) 'Seasonality and period-doubling bifurcations in an epidemic model', *J. Theor. Biol.* **110**, 665–679.

Bartlett, M.S. (1957) 'Measles periodicity and community size', *J. R. Statist. Soc. A* **120**, 48–70.

Bartlett, M.S. (1960) 'The critical community size for measles in the US'. *J. R. Statist. Soc. A* **123**, 37–44.

Black, F.L. (1966) 'Measles endemicity in insular populations: critical community size and its evolutionary implication', *J. Theor. Biol.* **11**, 207–211.

Black, F. L. (1984) 'Measles'. In *Viral Infections of Humans: Epidemiology and Control*, A.S. Evans (ed.), Plenum, New York, 397–418.

Bolker, B.M. and Grenfell, B.T. (1993) 'Chaos and biological complexity in measles dynamics', *Proc. R. Soc. Lond. Biol.* **251**, 75–81.

Bolker, B.M. and Grenfell, B.T., in preparation.

Brownlee, J. (1919) 'Periodicities of epidemics of measles in the large towns of Great Britain and Ireland', *Proc. R. Soc. Med. (Epid. State. Med.)* **12**, 77–117.

Campanella, N. and Tarantini, F. (1989) 'Health care organization and health in a region of Zaire', *Ann. Ig.* **1**, 1389–1417.

Chatfield, C. (1975) *The analysis of time series: theory and practice*, Chapman and Hall, London.

Clarkson, J.A. and Fine, P.E.M. (1985) 'The efficiency of measles and pertussis notification in England and Wales', *Int. J. Epidem.* **14**, 153–168.

Cliff, A. D. and Haggett, P. (1988) *Atlas of Disease Distributions: Analytic Approaches to Epidemiologic Data*, Basil Blackwell, Oxford.

Cliff, A.D. and Ord, J.K. (1978) 'Forecasting the progress of an epidemic'. In *Towards the Dynamic Analysis of Spatial Systems*, R.L. Martin, N.J. Thrift and R.J. Bennett, (eds.) Pion, London, 191–204.

Dietz, K. (1976) 'The incidence of infectious diseases under the influence of seasonal fluctuations', *Lecture Notes in Biomathematics* 11, 1–15.

Dietz, K. and Schenzle, D. (1985) 'Mathematical models for infectious disease statistics'. In *A Celebration of Statistics*, A.C. Atkinson and S.E. Feinberg (eds.), Springer, New York, 167–204.

Engbert, R. and Drepper, F.R. (1994) 'Qualitative analysis of unpredictability: a case study from childhood epidemics'. In *Predictability and nonlinear modelling in natural sciences and economics*, April 4–7, 1993, Wageningen (NL), *Chaos, Solitons and Fractals* 4, 1147–1169.

Fine, P.E.M. and Clarkson, J.A. (1982 'Measles in England and Wales I: an analysis of factors underlying seasonal patterns', *Int. J. Epidem.* 11, 5–15.

Grenfell, B.T. (1992) 'Chance and chaos in measles dynamics', *J. R. Statist. Soc. B.* 54, 383–398.

Grenfell, B.T. and Anderson, R.M. (1985) 'The estimation of age-related rates of infection from case notifications and serological data', *J. Hyg. (Camb.)* 95, 419–436.

Grenfell, B.T. *et al.*, in preparation.

Grossman, Z. (1980) 'Oscillatory phenomena in a model of infectious diseases', *Theor. Popul. Biol.* 18, 204–243.

Hamer, W.H. (1906) 'Epidemic disease in England-the evidence of variability and of persistency of type', *Lancet* 1, 733–739.

Kharat, I., Cheirmaraj, K., Prasad, G.B. and Harinath, B.C. (1989) 'Antigenic analysis of excretory-secretory products of Wuchereria bancrofti and Brugia malayi infective larval forms by SDS-PAGE', *Indian J. Exp. Biol.* 27, 681–684.

Kot, M., Graser, D.J., Truty, G.L., Schaffer, W.M. and Olsen, L.F. (1988) 'Changing criteria for imposing order', *Ecol. Modelling* 43, 75–110.

London, W.P. and Yorke, J.A. (1973) 'Recurrent outbreaks of measles, chickenpox and mumps. I. Seasonal variation in contact rates', *Am. J. Epidem.* 98, 453–468.

May, R.M. (1986) 'Population biology of microparasitic infections'. In *Biomathematics* 17, T.G. Hallam and S.A. Levin (eds.), Springer-Verlag, Berlin, 405–442.

McLean, A.R. and Anderson, R.M. (1988a) 'Measles in developing countries. Part I. Epidemiological parameters and patterns', *Epidemiol. Infect.* 100, 111–133.

McLean, A.R. and Anderson, R.M. (1988b) 'Measles in developing countries. Part II. The predicted impact of mass vaccination', *Epidemiol. Infect.* 100, 419–442.

Murray, G.D. and Cliff, A.D. (1975) 'A stochastic model for measles epidemics in a multi-region setting', *Inst. Brit. Geog.* **2**, 158–174.

Nychka, D., Ellner, S., Gallant, A.R. and McCaffrey, D. (1992) 'Finding chaos in noisy systems', *J. R. Statist. Soc. B* **54**, 399–426.

Olsen, L.F., Truty, G.L. and Schaffer, W.M. (1988) 'Oscillations and chaos in epidemics: a nonlinear dynamic study of six childhood diseases in Copenhagen, Denmark', *Theor. Pop. Biol.* **33**, 344–370.

Olsen, L.F. and Schaffer, W.M. (1990) 'Chaos versus noisy periodicity: alternative hypotheses for childhood epidemics', *Science* **249**, 499–504.

Pool, R. (1989) 'Is it chaos, or is it just noise?', *Science* **243**, 25–28.

Priestley, M.B. (1982) *Time series analysis and forecasting*, second edition, Academic Press, London.

Rand, D.A. and Wilson, H. (1991) 'Chaotic stochasticity: a ubiquitous source of unpredictability in epidemics', *Proc. R. Soc. Lond. Biol.* **246**, 179–184.

Schaffer, W.M. (1985a) 'Order and chaos in ecological systems', *Ecology* **66**, 93–106.

Schaffer, W.M. (1985b) 'Can nonlinear dynamics elucidate mechanisms in ecology and epidemiology?', *IMA. J. Math. Appl. Med. Biol.* **2**, 221–252.

Schaffer, W.M. and Kot, M. (1985) 'Nearly one dimensional dynamics in an epidemic', *J. Theor. Biol.* **112**, 403–427.

Schenzle, D. (1984) 'An age-structured model of pre- and post-vaccination measles transmission', *IMA. J. Math. Appl. Med. Biol.* **1**, 169–191.

Soper, M.A. (1929) 'The interpretation of periodicity in disease prevalence', *J. R. Statist. Soc. A* **92**, 34–61.

Stocks, P. (1942) 'Measles and whooping cough incidence before and during the dispersal of 1939–1941', *J. R. Statist. Soc.* **105**, 259–291.

Sugihara, G. and May, R.M. (1990) 'Nonlinear forecasting as a way of distinguishing chaos from measurement error in time series', *Nature* **344**, 734–741.

Yorke, J.A., Nathanson, N., Pianigiani, G. and Martin, J. (1979) 'Seasonality and the requirements for perpetuation and eradication of viruses in populations', *Am. J. Epidem.* **109**, 103–123.

Part 4
Heterogeneity in Human Diseases

Grouping in Population Models

Simon Levin

Summary

The key element in any model for the dynamics of infectious diseases is the transmission term, the major source of nonlinearity and hence the central determinant of dynamical behavior. Errors or modifications in this term can propagate, creating sensitivity to initial conditions and difficulty in prediction. In this regard, the usual null assumption, homogeneous mixing, is problematical, because conclusions based on it may not be robust.

Numerous recent efforts have considered how the details of population structure can alter the assumption of homogeneous mixing, with special attention to age structure, social structure, and spatial heterogeneity.

Spatial heterogeneity affects mixing rates in complicated ways, but ones amenable to study. In some cases, it is sufficient to represent heterogeneity through measures such as degree of aggregation (Hassell and May 1974). More generally, however, it may be essential to study the dynamics directly through mechanistic, individual-based models. This is the focus of this paper.

1 The General Mixing Problem

Busenberg and Castillo-Chavez (1989, 1991), among others, have directed attention to the problem of mixing through pair formation, because of its importance in the study of sexually-transmitted diseases. In particular, suppose a population is broken into n groups, $i = 1, ..., n$, and let $T_i(t)$ be the size of the ith group at time t. Furthermore, let c_i = rate of pair formation for individuals in group i, and define $\omega_i = c_i T_i$. Assume that the sex ratio is 1:1 within each group, (Alternatively, one can break each group into a male group and a female group, but I explicitly do not treat the two sex problem in this paper.) Then the *general mixing problem* is to find a matrix $p_{ij}(t)$, $i, j = 1, ..., n$, such that

$$0 \le p_{ij} \le 1, \tag{1.1}$$

$$\sum_{j=1}^{n} p_{ij} = 1, \tag{1.2}$$

and

$$\omega_i \, p_{ij} = \omega_j \, p_{ji}, \tag{1.3}$$

271

where p_{ij} may be interpreted as the probability that an individual in group i who is pairing will pair with an individual in group j. Condition (1.3) simply embodies a principle of conservation, namely that each i,j mating must involve an individual from i as well as an individual from j. One corollary of (1.3) is that

$$\omega_j = 0 \Rightarrow p_{ij} = 0 \text{ for all } i \text{ for which } \omega_i \neq 0. \tag{1.4}$$

This formulation (1.1-4) is slightly different from that in Busenberg and Castillo-Chavez (1989, 1991), but basically equivalent.

Define now the new quantities q_{ij} by

$$p_{ij} = \omega_j q_{ij}, \tag{1.5}$$

so that

$$0 \leq q_{ij} \leq 1/\omega_j \text{ if } \omega_j \neq 0. \tag{1.6}$$

For completeness, set $q_{ij} = 0$ if $\omega_j = 0$. Define further

$$Q_{ij} = q_{ij}\left(\sum \omega_k\right) - 1. \tag{1.7}$$

Then Q_{ij} satisfies the properties

$$Q_{ij} = Q_{ji} \quad \text{(from 1.3)}, \tag{1.8}$$

$$Q_{ij} \geq -1 \quad \text{(by definition)}, \tag{1.9}$$

$$Q_{ij} \leq \sum_{k \neq j} \omega_k/\omega_j \quad \text{(from 1.6)}, \tag{1.10}$$

and

$$0 = \sum_j \omega_{ji} Q_{ij} \quad \text{(from 1.5)}. \tag{1.11}$$

Recall that the explicit dependence of Q_{ij} and p_{ij} on t has been suppressed. Q_{ij} may be thought of as a measure of selectivity, with $Q_{ij} > 0(< 0)$ corresponding to positive (negative) selectivity, and $Q_{ij} = 0$ to proportionate mixing.

Because the steps taken to this point are all invertible, the mixing problem is reduced to one of finding a set of Q_{ij} that satisfy (1.8-11). The approach in this paper is to find a basis for the space of solutions to the linear system (1.8) and (1.11), and then to use (1.9) and (1.10) as constraints on the coefficients in linear combinations of the basis solutions. Thus, symmetry assumption (1.8) leaves $n(n+1)/2$ independent quantities to be determined, and equation (1.11) imposes n equations to be satisfied. Hence, there are $n(n-1)/2$ degrees of freedom, exactly equal to the number of off-diagonal terms that can be chosen independently (in light of 1.8). Therefore, fix a pair of indices $i \neq j$. Set $\tilde{Q}_{lk} = \tilde{Q}_{kl} = 0$ unless k and l both are chosen from the pair i,j, leaving 3 quantities $(\tilde{Q}_{ii}, \tilde{Q}_{jj}, \tilde{Q}_{ij} = \tilde{Q}_{ji})$ to be determined subject to the two equations (1.11). Clearly, the general solution is

$$
\begin{pmatrix} \tilde{Q}_{ii} & \tilde{Q}_{ij} \\ \tilde{Q}_{ji} & \tilde{Q}_{jj} \end{pmatrix} = k_{ij} \begin{pmatrix} -\omega_j^2 & \omega_i \omega_j \\ \omega_i \omega_j & -\omega_i^2 \end{pmatrix} \tag{1.12}
$$

where $k_{ij} = k_{ji}$ is a scaling factor that represents the remaining degree of freedom. The complete solution to the full system (1.8), (1.11) is thus

$$
Q_{ij} = \left\{ \begin{array}{ll} k_{ij}\omega_i\omega_j, & i \neq j \\ -\sum\limits_{l \neq i} k_{il}\omega_l^2, & i = j \end{array} \right\}, \tag{1.13}
$$

corresponding to linear combinations of the basis solutions. Note that the k_{ij} may be negative. (1.13) specifies the full set of solutions to (1.8) and (1.11), parametrized by the $n(n-1)/2$ coefficients $k_{ij}(= k_{ji})$. It remains to impose the constraints (1.9) and (1.10).

Based on (1.5), (1.7), and (1.13), one has

$$
\begin{aligned}
p_{ij} &= \frac{\omega_j}{\sum \omega_k}[1 + k_{ij}\omega_i\omega_j] = V_j(1 + Q_{ij}), i \neq j \\
p_{ii} &= \frac{\omega_i}{\sum \omega_k}\left[1 - \sum_{j \neq i} k_{ij}\omega_j^2\right] = V_i(1 + Q_{ii}) \text{ if } \omega_i \neq 0,
\end{aligned} \tag{1.14}
$$

where again $k_{ij} = k_{ji}$ are chosen arbitrarily, and where

$$
V_j = \omega_j / \sum \omega_k. \tag{1.15}
$$

For the system (1.14) the constraints (1.9) and (1.10) translate into $0 \leq p_{ij} \leq 1 \; \forall \; i, j$ (see 1.1). The coefficients k_{ij} may be intepreted as assortative mating parameters; in particular $k_{ij} \equiv 0$ corresponds to random mating.

It is instructive to consider as a special case $n = 2$, corresponding to two groups. Then the matrix $P = ((p_{ij}))$ can be rewritten

$$
P = \frac{1}{\omega} \begin{pmatrix} \omega_1 & \omega_2 \\ \omega_1 & \omega_2 \end{pmatrix} - k^* \begin{bmatrix} \omega_2 & -\omega_2 \\ -\omega_1 & \omega_1 \end{bmatrix},
$$

where $\omega = \omega_1 + \omega_2$ and $k^* = k\omega_1\omega_2/\omega$. If the groups are of the same size $(\omega_1 = \omega_2)$, then

$$
P = \frac{1}{2}\begin{pmatrix} 1 & 1 \\ 1 & 1 \end{pmatrix} + c\begin{pmatrix} 1 & -1 \\ -1 & 1 \end{pmatrix} \tag{1.16}
$$

for some parameter $c \; \varepsilon \left[-\frac{1}{2}, \frac{1}{2}\right]$. (Note that c, just as k_{ij}, can depend on t.) When $c = 0$, one obtains the Ross solutions (proportionate mixing, Busenberg and Castillo-Chavez 1989, 1991).

As an alternative formulation in the general case, set

$$
l_{ij} = k_{ij}\left(\sum \omega_k\right)^2 \tag{1.17}
$$

and
$$V_j = \omega_j / (\textstyle\sum \omega_k). \tag{1.18}$$

Then
$$p_{ij} = V_j(1 + l_{ij} V_i V_j), i \neq j \tag{1.19}$$

$$p_{ii} = V_i(1 - \sum_{j \neq i} l_{ij} V_j^2), \tag{1.20}$$

where the matrix $L = ((l_{ij}))$ measures assortativity.

2 Grouping

The epidemiologically important consequences of mixing through pair formation can be separated into the dynamics of mixing itself, and risk enhancing
behaviors such as sexual activity or needle sharing while individuals are members of a pair. The same comment applies to other forms of mixing through
group formation and dissolution. The frequencies of certain activities, with
consequent measures of risk, can be described by rates applied to individuals in groups (and out of groups); hence, I confine attention henceforth to
the dynamics of mixing. In this regard, the "general mixing problem" discussed in the previous section addresses only pair formation. To understand
the complete dynamics, one also must consider rates of dissolution of pairs
(Kendall 1949, Dietz and Hadeler 1988).

Now, let $x_{ij}(t)$ be the number of individuals in group i that are paired
with individuals in group j, and let

$$S_i(t) = T_i(t) - \sum_{j=1}^{n} x_{ij}(t) \tag{2.1}$$

be the number of solitary individuals in group i. Note that the pairing process
itself is a special case of group formation, in which solitary individuals are in
groups of size 1, and paired individuals in groups of size 2. Note further that
x_{ij} = the number of (i, j) pairs if $i \neq j$, and that $x_{ii}/2$ = the number of (i, i)
pairs. Then

$$\frac{d}{dt} S_i = R_i - \mu_i S_i - \omega_i + \Sigma d_{ij} x_{ij} \tag{2.2}$$

and

$$\frac{d}{dt} x_{ij} = R_{ij} - \mu_{ij} x_{ij} + \omega_i p_{ij} - d_{ij} x_{ij} \tag{2.3}$$

Here, if $i \neq j$, d_{ij} = rate of dissolution of (i, j) groups. For $i = j$, $d_{ii}/2$
is the dissolution rate. R_i and $R_{ij}(R_{ii}/2$ if $i = j)$ are immigration rates for
individuals and groups; μ_i and $\mu_{ij}(\mu_{ij}/2$ if $i = j)$, possibly negative, represent
the cumulative effects of emigration, and deaths minus births. All coefficients

can vary with time. Furthermore, recall that the p_{ij} will depend on the vector of ω_i's, and now $\omega_i = c_i S_i$, so that the system (2.2-3) is nonlinear.

For simplicity, I have ignored emigration or death of single individuals from pairs, treating any such event as a dissolution followed by death or emigration. More correctly, appropriate terms should be added to (2.2) and (2.3). Note that when recruitment, death, and emigration are set equal to 0, one obtains

$$\frac{d}{dt} S_i = -\omega_i + \sum_j d_{ij} x_{ij} \qquad (2.4)$$

$$\frac{d}{dt} x_{ij} = \omega_i p_{ij} - d_{ij} x_{ij}, \qquad (2.5)$$

so that $T_i = S_i + \sum_{j=1}^{n} x_{ij}$ is constant. Let

$$S = \sum S_i \qquad (2.6)$$

be the total number of solitary individuals. Assume further that $c_i = c$ for all i. Then

$$\frac{dS}{dt} = -\omega + \sum_i \sum_j d_{ij} x_{ij} = -cS + \sum_i \sum_j d_{ij} x_{ij}, \qquad (2.7)$$

where $\omega = \Sigma \omega_i$. If $d_{ij} = d$ for all i, j, this reduces to

$$\frac{dS}{dt} = dT - (d + c)S. \qquad (2.8)$$

Recall that $c = c(t)$. If $c(t)$ is a constant, and if population size T is constant, then the fraction of individuals that are solitary will tend to the limit

$$S/T = d/(d + c); \qquad (2.9)$$

alternatively, under the mass action assumption $c(t) = rS(t)$, r constant, the solitary fraction will tend to

$$S/T = (-d + \sqrt{d^2 + 4rdT})/2rT \qquad (2.10)$$

if T is constant. Note that $S/T \to 0$ as $d \to 0$, and $\to 1$ as $d \to \infty$.

As mentioned earlier, pairing is just one form of group formation, and reasoning such as that given above can be applied to groups of arbitrary type and size. The discussion recognizes that the population may be cross-classified according to a variety of criteria, with dynamics particular to each. For simplicity, in the rest of this section I will focus only on the dynamics of grouping within a particular class, or summed over all classes (as in 2.8), ignoring the within-class heterogeneity. Through methods such as those discussed earlier in this section, it will be obvious how such approaches can be generalized to deal with heterogeneity and cross-classification.

The general problem of group formation involves fusion and fission of groups of arbitrary sizes. This problem is analogous to one in polymer kinetics (Aizenman and Bak 1979), and I have been investigating it jointly with Shay Gueron. A related approach (Cohen 1971) allows group size to change only by individual decisions, so every fusion or splitting involves at least one group of size 1. The general approach is to consider the distribution function $\Pi(t, N)$ for groups of size N at time t, and to write a convolution equation for the change in group size. Thus (compare Aizenman and Bak (1979), van Dongen and Ernst (1984), Gueron and Levin (1994)), one obtains a system of equations of the form

$$
\begin{aligned}
\frac{d}{dt}\Pi(t, N) = {} & \sum_{M=N+1}^{\infty} \Pi(t, M)\phi(M, N) - K(N)\Pi(t, N) \\
& + \frac{1}{2}\sum_{M=1}^{N-1} \Psi(M, N - M)\Pi(t, N - M)\Pi(t, M) \\
& - \Pi(t, N)\sum_{M=1}^{\infty} \Psi(M, N)\Pi(t, M), N = 1, ...\infty \quad (2.11)
\end{aligned}
$$

Because the second argument is discrete-valued, the derivative clearly refers to the first argument. Here, $\phi(M, N) = \phi(M, M - N)$ is the rate at which groups of size N (or of $M - N$) are created from the splitting of groups of size M. If $N \neq M/2$, $\phi(M, N)$ is the rate that groups of size M split into groups of sizes N and $M - N$; if $N = M/2$, the splitting rate is $\phi(M, N)/2$. Thus $K(N)$, the rate at which groups of size N split, is given by

$$
K(N) = \frac{1}{2}\sum_{M=1}^{N-1} \phi(N, M). \quad (2.12)
$$

Furthermore, $\Psi(M, N) = \Psi(N, M)$ is the rate per M group per N group that groups of size M and N fuse.

For the case considered earlier in this section, the only feasible group sizes are 1 and 2, and

$$
\Pi(t, 1) = S(t), \quad \Pi(t, 2) = (T - S(t))/2. \quad (2.13)
$$

Since births, deaths, and migration have been ignored in (2.11), T is constant. Furthermore, ϕ and Ψ are zero, except for

$$
\phi(2, 1) = d, \ \Psi(1, 1)S^2 = \omega = cT. \quad (2.14)
$$

With these simplifications, the system (2.11) reduces to the single equation (2.8). Note that, more generally,

$$T = \sum_{N=1}^{\infty} N\Pi(t, N) \qquad (2.15)$$

must be constant.

Aizenman and Bak (1979) and Gueron and Levin (1994) treat generalizations, special cases, and a continuous approximation of (2.11), with the goal of obtaining the equilibrium distribution of group sizes. The problem is nontrivial. For example, if group sizes of 1, 2, and 3 represent the total feasible set, then the steady state distribution has

$$\frac{\Pi(3)}{\Pi(2)} = \gamma \frac{\Pi(2)}{\Pi(1)}, \qquad (2.16)$$

where

$$\gamma = \Psi(2,1)\phi(2,1)/\Psi(1,1)\phi(3,1) \qquad (2.17)$$

In Gueron and Levin (1994), steady-state distributions are given for a number of special cases, and limited stability results are obtained.

3   Swarms and Schools

The previous sections treat individuals as randomly mixing, ignoring relative spatial positions. In related work (Durrett and Levin 1994), this mean field approach is compared with spatially explicit approaches, in particular reaction-diffusion models and interacting particle models. Each of these approaches embodies qualitatively unique assumptions; and each has unique consequences for group formation, and indeed for persistence of species. These implications are substantial for problems in epidemiology, in which spatial (or other) localization determines the field of contact of an individual. See Okubo (1986) for a review of approaches to grouping.

Once aggregations form, their collective movements assume importance in determining how infections are spread through a population. Although the classical diffusion theory associated with fronts is the usual approach to characterizing the asymptotic spread of advance, (Levin 1986, Andow *et al.* 1992) such models suffer from the assumption of independence of individual movements. Other approaches, such as the interacting particle models considered by Durrett (1988 and this volume) or the models for front movement discussed by Gueron and Levin (1993), are better able to account for the irregular and wavy fronts often observed in nature. Given the huge and immensely influential literature on diffusion models of spread, dating back nearly a century, the liberating development of such new approaches is of great mathematical interest, and of significant potential application in epidemiology.

Acknowledgments

I gratefully acknowledge support from a University Research Initiative Program grant to the Woods Hole Oceanographic Institution from the Department of Defense, Office of Naval Research under Grant ONR-URIP N00014-92-J-1527. I also acknowledge the helpful comments of Jonathan Dushoff, Denis Mollison, Carlos Castillo-Chavez, and two referees.

References

Aizenman, M. and Bak, T.A. (1979) 'Convergence to equilibrium in a system of reacting polymers', *Commun. Math. Phys.* **65**, 203–230.

Andow, D.A., Kareiva, P.M., Levin, S.A. and Okubo, A. (1992) 'Spread of invading organisms', *Landscape Ecology* **4**, 177–188.

Busenberg, S. and Castillo-Chavez, C. (1989) 'Interaction, pair formation and force of infection terms in sexually-transmitted diseases'. In *Mathematical and statistical approaches to AIDS epidemiology*, C. Castillo-Chavez (ed.), *Lecture Notes in Biomathematics* **83**, Springer-Verlag, Berlin, Heidelberg, 289–300.

Busenberg, S., and Castillo-Chavez, C. (1991) 'A general solution of the problem of mixing subpopulations, and its application to risk- and age- structured epidemic models for the spread of AIDS', *IMA J. Math. Appl. in Med. and Biol* **8**, 1–29.

Cohen, J.E. (1971) *Casual groups of monkeys and men: Stochastic models of elemental social systems*, Harvard University Press, Cambridge, MA.

Dietz, K. and Hadeler, K.P. (1988) 'Epidemiological models for sexually transmitted diseases', *J. Math. Biol.* **26**, 1–25.

Durrett, R. (1988) 'Crabgrass, measles, and gypsy moths: an introduction to interacting particle systems', *Math. Intelligencer* **10**(2), 37–47.

Durrett, R. and Levin, S.A. (1993) 'On the importance of being discrete', *Theoret. Popul. Biol.*, in press.

Gueron,, S. and Levin, S.A. (1993) 'Self organization of front patterns in large wildebeest herds', *Journal of Theoretical Biology* **165**(4), 541–552.

Gueron, R. and Levin, S.A. (1994) 'The dynamics of group formation', *Math. Biosci.*, to appear.

Hassell, M. and May, R. (1974) 'Aggregation in predators and insect parasites and its effects on stability', *J. Anim. Ecol.* **43**, 567–94.

Kendall, D.G. (1949) 'Stochastic processes and population growth', *J. R. Statist. Soc. Ser. B.* **11**, 230–264.

Levin, S.A. (1986) 'Random walk models of movement and their implications'. In *Mathematical Ecology, an Introduction*, T.G. Hallam and S.A. Levin, (eds.) Springer-Verlag, Berlin, Heidelberg, 149–154.

Okubo, A. (1986) 'Dynamical aspects of animal grouping: swarms, schools, flocks, and herds', *Adv. in Biophys.* **22**, 1–94.

Core Groups and the R_0s for Subgroups in Heterogeneous SIS and SI Models

John Jacquez

Carl Simon

James Koopman

Summary

First, we examine closed SIS models for heterogeneous populations with subgroups of constant size. In order to define the core groups, we compare the relations between the epidemic threshold for the population as a whole, $R_0 = 1$, the basic reproduction numbers for contacts of infecteds in subgroup j with subgroup i, R_{0ij}, and the basic reproduction numbers for the subgroups, the R_{0j}. At the threshold $R_0 = 1$, the expression for $R_0 = 1$ in terms of the R_{0ij} reduces to a simpler expression $T_0 = 1$, which we develop. For populations with 2 or 3 subgroups, the plot of the threshold as a surface in R_{0i}-space is very useful for seeing the implications for epidemic take-off and for the definition of core groups. We compare results for assortative mixing in 1-sex models with those for disassortative mixing in 2-sex models. For some examples of 2 and 3 subgroup models we relate the analysis in terms of basic reproduction numbers to properties of the phase space plots. Then we extend the analysis to SI models with recruitment and deaths where the subgroups are no longer constant in size.

$R_{0ii} > 1$ is a sufficient condition for subgroup i to act as a core group, but it is not necessary. The general condition for i to be a core group is that $R_{0i} > 1$ and $R_0 > 1$, while $R_{0j} < 1$ for many other subgroups $j \neq i$.

1   Introduction

A basic problem in epidemic theory is to derive (in terms of the parameters of the model) thresholds for spread of an epidemic after a disease is introduced into a population.

For homogeneous populations with random mixing the results are simple and intuitively reasonable. An epidemic occurs if a dimensionless number

R_0, the basic reproduction number or ratio is greater than one (Anderson and May 1982, Diekmann *et al.* 1990, 1991, Dietz, 1975, 1993, Hethcote 1976, Heesterbeek 1992). If R_0 is less than or equal to one, the epidemic dies out. To specify R_0, let c be the number of contacts per unit time per person in the population; these are contacts of the type that have the potential of transmitting the disease. Let β be the probability of transmission in such a contact between a susceptible and an infected person, and let D be the mean duration of the infectious period. Then, cD is the total number of contacts made by an infected person over the period of infectiousness, and

$$R_0 = c\beta D \qquad (1.1)$$

is the number of individuals that would be infected per infectious person if all of the contacts of the infected person were susceptible. Obviously, the infection will spread if $R_0 > 1$ and die out if $R_0 < 1$.

For heterogeneous populations, the problem of finding a threshold is more complex (Diekmann *et al.* 1990, Simon and Jacquez 1992). To examine it in a sharp and simple manner, we assume the population is divided into a finite number of homogeneous subgroups which differ in characteristics important for transmission of the disease (rather than assume that these characteristics are continuously distributed in the population). Each subgroup i has its own R_{0i}, depending on the contacts made by members of subgroup i. In addition there is an R_0 for the population as a whole (Diekmann *et al.* 1990) and a threshold for epidemic take-off for the population as a whole, $R_0 = 1$. At that threshold, the expression for R_0 reduces to a simpler expression which we call T_0, giving $T_0 = 1$ at the threshold. The population R_0 depends on the distribution of contacts among the subgroups as well as on the subgroup R_{0i}'s. Thus the difficult problem of specifying the mixing between subgroups has to be addressed (Blythe *et al.* 1991, jacquez *et al.* 1989, Koopman *et al.* 1989).

For heterogeneous populations, it is possible that one or more subgroups are highly active as spreaders of the infection to the population as a whole. Such subgroups are now called core groups. The idea of core subgroups was first developed in the context of sexually transmitted diseases (Hethcote 1982, Hethcote and Yorke 1984, Yorke *et al.* 1978) and is now used in the medical and epidemiological literature (Brunham and Plummer 1990, Rice *et al.* 1991, Rothenberg 1983), and the modeling literature (Hethcote 1982, Hethcote and Yorke 1984, Stigum *et al.* 1994, Yorke *et al.* 1978). It has important implications; for example, for a treatable disease such as syphilis, it has been shown (Jaffe *et al.* 1979) that intense treatment of a core group of prostitutes markedly decreased the level of syphilis in a population of farm workers in an area. Martini (1928) used the idea and the term back in 1928. However, the concept of a core subpopulation was first developed in detail by Yorke, Hethcote and Nold (1978) and used in their work (Hethcote 1982, Hethcote and Yorke 1984) on the analysis of spread of gonorrhea which is in the main an SIS disease. They pointed out that subgroups with a high prevalence of gonorrhea were the spreaders and had an infector number, i.e. a reproduction number, greater than one. However, they did not provide precise criteria for a group to be a core group. Thus it is of interest to work out the relations between core group R_{0i}'s, non-core group R_{0i}'s, mixing between subgroups and R_0. That is our goal in this paper.

2 The problem for a heterogeneous population

In this paper, we focus on the spread of a disease in a heterogeneous population. We assume that the population is partitioned into n subgroups that differ - among other factors - in contact rates per person, c_i. We use a general description of arbitrary mixing between subgroups. Let r_{ij} denote the fraction of subgroup i's contacts that are with subgroup j; $\sum_j r_{ij} = 1$. In general, the r_{ij} may be functions of time, subgroup sizes, and of fractions infected in the subgroups; for simplicity of notation, we use the r_{ij} without arguments. Most of the developments that follow depend only on the initial values of the r_{ij}'s.

Let X_i, Y_i and N_i denote the number of susceptibles, the number of infectious and the total number in subgroup i for $i = 1, \ldots, n$. Since we are assuming no periods of latency or immunity, $X_i + Y_i = N_i$ for each i. Let β_{ij} denote the probability of transmission in a contact between a susceptible in group i and an infective in group j.

The rate at which susceptibles in i become infected may be obtained by following the contacts of the susceptibles in i with infecteds in all groups, or alternatively, by following the contacts of infecteds in all groups with susceptibles in i. We illustrate the latter first. Infecteds in j make $c_j Y_j$ contacts per unit time; $c_j Y_j r_{ji}$ of these are with members of group i. Thus, $c_j Y_j r_{ji} X_i / N_i$ are with susceptibles in i and of those the fraction β_{ij} become infected. Summing over all groups j, we obtain the rate susceptibles in i become infected,

$$\frac{X_i}{N_i} \sum_j c_j \beta_{ij} r_{ji} Y_j. \tag{2.1}$$

Taking the other approach, the susceptibles in group i make $c_i X_i$ contacts per unit time; $c_i X_i r_{ij}$ of these are with members of group j. Thus, $c_i X_i r_{ij} Y_j / N_j$ are with infecteds in group j. The fraction β_{ij} become infected, so summing over j we again obtain the rate susceptibles in i become infected,

$$c_i X_i \sum_j r_{ij} \beta_{ij} \frac{Y_j}{N_j}. \tag{2.2}$$

If the description of disease transmission by contacts is to be reasonable, these two expressions must be identical, term by term. That is assured by the standard symmetry condition obtained from the conservation of contacts between groups,

$$c_i N_i r_{ij} = c_j N_j r_{ji}. \tag{2.3}$$

Equation (2.3) states that the number of contacts that group i has with group j equals the number of contacts that group j has with group i. This conservation condition for contacts is often associated with diseases that are transmitted by close personal contact, such as sexually transmitted diseases. However, it holds more widely. For example, if transmission requires that one be within a certain distance of the infected person, or at some site with the infected person, as for droplet transmission of respiratory diseases, the symmetry condition holds. In particular, we assume it holds for diseases modeled by the SI and SIS systems we use in this paper. For diseases for which contacts of these types are not involved in the transmission process, other models will apply.

This paper explores the relationship between three basic reproduction numbers - one for the spread of the disease in group i attributable to infections in group j, one for all the infections attributable to group j and one for the entire population. The first two of these can be defined directly by extension of the ideas leading to equation (1.1); the last is a function of the R_{0ij} and depends on the specific dynamic model.

Let γ be the recovery rate of infecteds so that $1/\gamma$ is the mean duration of the infection. The expression

$$R_{0ij} \equiv \frac{c_j r_{ji} \beta_{ij}}{\gamma}, \tag{2.4}$$

is the number of infections in subgroup i caused by an infective in subgroup j during the course of infection when all of the contacts in group i are with susceptibles. We call R_{0ij} the **basic reproduction number for the group i contacts of an infected in group j.**

If we sum over the subgroups i, we obtain the **basic reproduction number R_{0j} for all the contacts of a group j infected:**

$$R_{0j} = \sum_{i=1}^{n} \frac{c_j r_{ji} \beta_{ij}}{\gamma}. \tag{2.5}$$

We can write R_{0j} as

$$R_{0j} = \frac{c_j \overline{\beta}_j}{\gamma}$$

where

$$\overline{\beta}_j \equiv \sum_{i=1}^{n} r_{ji}\beta_{ij}$$

is a weighted average of the β_{ij} for an infected in j, weighted by the fractions of contacts with the different groups i. If the transmission probabilities are independent of the subgroups of the susceptibles, i.e., uniform susceptibility $\beta_{ij} = \beta_{.j}$ for all i,j, then

$$R_{0j} = \frac{c_j\beta_{.j}}{\gamma} \sum_{i} r_{ji} = \frac{c_j\beta_{.j}}{\gamma}. \tag{2.6}$$

Finally, let R_0 be the basic reproduction number of the whole population. From an epidemiologic standpoint, R_0 is the average number of infections caused by an infective during the course of his infection if all contacts are with susceptibles. As we have seen, for a homogeneous population, R_0 is simply $c\beta/\gamma$. In a model with a heterogeneous population, the mathematical expression for R_0 (Diekmann *et al.* 1990) in terms of the R_{0ij} can be rather complex. In particular, the expression for R_0 depends strongly on the underlying mixing parameters, r_{ij}. See Jacquez *et al.* (1991) and Simon and Jacquez (1992) for examples.

Once properly defined, the basic reproduction number acts as a *threshold* for the spread of the disease in that:

1) if $R_0 < 1$, the disease free equilibrium should be at least locally stable,

2) if $R_0 > 1$, the disease free equilibrium should be unstable. In that case, in simple models, there will be a globally stable endemic equilibrium toward which all orbits of the model tend.

More generally, suppose that $T_0(r_{ij}, \beta_{ij}, c_i, \gamma)$ is a function of the parameters of the model with the property that the disease-free equilibrium is asymptotically stable if $T_0 < 1$ and unstable if $T_0 > 1$. Then, the function T_0 is called a *threshold* for the model and we will call the equation

$$T_0(\mathbf{r}, \beta, \mathbf{c}, \gamma) = 1,$$

the *threshold condition*.

The goal of this paper is to relate the spread of the disease in each subgroup to the spread of the disease in the whole population. Specifically, we want to find an expression for the threshold for endemicity in terms of the basic reproduction numbers R_{0i} and R_{0ij} of the subgroups. In the process, we obtain a threshold $T_0 = 1$, which is directly derived from the condition $R_0 = 1$, and will quantify the definition of core subgroups.

To operationalize the concept of a core group, we propose the following definition. In a dynamic model of disease spread, suppose the population is partitioned into n mutually disjoint subgroups. Suppose also that the model is irreducible or connected in the sense that the system cannot be divided into disjoint, noninteracting subsystems. Subgroup i is in the **core** for the spread of the disease if

1) the disease persists, i.e., $R_0 > 1$,

2) $R_{0i} > 1$,

We will prove the following relationships between the R_{0i}'s and the core:

1) if $R_0 > 1$, some $R_{0i} > 1$;

2) if $R_{0i} > 1$, R_0 need not be > 1;

3) if $R_{0ii} > 1$, then $R_{0i} > 1$ and $R_0 > 1$.

At the threshold, $R_0 = 1$ reduces to a simpler threshold condition, $T_0 = 1$. Of course, the concepts of endemicity, the threshold T_0 and the population basic reproduction number R_0 depend on the underlying dynamic: on both the type of disease (SI, SIR, SIS, etc.) and the type of mixing (the r_{ij}'s). In Simon and Jacquez (1992) and Jacquez et al. (1991) we proved that for an SI-model with *proportionate mixing* the population threshold $R_0 = 1$ gives a (linear) convex combination of the R_{0i}'s:

$$T_0 = \sum_{j=1}^{n} \alpha_j R_{0j}, \tag{2.7}$$

where $\alpha_j \geq 0$ and $\sum \alpha_j = 1$. This result holds even when the model includes constant recruitment to the susceptible population, disease-related death, background death and multiple stages of the disease.

3   Closed SIS model with no vital dynamics

We begin by examining the simplest model of disease spread in a heterogeneous population - each subgroup is a closed SIS model with no vital dynamics. This model has been used, for example, to study the spread of gonorrhea (Hethcote 1982, Hethcote and Yorke 1984, Lajmanovich and Yorke 1976, Nold 1980, Yorke et al. 1978). Using (2.1), we note that the equations for subgroup i are:

$$\frac{dX_i}{dt} = -\frac{X_i}{N_i} \sum_j c_j \beta_{ij} r_{ji} Y_j + \gamma Y_i \tag{3.1}$$

$$\frac{dY_i}{dt} = +\frac{X_i}{N_i} \sum_j c_j \beta_{ij} r_{ji} Y_j - \gamma Y_i \qquad (3.2)$$

Since $\dot{N}_i = \dot{X}_i + \dot{Y}_i = 0$ for each i, each N_i is constant. Substituting $X_i = N_i - Y_i$ into (3.2) yields a system of n equations in the n variables $Y_1, \ldots, Y_n$:

$$\frac{dY_i}{dt} = \gamma \left[\left(1 - \frac{Y_i}{N_i}\right) \sum_j \left(\frac{c_j \beta_{ij} r_{ji}}{\gamma} Y_j\right) - Y_i \right]. \qquad (3.3)$$

Lajmanovich and Yorke (1976) have shown that there are exactly two possible scenarios for the closed SIS system (3.3):

1) the disease-free equilibrium is *globally* asymptotically stable;

2) the disease-free equilibrium is unstable, and there is a unique endemic equilibrium and it is globally asymptotically stable.

The disease-free equilibrium (DFE) for system (3.3) is $Y_1^0 = \ldots = Y_n^0 = 0$. The linearized system about $\mathbf{Y} = \mathbf{0}$ is

$$\frac{d}{dt}\begin{pmatrix} y_1 \\ \vdots \\ y_n \end{pmatrix} = \gamma \begin{pmatrix} \frac{c_1 r_{11} \beta_{11}}{\gamma} - 1 & \frac{c_2 r_{21} \beta_{12}}{\gamma} & \cdots & \frac{c_n r_{n1} \beta_{1n}}{\gamma} \\ \vdots & \vdots & \ddots & \vdots \\ \frac{c_1 r_{1n} \beta_{n1}}{\gamma} & \frac{c_2 r_{2n} \beta_{n2}}{\gamma} & \cdots & \frac{c_n r_{nn} \beta_{nn}}{\gamma} - 1 \end{pmatrix}\begin{pmatrix} y_1 \\ \vdots \\ y_n \end{pmatrix}. \qquad (3.4)$$

Introducing the definition for R_{0ij}, the coefficient matrix for (3.4) becomes

$$A = \gamma(B - I) \equiv \gamma \begin{pmatrix} R_{011} - 1 & R_{012} & \cdots & R_{01n} \\ R_{021} & R_{022} - 1 & \cdots & R_{02n} \\ \vdots & \vdots & \ddots & \vdots \\ R_{0n1} & R_{0n2} & \cdots & R_{0nn} - 1 \end{pmatrix}, \qquad (3.5)$$

where the $(i,j)^{th}$ entry of B is R_{0ij} and R_0 is the dominant eigenvalue of B (Diekmann *et al.* 1990).

The matrix A is a **Metzler** matrix (Luenberger 1979, Takayama 1974) in that all its off-diagonal terms are ≥ 0. In general, Metzler matrices may have positive or negative entries on the diagonal. If all of the diagonal entries are non-positive and if all of the column sums are non-positive, the matrix is a compartmental matrix (Jacquez and Simon 1993) and cannot have eigenvalues with positive real part or purely imaginary eigenvalues.

Metzler and compartmental matrices arise naturally in many of the sciences, especially in economics and biology, and there is a rich theory specifying conditions under which $\mathbf{y} = \mathbf{0}$ is asymptotically stable for system (3.4), and therefore $\mathbf{Y} = \mathbf{0}$ is asymptotically stable for system (3.3). We summarize these results in the following theorem. For proofs and further discussion, see Takayama (1974) or Berman and Plemmons (1979). The latter lists fifty equivalent conditions for the stability of $\mathbf{y} = \mathbf{0}$ for a linear system with a Metzler matrix.

Theorem. Let $A = ((a_{ij}))$ be an $n \times n$ Metzler matrix, so that $a_{ij} \geq 0$ for all $i \neq j$. The following statements are equivalent for a Metzler or a compartmental matrix:

a) every eigenvalue of A has negative real part

b) every $k \times k$ principal submatrix of A has a determinant with sign $(-1)^k$.

c) each $a_{ii} < 0$ and there exist positive numbers $d_1, \ldots, d_n$ so that

$$-d_i a_{ii} > \sum_{j \neq i} a_{ij} d_j.$$

for $i = 1, \ldots, n$ (diagonal dominance).

An irreducible Metzler matrix A has a dominant (or Perron-Frobenius) eigenvalue $\lambda^*(A)$: an eigenvalue with the property that

i) $\lambda^*(A)$ is real

ii) every other eigenvalue λ of A satisfies $Re(\lambda) < \lambda^*(A)$.

In particular, $\mathbf{y} = \mathbf{0}$ is asymptotically stable for system (3.4) if and only if all the eigenvalues of the matrix A in (3.4) have negative real part if and only if $\lambda^*(A) < 0$. So,

$$\lambda^*(A) = 0$$

is a threshold condition for system (3.4) and therefore system (3.3), and $\lambda^*(A) = 0$ yields $R_0 = 1$ (Diekmann *et al.* 1990).

In particular, if some $R_{0ii} > 1$ in (3.4), then A has a positive i'th diagonal entry (1×1 principal minor). By the Theorem, $\lambda^*(A)$ must be positive and the DFE is an unstable equilibrium of (3.3). Since $R_{0i} = \sum_j R_{0ji}$, R_{0i} must be > 1 too. So, group i is in the core. This shows that at least for closed SIS models $R_{0ii} > 1$ is a sufficient condition for group i to be a core subgroup.

Finally, we want to write A in terms of the subgroup reproduction numbers, the R_{0i}'s.

By their definitions,

$$\frac{R_{0ij}}{R_{0j}} = \frac{c_j \beta_{ij} r_{ji}}{\sum_i c_j \beta_{ij} r_{ji}} = \frac{\beta_{ij} r_{ji}}{\sum_i \beta_{ij} r_{ji}} \equiv \alpha_{ij}. \tag{3.6}$$

where $\alpha_{ij} \geq 0$ and $\sum_i \alpha_{ij} = 1$ for each j. If the transmission probability does not depend on the susceptibles, $\beta_{ij} = \beta_{.j}$, then

$$\frac{R_{0ij}}{R_{0j}} = \frac{r_{ji}}{\sum_i r_{ji}} = r_{ji} = \alpha_{ij}.$$

In either case, we can write A in terms of the R_{0j}'s as

$$A = \gamma \begin{pmatrix} \alpha_{11}R_{01} - 1 & \alpha_{12}R_{02} & \cdots & \alpha_{1n}R_{0n} \\ \alpha_{21}R_{01} & \alpha_{22}R_{02} - 1 & \cdots & \alpha_{2n}R_{0n} \\ \vdots & \vdots & \ddots & \vdots \\ \alpha_{n1}R_{01} & \alpha_{n2}R_{02} & \cdots & \alpha_{nn}R_{0n} - 1 \end{pmatrix}. \qquad (3.7)$$

Notice that $\lambda^*(A) = \gamma(R_0 - 1)$ is obtained as the dominant root of,

$$|A - \lambda I| = \lambda^n + a_1\lambda^{n-1} + \cdots + a_{n-1}\lambda + a_n = 0. \qquad (3.8)$$

At the threshold $R_0 = 1$, $\lambda^*(A) = 0$ so (3.8) reduces to $a_n = 0$ which can be written in the form $T_0 - 1 = a_n = 0$. Thus we can obtain the threshold condition $T_0 = 1$, directly from $det A = 0$ and do not have to obtain the dominant eigenvalue and R_0 as functions of the R_{0ij} and then set $R_0 = 1$.

Since γ is a multiplier of all terms in $det A$ and $det A/\gamma^n$ has a term in $(-1)^n$, we use $[(-1)^{n-1}/\gamma^n]det A$ to obtain the threshold condition in the form,

$$\frac{(-1)^{n-1}}{\gamma^n} det A = P_n(R_{01}, R_{02}, \ldots, R_{0n}) - 1 = T_0 - 1 = 0, \qquad (3.9)$$

or,

$$T_0 = P_n(R_{01}, R_{02}, \ldots, R_{0n}) = 1, \qquad (3.10)$$

where P_n is an nth degree polynomial in the R_{0i}'s.

Odo Diekmann has pointed out that letting the recovery rate depend on the subgroup, i.e. using γ_j in equations (3.3), does not make the problem much more difficult. In that case, instead of a common multiplier, γ, for all elements of A, γ_j becomes the multiplier of all elements of the jth column. Then, we use $(-1)^{n-1}det A/\prod \gamma_j$ to obtain the result (16a).

To develop our intuition for the threshold (3.9), we examine in some detail models with 2 or 3 subgroups.

4 Two and three subgroup models

4.1 Two Subgroups

The simplest heterogeneous model is one with just two subgroups. Equations (3.3) then become

$$\frac{dY_1}{dt} \equiv \gamma[(1 - \tfrac{Y_1}{N_1})(\tfrac{c_1 r_{11}\beta_{11}}{\gamma}Y_1 + \tfrac{c_2 r_{21}\beta_{12}}{\gamma}Y_2) - Y_1] \qquad (4.1)$$

$$\frac{dY_2}{dt} \equiv \gamma[(1 - \tfrac{Y_2}{N_2})(\tfrac{c_1 r_{12}\beta_{21}}{\gamma}Y_1 + \tfrac{c_2 r_{22}\beta_{22}}{\gamma}Y_2) - Y_2] \qquad (4.2)$$

The linearization at the DFE has matrix

$$A = \gamma \begin{pmatrix} \alpha_{11}R_{01} - 1 & \alpha_{12}R_{02} \\ \alpha_{21}R_{01} & \alpha_{22}R_{02} - 1 \end{pmatrix}. \qquad (4.3)$$

To keep our example simple, assume β_{ij} is independent of the susceptible subgroup so $\alpha_{ij} = r_{ji}$. The threshold $T_0 - 1 = -det A/\gamma^2 = 0$ becomes

$$T_0 \equiv r_{11}R_{01} + r_{22}R_{02} + R_{01}R_{02}(r_{12}r_{21} - r_{11}r_{22}) = 1. \qquad (4.4)$$

Since $r_{11} + r_{12} = 1$ and $r_{21} + r_{22} = 1$, we can rewrite (4.4) as:

$$T_0 \equiv r_{11}R_{01} + r_{22}R_{02} + R_{01}R_{02}(1 - r_{11} - r_{22}) = 1. \qquad (4.5)$$

Equation (4.5) is a quadratic that passes through the points $(1,1)$, $(0, 1/r_{22})$ and $(1/r_{11}, 0)$ in the $R_{01} - R_{02}$ plane. As Figure 1 shows, there are two possible shapes for (4.5) – one convex to the origin and one concave to the origin – depending on whether $r_{22} < r_{12}$ or $r_{22} > r_{12}$.

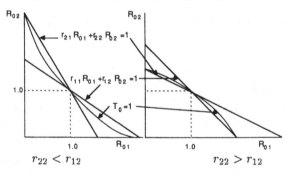

Figure 1. Plot of threshold, $T_0 = 1$, in the $R_{01} - R_{02}$ plane for a 2-subgroup SIS model for general assortative mixing. The lines, $r_{21}R_{01} + r_{22}R_{02} = 1$ and $r_{11}R_{01} + r_{12}R_{02} = 1$, come together to form one line as the mixing approaches proportional mixing; that line is $T_0 = 1$ for proportional mixing.

Note that the locus (4.5) lies between the lines $r_{11}R_{01} + r_{12}R_{02} = 1$ (which goes through $(1,1)$ and $(1/r_{11}, 0)$) and $r_{21}R_{01} + r_{22}R_{02} = 1$ (which goes through $(1,1)$ and $(0, 1/r_{22})$). In particular, the unit box $[0,1] \times [0,1]$ lies below the threshold curve (4.5). This implies that if $T_0 > 1$, at least one R_{0i} must be greater than 1.

On the other hand, $R_{0i} > 1$ is not sufficient for group i to be a core group. For example, in Figure 1 consider a point where $R_{01} < 1$ and $R_{02} > 1$. Then for R_{02} to be a core subgroup, R_{02} must be sufficiently greater than 1 that the point (R_{01}, R_{02}) falls above the threshold curve, $T_0 = 1$. If it falls between $R_{02} = 1$ and $T_0 = 1$, the disease must die out. The reason for that is clear. Because $R_{01} < 1$ the disease tends to die out in subgroup 1. Thus, infections transmitted to 1, whether from 1 or 2, tend to die out and R_{02} must be sufficiently greater than one to compensate for the transmissions lost in subgroup one; the condition for that is $T_0 > 1$. These observations should help to clarify our definition of a core subgroup.

In *proportionate mixing*, r_{ij} is independent of i since the number of contacts with subgroup j depends only on the fraction of total number of contacts attributable to group j. In other words,

$$r_{11} = r_{21} \quad \text{and} \quad r_{12} = r_{22}. \tag{4.6}$$

In that case, the $R_{01}R_{02}$-term in (4.5) vanishes and we recapture the result in Simon and Jacquez (1992) and Jacquez *et al.* (1991) that for proportionate mixing, the threshold condition is a weighted average of the subgroup reproduction numbers:

$$T_0 = r_{11}R_{01} + r_{12}R_{02} = r_{21}R_{01} + r_{22}R_{02}. \tag{4.7}$$

Geometrically, when (4.6) occurs, the two lines in Figure 1 collapse to one.

We can compute the dominant eigenvalue of a 2×2 matrix A using the quadratic formula:

$$\lambda^*(A) = \gamma \left[\frac{\sqrt{(R_{011} - R_{022})^2 + 4R_{012}R_{021}} + R_{011} + R_{022}}{2} - 1 \right] \tag{4.8}$$

$$= \gamma \left[\frac{\sqrt{(r_{11}R_{01} - r_{22}R_{02})^2 + 4r_{12}r_{21}R_{01}R_{02}} + r_{11}R_{01} + r_{22}R_{02}}{2} - 1 \right]. \tag{4.9}$$

From Diekmann, Heesterbeek and Metz (1990), the expression in the square brackets in (4.9) is $R_0 - 1$, where R_0 is the population basic reproduction number, and it provides a natural threshold for endemicity. We think that the determinant gives a simple condition which is often easier to use. Let us compare values of the threshold expressions, R_0 from (4.9), and T_0 calculated from (4.5), for some special cases:

Mixing	R_0	T_0
Disassortative Mixing: $R_{011} = R_{022} =$	$\sqrt{R_{012}R_{021}}$	$R_{012}R_{021}$
Proportionate Mixing: $r_{ij} = r_j$	$r_{11}R_{01} + r_{22}R_{02}$	$r_{11}R_{01} + r_{22}R_{02}$

Figure 2 shows the plot in the $R_{01} - R_{02}$ plane for disassortative mixing for comparison with Figure 1.

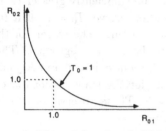
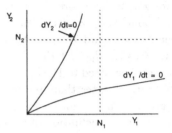

Figure 2. Plot of the threshold for a two subgroup SIS model with disassortative mixing.

Figure 3. One possible plot for the isoclines, $\dot{Y}_1 = 0$ and $\dot{Y}_2 = 0$, for the two subgroup SIS model with assortative mixing when the disease-free equilibrium is stable.

Of course, the determinant as the product of the eigenvalues is not as sharp a threshold as the dominant eigenvalue. Indeed, the determinant changes sign as the dominant eigenvalue changes sign; however, the determinant also changes sign when a non-dominant eigenvalue changes sign. Geometrically, we would expect the threshold curve (3.9) defined from det $A = 0$ to have more branches than the locus 'dominant eigenvalue = 0'. In fact, in Figure 1 we are seeing just one of two branches of the *hyperbola* $T_0 = 1$. In the first case of Figure 1, the second branch lies in the negative quadrant. In the second case, the second branch lies entirely in the positive quadrant - in fact, inside the quadrant $[1, \infty) \times [1, \infty)$. Therefore, we can use the determinant threshold by stating that the disease will die out if and only if $T_0(R_{01}, \ldots, R_{0n}) < 1$.

(a) The Phase Plane

Examination of the phase plane gives further insight into the two subgroup case. Consider the isoclines for (4.2). The zeros of dY_1/dt are given by the relation

$$Y_2 = \frac{Y_1}{R_{012}(1 - Y_1/N_1)} - \frac{R_{011}}{R_{012}}Y_1, \tag{4.10}$$

and those for dY_2/dt by

$$Y_1 = \frac{Y_2}{R_{021}(1 - Y_2/N_2)} - \frac{R_{022}}{R_{021}}Y_2. \tag{4.11}$$

Recall that $0 \leq Y_1 \leq N_1$ and $0 \leq Y_2 \leq N_2$. The right side of (4.10) goes from zero to infinity as Y_1 goes from zero to N_1. Interchanging the roles of Y_1 and Y_2, similar results hold for equation (4.11). Figures 3 to 5 show the range of plots obtainable. The plots for the trajectories in Figures 3 and 4 have been reported by Hethcote (1976) for the phase plane plots in

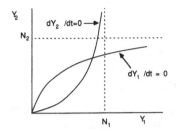

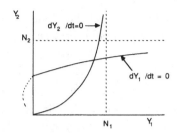

Figure 4. Another possible isocline plot for the two subgroup SIS model when the endemic equilibrium is stable.

Figure 5. Another possible isocline plot for the two subgroup SIS model when the endemic equilibrium is stable.

terms of infected fractions in his Figures 4 and 5. Notice that for the isocline $dY_1/dt = 0$, Y_2 is an increasing function of Y_1 and the derivative dY_2/dY_1 increases on the isocline as Y_1 increases. Thus the isocline dY_1/dt is concave upwards. The reverse is true for the isocline $dY_1/dt = 0$. Consequently, in the box $0 \le Y_1 \le N_1$ and $0 \le Y_2 \le N_2$, either the two isoclines cross at only one point, $(0,0)$, or they cross at two points; if the latter, one point is $(0,0)$, which is an unstable equilibrium, the other is an endemic equilibrium which is globally asymptotically stable. The threshold between these two situations occurs when the initial slopes of the two isoclines are equal. The initial slope for isocline (4.10) is

$$\left.\frac{dY_2}{dY_1}\right|_0 = \frac{1 - R_{011}}{R_{012}}, \tag{4.12}$$

and that for (4.11) is

$$\left.\frac{dY_2}{dY_1}\right|_0 = \frac{R_{021}}{1 - R_{022}}. \tag{4.13}$$

Equating (4.12) and (4.13), we obtain equation (4.4). Thus the phase plane approach directly gives the threshold condition $T_0 = 1$.

4.2 Three Subgroups

Again we assume β_{ij} does not depend on the subgroups of the susceptibles. The equations for the infecteds for three subgroups are

$$\frac{dY_1}{dt} = \gamma[(1 - \frac{Y_1}{N_1})(R_{011}Y_1 + R_{012}Y_2 + R_{013}Y_3) - Y_1] \tag{4.14}$$

$$\frac{dY_2}{dt} = \gamma[(1 - \frac{Y_2}{N_2})(R_{021}Y_1 + R_{022}Y_2 + R_{023}Y_3) - Y_2] \tag{4.15}$$

$$\frac{dY_3}{dt} = \gamma[(1 - \frac{Y_3}{N_3})(R_{031}Y_1 + R_{032}Y_2 + R_{033}Y_3) - Y_3]. \tag{4.16}$$

The determinant of the coefficient matrix from the linearized equations provides the threshold condition:

$$
\begin{vmatrix}
R_{01}r_{11} - 1 & R_{02}r_{21} & R_{03}r_{31} \\
R_{01}r_{12} & R_{02}r_{22} - 1 & R_{03}r_{32} \\
R_{01}r_{13} & R_{02}r_{23} & R_{03}r_{33} - 1
\end{vmatrix} = 0.
\tag{4.17}
$$

This gives a cubic surface in the space of R_{01}, R_{02} and R_{03} for the threshold $T_0 = 1$, as is shown in Figure 6. To illustrate the definition of a core group, suppose $R_{01} > 1$ and $R_{02} < 1$ and $R_{03} < 1$. Then, R_{01} must fall outside of the surface $T_0 = 1$ for subgroup 1 to be a core group.

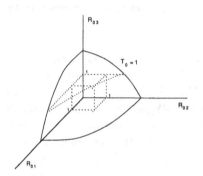

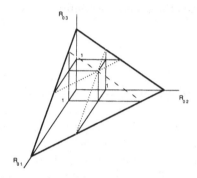

Figure 6. The threshold surface, $T_0 = 1$, for the 3-subgroup SIS model in $R_{01} - R_{02} - R_{03}$ space.

Figure 7. The threshold surface, $T_0 = 1$, for the 3-subgroup SIS model when the mixing is proportional mixing.

For proportional mixing, the cubic surface of equation (4.17) reduces to the plane

$$
T_0 = r_{11}R_{01} + r_{12}R_{02} + r_{13}R_{03} = 1,
\tag{4.18}
$$

where $r_{11} = r_{21} = r_{31}$, $r_{12} = r_{22} = r_{32}$ and $r_{13} = r_{23} = r_{33}$. That is shown in Figure 7.

(a) Phase Space

The isoclines are similar in structure to equations (4.10) and (4.11):

$$
R_{012}Y_2 + R_{013}Y_3 = \frac{Y_1}{(1 - Y_1/N_1)} - R_{011}Y_1
\tag{4.19}
$$

$$
R_{021}Y_1 + R_{023}Y_3 = \frac{Y_2}{(1 - Y_2/N_2)} - R_{022}Y_2
\tag{4.20}
$$

$$
R_{031}Y_1 + R_{032}Y_2 = \frac{Y_1}{(1 - Y_3/N_3)} - R_{033}Y_3.
\tag{4.21}
$$

Figure 8 shows two of these surfaces; they intersect in a line. If the other surface intersects the first two, it intersects that line in one point giving a stable endemic equilibrium. If any two of the surfaces do not intersect, the only stable equilibrium is $(0, 0, 0)$.

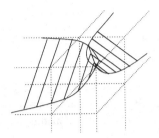 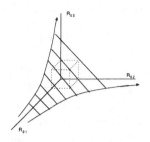

Figure 8. The plot of two of the surfaces, $\dot{Y}_1 = 0$ and $\dot{Y}_2 = 0$, for the 3-subgroup SIS model. They may or may not intersect; in the case shown they intersect in a curve.

Figure 9. Plot of $T_0 = 1$ surface for a 3-subgroup SIS model with mixing only between subgroup 1 and subgroup 2 or subgroup 3, i.e. disassortative mixing.

5 Disassortative mixing

Strict disassortative mixing is a selective mixing in which members of one subgoup only contact members of certain other subgroups. Then the A matrix has a particular structure in that $r_{ii} = 0$ for all i; in addition it may be that $r_{ij} = r_{ji} = 0$ for some combinations of $i \neq j$. Of particular interest for sexually transmitted diseases is the two-sex model with only heterosexual contacts.

Assume there are two sexes, G and H. Let $G = \{1,\ldots,g\}$ be the set of indexes for the subgroups of sex G and $H = \{g+1,\ldots,g+h\}$ be the indexes for the subgroups of sex H. The A matrix has the following structure:

$$A = \left(\begin{array}{cc} A_{11} & A_{12} \\ A_{21} & A_{22} \end{array} \right). \tag{5.1}$$

A_{11} is a $g \times g$ diagonal matrix with $-\gamma$ in all diagonal positions, and A_{22} is the corresponding $h \times h$ diagonal matrix. A_{12} and A_{21} are shown below.

$$A_{12} = \gamma \left(\begin{array}{cccc} R_{01,g+1} & R_{01,g+2} & \cdots & R_{01,g+h} \\ R_{02,g+1} & R_{02,g+2} & \cdots & R_{02,g+h} \\ \vdots & \vdots & \ddots & \vdots \\ R_{0g,g+1} & R_{0g,g+2} & \cdots & R_{0g,g+h} \end{array} \right)$$

$$A_{21} = \gamma \left(\begin{array}{cccc} R_{0,g+1,1} & R_{0,g+1,2} & \cdots & R_{0,g+1,g} \\ R_{0,g+2,1} & R_{0,g+2,2} & \cdots & R_{0,g+2,g} \\ \vdots & \vdots & \ddots & \vdots \\ R_{0,g+h,1} & R_{0,g+h,2} & \cdots & R_{0,g+h,g} \end{array} \right)$$

This is quite different from the structure for assortative mixing. In addition, the constraints of equation (2.3) reduce to

$$c_i N_i r_{ij} = c_j N_j r_{ji}, \qquad i \in G, j \in H. \tag{5.2}$$

1. One G and Two H Subgroups

Suppose $G = \{1\}$ and $H = \{2, 3\}$. Now $r_{21} = r_{31} = 1$ and $r_{12} + r_{13} = 1$. In this example, we let the transmission probability depend on the subgroups of the susceptibles as well as the infectives, i.e. β_{ij}. The equations for the rates of change of the infecteds are now

$$\frac{dY_1}{dt} = \gamma \left[(1 - \frac{Y_1}{N_1})(R_{02}Y_2 + R_{03}Y_3) - Y_1 \right] \tag{5.3}$$

$$\frac{dY_2}{dt} = \gamma \left[(1 - \frac{Y_2}{N_2})\alpha_{21}R_{01}Y_1 - Y_2 \right] \tag{5.4}$$

$$\frac{dY_3}{dt} = \gamma \left[(1 - \frac{Y_3}{N_3})\alpha_{31}R_{01}Y_1 - Y_3 \right]. \tag{5.5}$$

The threshold condition is

$$\begin{vmatrix} -1 & R_{02} & R_{03} \\ \alpha_{21}R_{01} & -1 & 0 \\ \alpha_{31}R_{01} & 0 & -1 \end{vmatrix} = 0, \tag{5.6}$$

which is:

$$T_0 = R_{01}(\alpha_{21}R_{02} + \alpha_{31}R_{03}) = 1. \tag{5.7}$$

The plot showing how core groups can be defined is Figure 9. The surface intersects coordinate plane 1-2 and 1-3 in hyperbolas and the rest of the surface consists of straight lines connecting the hyperbolas.

6   At least one R_{0i} must be greater than one

We now use the intuition we have developed from Figures 1 to 9 to prove for a general closed SIS model that

$$R_{0i} < 1 \text{ for all } i \Rightarrow T_0 < 1, \tag{6.1}$$

and the DFE is (globally) asymptotically stable.

Recall that the threshold condition is given by

$$(-1)^{n-1} det \begin{bmatrix} \alpha_{11}R_{01} - 1 & \alpha_{12}R_{02} & \cdots & \alpha_{1n}R_{0n} \\ \alpha_{21}R_{01} & \alpha_{22}R_{02} - 1 & \cdots & \alpha_{2n}R_{0n} \\ \vdots & \vdots & \ddots & \vdots \\ \alpha_{n1}R_{01} & \alpha_{n2}R_{02} & \cdots & \alpha_{nn}R_{0n} - 1 \end{bmatrix} \tag{6.2}$$

$$\equiv \; T(R_{01}, \dots, R_{0n}) - 1 \qquad (6.3)$$

$$= \; 0. \qquad (6.4)$$

One checks easily that (6.2) is satisfied at the following $(n+1)$ points in $(R_{01}, \dots, R_{0n})$ -space:

$$\begin{pmatrix} 1 \\ 1 \\ \vdots \\ 1 \end{pmatrix}, \begin{pmatrix} \frac{1}{\alpha_{11}} \\ 0 \\ \vdots \\ 0 \end{pmatrix}, \begin{pmatrix} 0 \\ \frac{1}{\alpha_{22}} \\ \vdots \\ 0 \end{pmatrix}, \dots, \begin{pmatrix} 0 \\ 0 \\ \vdots \\ \frac{1}{\alpha_{nn}} \end{pmatrix}.$$

The threshold locus is the level set of the of nth degree polynomial in $\mathbf{R}^n$ which passes through these $(n+1)$-points.

To show that statement (6.1) holds, we show that (6.2) has no solution $(R_{01}, \dots, R_{0n})$ in $[0,1)^n$. For, if each R_{0i} satisfies $0 < R_{0i} < 1$, then the matrix of the determinant in (6.2) is a strictly diagonal dominant matrix with nonnegative off-diagonal entries, strictly negative diagonal entries and for which each column j sums to $\sum_i \alpha_{ij} R_{0j} - 1$, which is $< \sum_i \alpha_{ij} - 1 = 0$. By our theorem on Metzler matrices, all eigenvalues of the matrix have negative real part. In particular, none are zero and the determinant in (6.2) is not zero.

We conclude that if the population is above threshold, some groups have to have $R_{0i} > 1$ and hence are part of the core.

7   The SI model

As shown in Figure 10, the SI model considered here differs considerably from the closed SIS model. Because there is recruitment and deaths, the subgroups and the population as a whole are no longer constant in size.

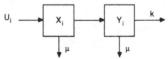

Figure 10. Compartmental diagram of SI model with constant recruitment into the susceptible class, background deaths with rate constant μ, and extra deaths due to the infection with rate constant k.

The equations for the numbers susceptible and infected in subgroup i are

$$\frac{dX_i}{dt} = -\frac{X_i}{N_i} \sum_j c_j r_{ji} \beta_{ij} Y_j - \mu X_i + U_i \qquad (7.1)$$

$$\frac{dY_i}{dt} = +\frac{X_i}{N_i} \sum_j c_j r_{ji} \beta_{ij} Y_j - (k + \mu) Y_i. \qquad (7.2)$$

In this system, U_i is the rate at which susceptibles join group i (the 'recruitment rate'), μ is the background death rate, and k is the rate for disease-related death.

The r_{ij} cannot be treated as constants since they will depend, at the minimum, on the relative sizes of the subgroups and these change as the process unfolds. However, the conservation condition for contacts still holds at all times. Because $X_i + Y_i = N_i$ is not constant, both equations (7.1) and (7.2) are required to completely describe the dynamics. An alternative description is given by equations (7.2) and the equations for the subgroup sizes.

$$\frac{dN_i}{dt} = U_i - \mu N_i - kY_i \qquad (7.3)$$

Now we assume that the r_{ij} are functions of the N_k; to simplify notation, we use $r_{ij}(U)$ for its value at $X_k = U_k/\mu$ and $Y_k = 0$, for all k.

Linearize (7.1) and (7.2) around the disease free equilibrium $X_i = U_i/\mu$ and $Y_i = 0$. Write x_i and y_i as the variables for the linearized system:

$$\frac{dx_i}{dt} = -\sum_j c_j r_{ji}(U)\beta_{ij}y_j - \mu x_i \qquad (7.4)$$

$$\frac{dy_i}{dt} = +\sum_j c_j r_{ji}(U)\beta_{ij}y_j - (k+\mu)y_i. \qquad (7.5)$$

These may be written as

$$\frac{dx_i}{dt} = -\mu x_i - (k+\mu)\sum_j R_{0ij}y_j \qquad (7.6)$$

$$\frac{dy_i}{dt} = (k+\mu)(\sum_j R_{0ij}y_j - y_i), \qquad (7.7)$$

where, $R_{0ij} = c_j\beta_{ij}r_{ji}(U)/(k+\mu)$.

Putting the variables in the order, $x_1,\ldots,x_n,y_1,\ldots,y_n$, the coefficient matrix has the form

$$A = \begin{pmatrix} A_{11} & A_{12} \\ A_{21} & A_{22} \end{pmatrix}. \qquad (7.8)$$

A_{11} is diagonal, $n \times n$, with $-\mu$ in the diagonal positions; A_{21} is an $n \times n$ null matrix; and A_{22} is

$$A_{22} = (k+\mu)\begin{pmatrix} R_{011}-1 & \cdots & R_{01n} \\ \vdots & \ddots & \vdots \\ R_{0n1} & \cdots & R_{0nn}-1 \end{pmatrix}. \qquad (7.9)$$

Furthermore, $|A| = 0$ implies $|A_{22}| = 0$.

Consequently, A_{22} has the same structure and properties as matrix (3.5), with $(k+\mu)$ playing the role of γ. The results for the SIS model carry over, with the important exception that only local asymptotic stability of $(U_1/\mu, \ldots, U_n/\mu, 0, \ldots, 0)$ is implied if $T_0 \leq 1$. Simon and Jacquez (1992) gave a number of situations in which $T_0 \leq 1$ implies the DFE is globally stable.

The analysis of two and three subgroup cases in terms of T_0 and the R_{0i} follows the same path as for the SIS model. For example, the two subgroup case gives equation (4.4) for the threshold condition so the plot of T_0 in (R_{01}, R_{02}) space is the same. However, since the results for the SI model are local results around $(U_1/\mu, \ldots, U_n/\mu, 0, \ldots, 0)$, the phase space plots are different from those for the SIS model, and in fact involve twice as many dimensions as the plots for the closed SIS model.

8 Preferred mixing

In specifying a model in which there is a preference for within group contacts, we defined **preferred mixing** (Jacquez *et al.* 1988) as an intermediate type of mixing between no mixing and proportional mixing. Also see Andreason and Christiansen (1989), Blythe and Castillo-Chavez (1989), Diekmann *et al.* (1990), Hethcote and Yorke (1984), Hyman and Stanley (1989) and Nold (1990) for work on models with preferred like-with-like mixing. In preferred mixing, each group reserves a portion r_i of its contacts for its own group and then uses proportional mixing for the rest of its contacts, so that

$$
r_{ij} = \left\{
\begin{array}{ll}
r_i + (1 - r_i)\dfrac{c_i(1 - r_i)N_i}{\sum_h c_h(1 - r_h)N_h} & \text{if } i = j \\[3mm]
(1 - r_i)\dfrac{c_j(1 - r_j)N_j}{\sum_h c_h(1 - r_h)N_h} & \text{if } i \neq j
\end{array}
\right.
$$

In Simon and Jacquez (1992), we computed the threshold for preferred mixing in terms of the R_{0j}'s as:

$$
T_0 = \sum_j \left(\frac{c_j(1 - r_j)U_j}{\sum_h c_h(1 - r_h)U_h} \right) \left(\frac{1 - r_j}{1 - r_j R_{0j}} \right) R_{0j}.
$$

It follows that if all $R_{0j} < 1$, then $T_0 < 1$ and the DFE is globally asymptotically stable. Therefore, $T_0 > 1 \Rightarrow \exists$ core group.

For more details on the properties of heterogeneous SI models for the specific types of mixing, restricted, preferred, proportional and structured, see Simon and Jacquez (1992).

9   Discussion and conclusions

Populations are heterogeneous and many diseases spread in spite of the fact that many subgroups in the population have their R_{0i}'s so low that the disease would die out in those subgroups if they were isolated from the rest of the population. Thus it is important to characterize the subgroups that act as sources (spreaders) for the population as a whole; those are the core groups.

It is clear that

$$R_{0ii} > 1$$

is sufficient but not necessary for i to be a core group. Furthermore,

$$R_{0i} > 1$$

is necessary but not sufficient to make group i a core group for the spread of a disease. For that to occur, the population R_0 must also be greater than 1.

We have given necessary and sufficient conditions for a population subgroup to be part of the core based on properties of the coefficient matrix of the linearized equations and the R_{0i} for the subgroups. For epidemiological applications, if more than one subgroup is in the core, it may also be important to distinguish the relative importance of the groups in the core. Some may be much more active as disease spreaders than others. For example, from Figures 6 or 7, for three subgroups, it is easy to imagine a case in which $R_{01} > 1$, $R_{02} > 1$ and $R_{03} < 1$ and $T_0 > 1$. Suppose $R_{01} >> 1$ but R_{02} is just slightly over one; that does not mean that subgroup 1 is necessarily the dominant subgroup of the core. It should be clear that a ranking of the R_{0i} that are greater than one is not necessarily a ranking by activity as spreaders to other groups!

First, we note that the basic reproduction numbers are measures of potential spread *per infective*, they do not take into account the sizes of the groups. We use the term potential for spread because a basic reproduction number would be the number of secondary cases if all contacts were with susceptibles. Secondly, a group may have a very high R_{0i} but have only a few contacts with other groups; such a group maintains a population endemic state primarily by maintaining a within group endemic state. Thus if a number of groups have their $R_{0i} > 1$, their relative roles per infective, in spreading infection to other groups depend on their relative R_{0ji}. Since R_{0ii} measures the within group spreading potential per infective in group i, a comparison of the

$$R_{0i} - R_{0ii} = \sum_{j \neq i} R_{0ji}$$

provides a better measure of the relative potentials per infective for spreading infection to other groups. But for heterosexual spread, $R_{0ii} = 0$, so in that case the R_{0i} provide a measure of potential per infective for spreading the infection to other groups. Relative to the point that R_{0ji}, R_{0ii} and R_{0i} are measures of potential activity in spreading *per infective* in i, a measure that takes into account the relative sizes of different groups would also be useful. At any time, such a measure would be the product of the R_{0ji}, R_{0ii} and R_{0i} with the number of infectives in group i.

An alternative approach, suggested by Odo Diekmann, is to define the groups for which $R_{0i} > 1$ as core groups (spreaders) whether or not $T_0 > 1$. Although we see that has some argument for it, for applications the issue is of interest primarily if there is spread, so we prefer to retain the requirement that the infection is actually spreading or endemic in the population, i.e. $T_0 > 1$. We do think it is useful to distinguish the two cases.

Finally, we wish to point to some other insights afforded by this approach. For a system of many subgroups that is near threshold, generally reasonable public health measures may, for special circumstances, give unexpected results. For example, consider Figure 1 for an STD with two subgroups, one is relatively inactive with $R_{01} \ll 1$ whereas the other is highly active with $R_{02} > 1$, giving a point far up in the left corner of Figure 1 that is just under the threshold so that the disease would eventually die out. Assume that the response to the standard public health message, to decrease the number of partners and to choose partners well, leads to little change in contact rates but the low activity group further restricts its partners to its own group, thus forcing the high activity group to also take a higher fraction of its partners from its own group. The change in distribution of contacts means $1/r_{11}$ and $1/r_{22}$ decrease with very little change in R_{01} and R_{02}. Thus the intercepts of the quadratic on the coordinate axes shift towards the origin and possibly push the threshold just below the point (R_{01}, R_{02}) so that the disease now has an endemic equilibrium. Of course, that would be a small endemic equilibrium, close to the disease-free equilibrium.

Acknowledgements

Stimulating conversations with many at the NATO workshop on Epidemic Models in Cambridge, Jan. 4-9, 1993, helped us sharpen our ideas on this problem. We particularly want to thank Odo Diekmann, Herb Hethcote and Hans Heesterbeek for their useful critiques of a prior version of this paper. This work was supported in part by grant R01 AI29876 from NIAID, DHEW and by RR02176 from the Natl. Center for Research Resources, DHEW.

References

Anderson, R.M. and May, R.M. (eds.) (1982) *Population Biology of Infectious Diseases: Dahlem Konferenzen*, Springer-Verlag.

Andreasen, V. and Christiansen, F.B. (1989) 'Persistence of an infectious disease in a subdivided population', *Math. Biosci.* 96, 239–53.

Berman, A. and Plemmons, R.J. (1979) *Nonnegative Matrices in the Mathematical Sciences*, Academic Press, New York.

Blythe, S.P. and C. Castillo-Chavez, C. (1989) 'Like-with-like preference and sexual mixing models', *Math. Biosci.* 96, 221–38.

Blythe, S.P., Castillo-Chavez,C., Palmer, J.S. and Cheng, M. (1991) 'Toward a unified theory of sexual mixing and pair formation', *Math. Biosci.* 107, 379–405.

Brunham, R.C. and Plummer, F.A. (1990) 'A general model of sexually transmitted disease epidemiology and its implications for control', *Medical Clinics of North America* 74, 1339–52.

Diekmann, O., Dietz, K. and Heesterbeek, J.A.P. (1991) 'The basic reproduction ratio for sexually transmitted diseases: I. Theoretical considerations', *Math. Biosci.* 107, 325–39.

Diekmann, O., Heesterbeek, J.A.P. and Metz, J.A.J. (1990) 'On the definition and the computation of the basic reproduction ratio R_0 in models for infectious diseases in heterogeneous populations', *J. Math. Biol.* 28, 365–82.

Dietz, K. (1975) *Epidemiology: Proceedings of a SIMS Conference on Epidemiology*, D. Ludwig and K.L. Cooke, (eds.) SIAM, Philadelphia, 104–21.

Dietz, K. (1993) 'The estimation of the basic reproduction number for infectious diseases', *Stat. Methods in Med. Res.* 2, 23–41.

Hethcote, H.W. (1976) 'Qualitative analysis of communicable disease models', *Math. Biosci.* 28, 335–56.

Heesterbeek, J.A.P. (1992) R_0. Thesis, Leiden.

Hethcote, H.W., Yorke, J.A. and Nold, A. (1982) 'Gonorrhea modeling: A comparison of control methods', *Math. Biosci.* 58, 93–109.

Hethcote, H.W., and Yorke, J.A. (1984) *Gonorrhea Transmission Dynamics and Control*, Lecture Notes in Biomathematics 56, Springer-Verlag, Berlin.

Hyman, J.M. and Stanley, E.A. (1989). 'Using mathematical models to understand the AIDS epidemic', *Math. Biosci.* 90, 415–73.

Jacquez, J.A. and Simon, C.P. (1993) 'Qualitative theory of compartmental systems', *SIAM Review* 35, 43–79.

Jacquez, J.A., Simon, C.P., Koopman, J. *et al.* (1988) 'Modeling and analyzing HIV transmission: The effect of contact patterns', *Math Biosci.* 92, 119–99.

Jacquez, J.A., Simon, C.P. and Koopman, J. (1989) 'Structured mixing: Heterogeneous mixing by the definition of activity groups'. In *Lecture Notes in Biomathematics* **83**, 301–315.

Jacquez, J.A., Simon, C.P., and Koopman, J. (1991) 'The reproduction number in deterministic models of contagious diseases', *Comments on Theor. Biol.* **2**, 159–209.

Jaffe, H.W., Rice, D.T., Voigt, R., Fowler, J. and St. John, R.K. (1979) 'Selective mass treatment in a venereal disease contact program', *Am. J. Publ. Hlth.* **69**, 1181–82.

Koopman, J.S., Simon, C.P., Jacquez, J.A. and Park, T.S. (1989) 'Selective contact within structured mixing with an application to HIV transmission risk from oral and anal sex', *Lecture Notes in Biomathematics* **83**, 316–48.

Lajmanovich, A. and Yorke, J.A. (1976) 'A deterministic model for gonorrhea in a nonhomogeneous population', *Math. Biosci.* **28**, 221–36.

Luenberger, D.G. (1979) *Introduction to Dynamic Systems*, Wiley, New York.

Martini, E. (1928) 'Betrachtungen zur Epidemiologie der Malaria und der Syphilis', *Dermatologische Wochenschrift* **19**, 640–43.

Nold, A. (1980) 'Heterogeneity in disease-transmission modeling', *Math. Biosci.* **52**, 227–40.

Rice, R.J., Roberts, P.L., Handsfield, H.H. and Holmes, K.K. (1991) 'Sociodemographic distribution of gonorrhea incidence:Implications for prevention and behavioral research', *Am. J. Publ. Hlth.* **81**, 1252–58.

Rothenberg, R.B. (1983) 'The geography of gonorrhea:Empirical demonstration of core group transmission', *Am. J. Epidem.* **117**, 688–94.

Stigum, H., Falck, W. and Magnus, P. (1994) 'The core group revisited, the effect of partner mixing and migration on the spread of gonorrhea, chlamydia and HIV', *Math. Biosci.* **120**, 1–23.

Simon, C.P. and Jacquez, J.A. (1992) 'Reproduction numbers and the stability of equilibria of SI models for heterogeneous populations', *SIAM J. Appl. Math.* **52**, 541–76.

Takayama, A. (1974) *Mathematical Economics.* Dryden Press, Hinsdale, Ill. Second edition 1985, Cambridge University Press, Cambridge.

Yorke, J.A., Hethcote, H.W. and Nold, A. (1978) 'Dynamics and control of transmission of gonorrhea', *Sexually Transm. Diseases* **5**, 51–56.

Data Driven Network Models for the Spread of Infectious Disease

Martina Morris

Summary

Infectious diseases spread by person-to-person contact may be strongly channeled by patterns of selective (or 'non-random') social mixing. The more intimate and extended the contact needed for disease transmission, the more impact selective mixing will have on the speed and direction of spread. Patterns of selective mixing at the population level are in turn the outcome of the heterogeneity in individual contact networks. This paper will provide an overview of the empirical and theoretical issues that such networks raise for epidemiological modeling, and some examples of the impact that networks can have on disease transmission dynamics. While network models have recently been an active area of research in mathematical epidemiology, the link between models and data has often been neglected. In keeping with the spirit of this volume, the focus here will be on the implications of alternative models for data collection and analysis.

1   Modeling Networks

A 'network' can be defined as a set of nodes connected by a set of links, and network analysis is generally concerned with specifying the probability of a link between two nodes. For infectious disease networks, the nodes are persons (or animals and vectors), and the links represent the relation needed for disease transmission, for example physical proximity, touching, or exchange of bodily fluids. The probability of a link is typically modeled as a function of nodal attributes, e.g. sex, age, or more abstractly 'degree', and sometimes also of higher-order properties such as transitivity or triad bias (if A knows B and B knows C then C is likely to know A, cf., Harary *et al.* (1965), Holland and Leinhardt (1970)).

There are two approaches that have been taken in analyzing such networks cf., Pattison (1993). The first has its roots in graph theory, and is based on a complete enumeration of all the nodes (and nodal attributes) and all the links in a network (Figure 1a). In epidemiology, this graph-theoretic approach has been shown to be consistent with the stochastic formulations of the Reed-Frost model (Mollison and Barbour 1989), and has been adopted by several

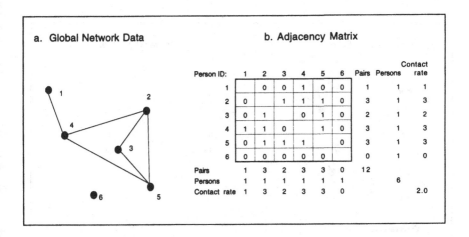

a. Global Network Data   **b. Adjacency Matrix**

Person ID:	1	2	3	4	5	6	Pairs	Persons	Contact rate
1		0	0	1	0	0	1	1	1
2	0		1	1	1	0	3	1	3
3	0	1		0	1	0	2	1	2
4	1	1	0		1	0	3	1	3
5	0	1	1	1		0	3	1	3
6	0	0	0	0	0		0	1	0
Pairs	1	3	2	3	3	0	12		
Persons	1	1	1	1	1	1		6	
Contact rate	1	3	2	3	3	0			2.0

Figure 1: Global network data. For a bounded network, all nodes and links are enumerated (panel (a)), and the data can be displayed in a socio- or adjacency matrix (panel (b)). The zeros and ones in the matrix represent the presence or absence of a link between two modes; the margins represent the total number of partnerships for each group ('pairs'), the number of persons in the group ('persons') and the average number of partnerships per per unit time ('contact group').

authors (Altmann 1993, Blanchard *et al.* 1988, Kretzschmar *et al.* 1993). In sociology, this approach is called global or 'sociocentric' network analysis, as the unit of analysis is the social group. Its origins are usually traced to the early work of Rapoport (Rapoport 1952, 1957, 1980), and it remains the dominant approach in network analysis; for overviews, see Berkowitz (1982), Burt and Minor (1983), Leinhardt (1977), Wasserman and Faust (1994).

The second approach is based on a sampling nodes from a network (Figure 2a). Here information is collected on the attributes of and links from the respondent node, and the respondent is also asked to report on the attributes of the nodes to which they are directly linked. This approach is called local or 'egocentric' network analysis in sociology, because the unit of analysis is 'ego', the respondent; see Burt and Minor (1983), Marsden (1981).

In epidemiology, this approach is most often used in conjunction with (though not limited to) deterministic compartmental modeling, and contact matrices (or their algebraic equivalents) have been used in these models by many analysts; see Anderson *et al.* (1990), Castillo-Chavez and Blythe (1989), Hethcote and Yorke (1984), Hyman and Stanley (1988), Jacquez *et al.* (1989), Sattenspiel (1987).

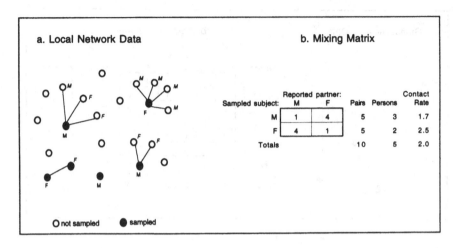

Figure 2: Local network data. For a bounded network, nodes and links are sampled (panel (a)), and the data can be displayed in a mixing or contact matrix (panel (b)). The cell entries of the matrix represent the number of partnerships between respondents in the row category with partners in the column category.

Because the global-local network split has coincided with the stochastic-deterministic split among modelers, a comparison of the two network approaches has been overshadowed by the debate over stochastic and deterministic representations. Local network data can, however, be modeled stochastically (Morris 1991) and there are other issues that determine the relative merits of the two network approaches. The most important of these, from the standpoint of applied epidemiology, are (1) the feasibility of data collection, and (2) the relevance for transmission dynamics.

The first issue for data collection is to identify the appropriate set of nodes. This has been called the 'boundary problem' in network analysis (Laumann, in Burt and Minor 1983). In the context of epidemiology, a reasonable answer would be the people who, by virtue of susceptibility and connectedness, are at risk for an infectious disease. If the life span of the disease agent is very short, or if suscesptibility is rare, this may sometimes be a small group, e.g., an isolated tribe of indigenous peoples. More often, however, the network at risk will be a very large group. With influenza or AIDS, for example, it is probably the majority of the world's population. A complete enumeration of nodes and links for such a network would be impossible. In such cases, the sampling strategy of the local network approach gives it a strong advantage over the global network approach.

Another issue that must be considered is intrusiveness. The global network approach requires that each person in the network identify their contacts, so that each contact can be uniquely matched. If the type of contact is relatively public, e.g., office sharing, there may be little difficulty in obtaining the information from the respondent. If the type of contact is intensely private, e.g., sexual relations, data collection will require questions like 'tell me the names of the people you had sex with in the last six months'. Such questions are likely to be viewed as highly intrusive by the respondent. They raise not only significant issues of privacy, but also of validity and reliability, as intrusive questions may be met with non-disclosure.[1]

By contrast, the local network approach requires a respondent to provide only a list of attributes for each partner, e.g., their age, race, and sex. The partner, otherwise, remains anonymous. While questions about sexual behavior will always be intrusive, the guarantee of partner anonymity reduces intrusiveness and may increase respondent cooperation. Here, again, the local network approach has strong advantages over the global network approach.

The tradeoff is that the local network approach loses information. It is not by virtue of sampling, per se, but rather because it is not possible from egocentric reports to collect specific information on higher order network properties, such as triad bias and chain length. In addition, there is clearly some error introduced by relying on respondent reports of their partners' attributes rather than collecting that information from the partners themselves. How serious these drawbacks are is an open question. The loss of information on higher order network properties is a question that can be explored with simulation. It is an important issue for future research and will be taken up in the conclusion. The magnitude of the measurement error introduced by relying on respondent reports, on the other hand, is an empirical question. There have been studies of the accuracy of such reports in friendship networks (Laumann 1973), which found generally high correlations between the respondent's report and the partner's actual characteristics. Not surprisingly, the degree of accuracy is highest for observable characteristics such as age, where there is about 86% agreement within 12 years, and lower for characteristics such as political party preference (53%). There were no systematic biases observed in the errors that were made, with the exception of political party preference, which respondents were more likely to report as similar to their own. The results of this analysis are encouraging, but not conclusive, because patterns observed for friendship networks may not hold in general.

---

[1]*Note:* This approach is used now for contact tracing in STD prevention, but non-infected cases are not followed, and among infected cases there is a compelling rationale to provide contact names: they are known to have been exposed and there is treatment available. A global network survey in the service of AIDS research is likely to face much more serious obstacles both at the level of political approval and respondent compliance.

2   Modeling Epidemics on Networks

If networks never changed, then the analysis of epidemic spread on a network would be relatively straightforward. Contact networks, however, are very dynamic. This raises two basic issues for modeling: summarizing the patterns of selective mixing over time, and solving the generalized two-sex problem.

The need for a parsimonious summary of selective mixing parameters can best be appreciated by a simple example of STD transmission. The types of attributes that are likely to influence sexual partner selection include such things as age, sex, race, sexual preference and marital status. Though by no means an exhaustive list, these five simple attributes generate 108 categories for respondents[2], a corresponding number for partners, and a mixing matrix with over ten thousand cells (or a similar number of link-specific probabilities for sociocentric data). Even if it were possible to use the cell counts directly to drive an epidemiological simulation (which it is not unless the vital dynamics and selection patterns are both in equilibrium), it would not be desirable. A model which captures the important selective dynamics in a limited number of parameters is therefore necessary.

In the local network tradition several simple models have been proposed, most focusing on the degree of assortative (Laumann 1973) or disassortative mixing (Gupta and Anderson 1989, Haraldsdottir *et al.* 1992). While the assortative-disassortative axis is likely to be the single most powerful summary of mixing, it is difficult to use such a summary for multiple attributes, e.g., mixing by both race (assortative) and sex (disassortative). For this, a more general modeling framework is needed. Several general frameworks have also been proposed (Blythe *et al.* 1991, Koopman *et al.* 1989, Morris, 1991). There is no consensus as yet on the criteria that should be used to evaluate the relative merits of these alternative frameworks, but some data-related criteria may be suggested.

One important criterion involves the estimation and interpretation of mixing parameters. While parameters can usually be calculated from data, estimation is most reliable when backed by a framework for statistical inference. Only then can one answer the central question of how well the model (with its reduced parameter space) fits the observed patterns. When the estimated parameters are also easy to interpret, they can provide insight into the complex impact of mixing on transmission.

The second criterion concerns the solution of multiple matching constraints over time. The constraints are imposed by the inherent symmetry in contact processes – if A meets B, then B has to meet A – and imply symmetry

---

[2]This is a conservative figure, calculated assuming 3 age groups, 2 sexes, 3 race categories, 3 sexual preference categories and 2 marital statuses. A full cross-tabulation of these categories produces an index with 108 different groups.

in a socio- or contact matrix. This is a generalized version of the 'two-sex problem' familiar to demographers (see Pollard 1948, Schoen 1982). In the context of disease transmission, the problem arises when the sizes, activity levels, or selection patterns of population subgroups change over time. These three basic factors drive the structure of a network. If one or more changes, the network must be reconfigured, and multiple matching constraints must be satisfied. There is more than one way to achieve this, but all involve changing the activity levels and/or preference patterns of other groups, and the assumptions made will clearly affect the disease projections. For this reason, it is important that the assumptions are explicitly stated.

In the local network tradition, log-linear models for the contact matrix provide the framework for estimation and inference (Morris 1991), and make it possible to explicitly solve the generalized two-sex problem when one or more of the three network factors changes (Morris 1995). In the global network tradition, estimation is more problematic. Models typically include higher-order effects such as triad bias and chain length which imply a dependence between pairs, i.e., one pair is more likely to be linked if it shares a node with another pair. This dependence among observations violates the assumptions of traditional methods of estimation. In the last 10 years some progress has been made on models for Markov random graphs, where the markovian property is interpreted to mean that two links are independent unless they share a node (Frank and Strauss 1986, Strauss and Ikeda 1990).

To summarize, recent work has generated several alternative approaches to modeling the role of networks in disease transmission. The title of this volume suggests that an important criterion for evaluating alternative models is how well they relate to data. From the standpoint of data collection, feasibility and intrusiveness are important considerations. The local network network approach has many advantages here, which are traded off against a loss of information on higher-order network properties. From the standpoint of data representation, the issues of parsimony, flexibility and goodness-of-fit measures become important criteria. Here, too, the local network approach can take advantage of existing statistical methods for estimation and inference. The tradeoff again is loss of higher-order network effects, but it is precisely such effects, and the dependencies they create among observations, which are problematic in the context of traditional statistical methods.

3   Some Examples

Does selective mixing really matter in the spread of disease? The answer is yes, and this section will present several examples based on the spread of HIV that show the strength and variability of these effects. The examples have been chosen to highlight two dimensions of selective mixing that are realistic and important for disease transmission dynamics: the assortative-disassortative continuum, and the stability of the attributes on which selection is based. Simulations in all cases use compartmental models for disease transmission and log-linear methods for incorporating local network mixing data. HIV-related biological parameters are the same in all cases: infectivity is varied from 0.01-0.1/partnership for gay and heterosexual populations respectively (Fischl *et al.* 1987, Peterman *et al.* 1988, Wiley *et al.* 1989), and for simplicity is modeled as constant throughout the infectious period (but see Longini *et al.* 1989), the incubation period is 10 years (Taylor *et al.* 1991), and time from AIDS to death is 2 years; both periods are modeled with simple exponential functions. Vital dynamics are included, though set to produce fairly stable populations in the absence of disease-induced mortality. In all but one case, the mixing matrices are based on observed behavioral data. Selective mixing is compared to proportional mixing using a 'prevalence ratio': the ratio of infection generated when the simulation is run using selective mixing to that generated when it is run using proportional mixing. When this ratio is larger than 1, selective mixing generates relatively more infection.

Case 1: Race/Ethnicity-matching among heterosexuals

Stable attributes with loose and variable assortative matching

Rates of HIV infection and clinical AIDS in the heterosexual population are much higher among Blacks and Hispanics in the US than among whites (Centers for Disease Control 1991a,b). Because the original focus of heterosexual infection was among IDUs, there is some question whether the epidemic will continue to spread sexually to non-IDUs, and whether patterns of race and ethnicity matching in sexual behavior are strong enough to decouple the HIV epidemics in the different subgroups. The AIDS in Multi-Ethnic Neighborhoods Survey (AMEN), a random sample of adults in 3 high-risk neighborhoods of San Francisco, has collected sexual network data that make it possible to examine parts of this question (Catania *et al.* 1992). The race and ethnicity mixing matrix of sexual partners from this study is presented in Figure 3. Given the sample neighborhoods, the contact rates here, about 2 new partners/year, are likely to be somewhat higher than in the general population.

The results of simulating the sexual transmission of HIV in this population are presented in the four panels of Figure 4. Simulations based on an infectivity of 0.01/partnership do not sustain the epidemic in this population (panels (a) and (b)). In order to raise the reproductive rate above threshold, infectivity would have to be on the order of 0.1/partnership (panels c and d). At this level, the effects of mixing can be clearly seen. Assortative mix-

Men:	Women:					Contact		Black	Latina	White	Other	Margins
	Black	Latina	White	Other	Pairs	Rate						
Black	506	32	69	26	633	2.61		36.23				1.00
Latino	23	308	114	38	483	1.61			8.24			3.16
White	26	46	599	68	739	2.01				3.97		5.70
Other	10	14	47	32	103	1.56					1.75	12.24
Pairs	565	400	829	164	1958			1.00	1.21	1.36	2.32	0.31
Contact rate	1.58	2.00	2.53	2.73	2.07	2.04						

Initial prevalence:
	Black	Latina	White	Other
males:	1.8%	2.4%	3.7%	2.2%
females:	0.5%	0.7%	0.3%	0.0%

Figure 3: Race and ethnicity matching among heterosexuals. The first table presents the mixing matrix observed in the AMEN study and the race and sex-specific seroprevalence, the second table schematically presents the exponentiated coefficients from the best fitting log-linear model.

ing lowers overall seroprevalence (panel c) but it turns out this is largely a composition effect, as it lowers prevalence among whites, the largest group. At the subgroup level, the effects of the assortative bias vary strongly, interacting with other characteristics of the transmission process (panel d). The initial effects depend on initial prevalence. Where initial prevalence is high, as among whites here, assortative mixing acts to intensify within-group spread, increasing rates of infection relative to proportional mixing. Where initial seroprevalence is low, as it is among blacks here, assortative mixing helps to keep it low. These initial effects may be transient, however. If the group has a relatively lower contact rate, as whites do here, transmission is reduced by within-group selection and eventually leads to lower levels of infection. If the group has a relatively higher contact rate, as Blacks do here, within-group selection amplifies transmission, leading to higher levels of infection. Where both initial prevalence and activity level are low, and the assortative bias is relatively strong, selective mixing always leads to lower levels of infection. This pattern can be seen in the Latin subgroup.

These simulations show that even when the effects of selective mixing are small at the aggregate level, they may be quite pronounced at the subgroup level. While overall seroprevalence is reduced by about 5%, subgroup prevalence may be as much as 20-40% higher (or lower).

Case 2: Sexual preference matching

Stable attributes, strong assortative and disassortative matching

One of the most frequently asked questions about the future of HIV trans-

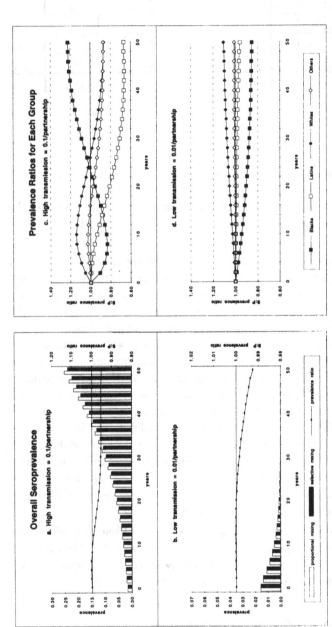

Figure 4: Effects of race and ethnicity matching on seroprevalence. Panels (a) and (b) display the overall seroprevalence in the population under different mixing and contact scenarios in the bars, and the ratio of selective to proportional mixing in the dashed line. Panels (c) and (d) display the four group-specific prevalence ratios for high and low infectivity scenarios. When infectivity is low, the epidemic dies out. When infectivity is high enough to sustain the epidemic, assortative mixing lowers overall seroprevalance, but either raises or lowers group-specific prevalence, depending on contact rates, the strength of the assortative bias, and initial levels of seroprevalence.

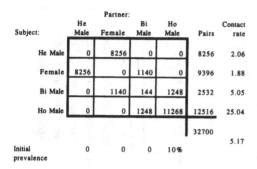

Subject:	Partner: He Male	Female	Bi Male	Ho Male	Pairs	Contact rate		He Male	Female	Bi Male	Ho Male	Margins
He Male	0	8256	0	0	8256	2.06		0		0	0	1.00
Female	8256	0	1140	0	9396	1.88			0		0	.91
Bi Male	0	1140	144	1248	2532	5.05						1.10
Ho Male	0	0	1248	11268	12516	25.04					1.0	9.97
					32700							4.53
						5.17						
Initial prevalence	0	0	0	10%								

Figure 5: Sexual preference matching (simulated data). The first table presents the mixing matrix of simulated data on sex and sexual preference matching for the high-activity, no assortative bias scenario. Initial prevalence was set at 10% of the homosexual male population. The second table schematically presents the exponentiated coefficients from the log-linear model used to produce the mixing matrix. The shaded cells indicate this is a model of symmetry, so the lower triangle and margins have the same parameters as the upper.

mission in the US is whether the epidemic will spread from gay males to the heterosexual population. The potential for this spread is a function of two things: the size and mixing patterns of the bisexual bridge population and the contact rates for the different subgroups. While some data exist on group-specific contact rates, there are no data on the prevalence and mixing patterns of bisexuals, making simulated data the only way to address this question. The example here uses a log-linear model to generate simulated contact matrices under various mixing and activity level conditions. Four conditions were simulated: high and low levels of activity among homosexual men (25 and 2 new partners/year) and two levels of mixing with bisexuals, regulated by setting the odds-ratio of the bottom right quadrant of the matrix. When this odds-ratio is 1, there is no assortative bias among homosexual and bisexual males. Figure 5 presents the contact matrix for the high activity, no assortative bias condition, and the corresponding exponentiated log-linear parameters.

The effects of the activity and mixing assumptions can be seen in Figure 6.

The activity effects dominate in this set of simulations, with the lower level generating substantially lower seroprevalence (panels a and b). Selective mixing, however, also has strong effects, as the heterosexual population

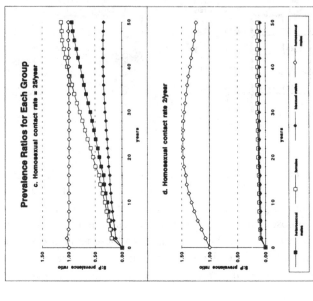

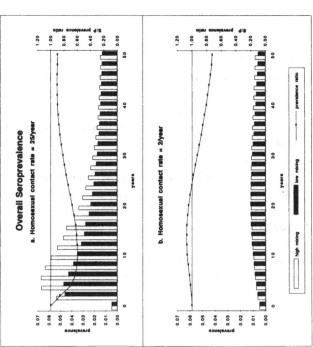

Figure 6: Effects of sexual preference mixing on seroprevalence. Panels (a) and (b) display the overall seroprevalence in the population under different mixing and contact scenarios in the bars, and the ratio of selective to 'proportional' mixing in the dashed line. Panels (c) and (d) display the four group-specific prevalence ratios for high and low contact scenarios. When contact rates are high, selective mixing reduces transmission from the initially infected group to the other three groups, but this shielding declines over time, especially for heterosexuals. When contact is low, there is little spread beyond the seeded group, and the shielding effect of selective mixing slightly increases over time.

is not infected under any of the four scenarios. Even in the high-contact simulations (panels c and d), which generate 50-70% infection rates among the homosexual and bisexual men, the combination of a limited bridge population and lower transmission in the heterosexual population prevents the epidemic from spreading further. When contact rates are low, assortative mixing displays the same patterns as in the race-matching example, raising within-group transmission among the initially infected group by about 50%, and shielding the other three groups, lowering their prevalence by around 90%. When contact rates are high, the story is a bit more complicated. Assortative mixing reduces overall prevalence, but these effects diminish over time. Among the individual subgroups, the assortative shielding effect is strongest for bisexuals. This effect is also initially strong for heterosexuals, but then, counterintuitively, it rises over time and actually becomes larger than 1 for females. The reason is because assortative homosexual mixing here increases bisexual-female contacts by more than it reduces the bisexual infection rate. Under assortative mixing, bisexual contacts with females rise by a factor of 3.7. Part of this is due to the mixing bias (46%), and part to the lower infection, and thus lower AIDS-related population depletion, for bisexuals (54%). The bisexual infection rate is roughly 1/3 lower under assortative mixing. As a result, the increase in contacts outweighs the decrease in prevalence, and there is eventually more spread from bisexuals to heterosexuals under the assortative mixing scenario. In neither case, however, does the prevalence among heterosexuals rise above 1%. Thus, the existence of a bridge population does not in itself guarantee that the epidemic will spread. If the level of activity in the uninfected population is below reproductive threshold, the infections transmitted by the bridge population will not be sustained.

In sum, selective mixing based on stable characteristics permits group isolation. It allows the disease to spread pervasively some groups without ever gaining a foothold elsewhere. One implication of this is that resources should be focused where they will have the most impact, not on a flank where the fear may be high but the the the risk is demonstrably low.

Case 3: Age-Matching among Heterosexuals

Changing attributes, strong assortative matching

Among heterosexuals, one of the strongest forms of assortative mixing is age-matching. If this matching were perfect, young cohorts would never become infected by older ones, and the disease would disappear from the population as the infected cohorts eventually died. Age-matching is not perfect, however, and contact rates tend to be higher among younger persons than among older. As in the examples above, assortative bias coupled with higher contact rates might instead raise infection rates for the younger cohorts. The

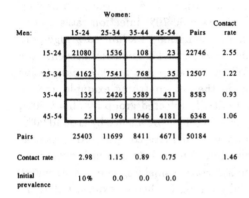
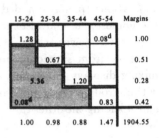

Figure 7: Age matching among heterosexuals. The first table presents the mixing matrix for heterosexuals constructed from 1991 US Census marriage tables and General Social Survey data on age-specific sexual contact rates. Initial prevalence was set at 10% of the youngest age group for both sexes. The second table schematically presents the exponentiated coefficients from the best fitting log-linear model. The shading identifies cells with the same selection effect, in this case a strong asymmetric bias towards older men-younger women. The distance effect is only shown in the upper right and lower left corners, but it affects all the off-diagonal cells. This effect requires only one parameter, and takes the form of a decrement, $\beta^{|d|}$, where d is the distance from the diagonal. Here, each step off the diagonal reduces the probability of a partnership by 92%.

strength of the assortative bias will therefore determine the degree of infection in younger cohorts and the future of the disease. There is one survey that has collected sexual network data on age-matching in the US adult population, but was is not publicly available when this analysis was performed. What is used as a proxy here comes from the US Census crosstabulations of age of husbands and wives (United States Bureau of the Census, 1991), supplemented by data from the General Social Survey on age-specific sexual contact rates (Davis and Smith 1992, Smith 1991, 1992). The resulting mixing matrix is presented in Figure 7.

The effects of age-matching on the epidemic can be seen in Figure 8. Here, as in the previous example, the contact rates are too low to support an epidemic when infectivity is at 0.01/partnership. The reproductive threshold occurs at around 0.05/partnership, and a sustained epidemic in the youngest group requires infectivity closer to 0.1/partnership. The results in Figure 8 are based on the 0.1 level. The effects of mixing are similar for each level of infectivity, but easier to see at higher levels.

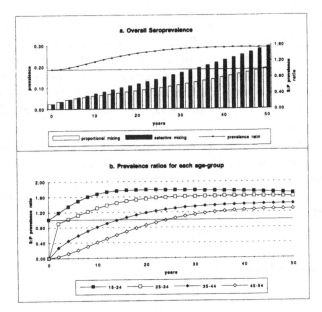

Figure 8: Effects of heterosexual age matching on seroprevalence. Panel (a) displays the overall seroprevalance in the population under proportional and selective mixing scenarios in the bars, and the prevalence ratio in the dashed line. Panel (b) displays the age-group specific prevalence ratios. Here assortative mixing raises seroprevalence in every age group.

In contrast to the two previous examples, selective mixing here increases overall seroprevalence by about 60% (panel a), and eventually increases the prevalence in every age group as well (panel b). The assortative bias generates higher levels of infection among the youngest group from the start, due, as in the previous examples, to the combination of assortative bias and higher contact rates. At its peak, assortative mixing raises prevalence by 80% over proportional mixing. The older groups, with lower contact rates and initially lower prevalence, are shielded by the assortative bias at first. But this effect is transitory because age, unlike race or sexual preference, is an attribute that changes over time. As a result, the infections are sent up the age chain in two ways: through sexual contacts between age groups, and by the aging process. While assortative mixing reduces the contacts between groups, it does not affect the aging process, so the higher prevalence it generates among the youngest group becomes, as they age, higher prevalence among the older groups.

The relative impact of aging and sexual transmission can be observed by comparing these results to models run without any sexual transmission (i.e., models where the infectivity is set to 0). The effects of aging are larger for the groups closer to the initially seeded group, as might be expected. Aging accounts for about 50% of the infections among the 25–34 year olds, 16% among the 35–44 year olds, and 6% among the 45–54 year olds. These effects are slightly stronger under selective mixing, as the assortative bias reduces the extent of sexual transmission between groups. When infectivity is too low to sustain the epidemic over time, the infection moves like a bulge through the age chain, and the highest rates of infection are eventually found among the older groups.

When the attributes that define mixing groups change over time, therefore, mixing may not isolate infection in groups but spread it more effectively. This has strong implications for the way in which HIV may spread in minority communities in the US. While race and ethnicity-matching may serve to decouple the epidemics, age-matching within racial and ethnic subgroups may serve to amplify within-group spread.

Case 4: Age-Matching among Gay Men

Changing attributes, loose assortative matching

As in the example above, the future of HIV among gay men in the US will be determined largely by the rates of new infection among its younger cohort. Age-matching again might be expected to provide a partial shield against the transmission of HIV from the higher prevalence older cohorts. The assortative bias is likely to be looser among gay men than among heterosexuals, however, and surveys suggest that young gay men continue to practice unsafe sex at higher rates than their older peers (Ekstrand and Coates 1990, Hays *et al.* 1990). Whether the interaction between mixing and contact rates is sufficient to sustain the epidemic in this population is thus an open question. Data from the Longitudinal AIDS Impact Project (LAIP), one of the few studies of gay men to collect any form of network data, will be used to examine this question. LAIP is a 7-year cohort study based on a stratified convenience sample of gay men in New York City (Martin and Dean 1990). The age-matching matrix for insertive and receptive anal intercourse partners from this study is presented below in Figure 9.

The infection is seeded into the 35–54 year olds (groups 3 and 4 in the matrix). Contact rates change over the simulation period from about 13/year to about 1/yr, based on LAIP data. Initial simulations were calibrated against AIDS surveillance data in New York City for the risk group 'men who have sex with men' to ensure that early patterns in the epidemic were matched. The calibrated model suggests that the current patterns of behavior are just on the boundary of reducing the epidemic spread below the reproductive threshold. If these data on behavior are accurate, and the patterns are maintained in the future, then the disease would eventually die out in the absence of other sources of infection (e.g., links with IDUs). If, on the other hand, respondents

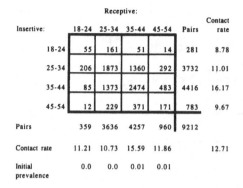
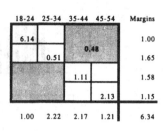

Insertive:	Receptive: 18-24	25-34	35-44	45-54	Pairs	Contact rate		18-24	25-34	35-44	45-54	Margins
18-24	55	161	51	14	281	8.78		6.14				1.00
25-34	206	1873	1360	292	3732	11.01			0.51	0.48		1.65
35-44	85	1373	2474	483	4416	16.17				1.11		1.58
45-54	12	229	371	171	783	9.67					2.13	1.15
Pairs	359	3636	4257	960	9212			1.00	2.22	2.17	1.21	6.34
Contact rate	11.21	10.73	15.59	11.86		12.71						
Initial prevalence	0.0	0.0	0.01	0.01								

Figure 9: Age-matching among gay men. The first table presents the age-mixing matrix observed in the LAIP study for 1981, and initial age-specific prevalence is set for both insertive and receptive groups as shown. The second table schematically presents the exponentiated coefficients from the best fitting log-linear model. The shading represents cells with the same selection effect, here a 'blocking' effect that reduces the probability of a partnership by 52% in the off-diagonal quadrants.

have under-reported the number of new partners they have, the result could be quite different. With about two new partners per year (instead of the one reported), the disease would instead become endemic, with seroprevalence levels of about 50% among the exposed population in the oldest group, and about 25% among the youngest.

The mixing effects can be seen in Figure 10. In contrast to the previous example, age-matching here initially raises seroprevalence, but eventually lowers it (panel a). This pattern is reproduced for each age-group (panel b), but the reasons are fairly complicated.

For the initially seeded groups, the assortative bias raises within-group contacts by 25-100%, leading to faster within-group spread at first. Within five years, however, the higher infection rates begin to lead to greater population depletion in these two groups. This translates into fewer infections passed down the age chain, and, by virtue of the aging process, eventually leads to lower seroprevalence among these older groups.

The key to the rest is what happens to the second group, the 25-34 year olds. The assortative bias here lowers contacts with the older two groups by 20-25%, but the 40-60% higher infection rates in the older groups offset the contact reduction, and the net result is 20-30% more infections transmitted to this group. During the first five years, while contact rates are still high, the assortative bias amplifies the higher rates of infection entering the group,

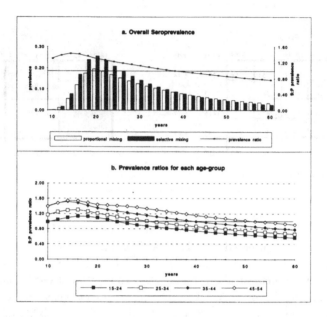

Figure 10: Effects of homosexual age matching on seroprevalence. Panel
(a) displays the overall seroprevalance in the population under selective and
proportional mixing scenarios in the bars, and the prevalence ratio in the
dashed line. Panel (b) displays the age-group specific prevalence ratios.
Age-matching again increases prevalence in all groups, but the effect declines
over time, and the assortative bias eventually acts as a shield.

and the result is prevalence levels 40% above those found under proportional
mixing. Eventually, however, the population depletion in the older two groups
reduces the number of contacts sufficiently that the assortative shielding effect
begins to dominate, and prevalence is lowered relative to proportional mixing.

The youngest group is initially the least active here, and the assortative
bias is strongest for them, so one might have expected selective mixing to
lower their prevalence from the beginning. The 'block' effect found in the
off-diagonal quadrants of the mixing matrix data, however, is strong enough
to raise the number of contacts between this group and their 25–34 year old
neighbors by about 25%. Coupled with the 25–30% higher rates of infection
among 25–34 year olds, these additional contacts translate into higher rates of
infection among the youngest group as well. Once prevalence begins to decline
in the 25–34 year olds (due to population depletion in the older groups), it
also begins to decline in this group. As in the heterosexual age-matching
example, the lower rates of infection for the young eventually work their way
up the age chain to become lower rates of infection for older groups, cf. Morris
and Dean (1994) for a more complete discussion.

Assortative age-matching can therefore have a shielding effect, but the timing of this effect depends on other parameters of the transmission process. Rates of contact and AIDS-related population depletion determine whether the assortative bias increases or reduces rates of infection over time.

4 Conclusion

These examples make it clear that network structures matter for disease transmission. The type of attributes that define network boundaries also matter, and can channel diffusion into markedly different paths. Where attributes like race and sexual preference form stable mixing groups, the potential for spread from a seeded population depends on bridges, initial seroprevalence, and eventually group-specific contact rates. With a small bridge, infection may remain isolated, even under fairly extreme conditions, provided contact rates in other groups are below the reproductive threshold. Where attributes like age instead form ordinal, fluid mixing groups, the potential for spread is much higher. Here the mixing structure is characterized by a dual transmission regime, with some infections carried up the age ladder along with each cohort, and others passed by sexual contact. This mixing structure makes the epidemic much more likely to spread, even with lower contact rates. Assortative age-matching can provide some shielding effect to younger cohorts, but the strength of this effect depends on the strength of the bias and on other aspects of the transmission process, especially disease-related population depletion.

Given the complicated way that mixing interacts with other factors, it may not be possible to develop simple descriptions of 'mixing effects'. Analytic results should continue to be sought, however, and this is an important area for future research. The initial explorations here suggest that the assortative/disassortative continuum and the stable/changing attributes distinction must be incorporated into any future analytic development.

The importance of stable and changing attributes has a parallel in spatial models: 'nearest neighbor' models can be thought of as forcing nodes to occupy a stable position, while models that permit long jumps allow for some notion of changing position. From this perspective, people can be thought of as inhabiting a multidimensional space. Some of these dimensions describe their coordinates in the physical world, but the remainder describe their position in social terms, and their 'distance' from others. The integration of spatial and social networks is necessary to provide a comprehensive framework for non-random mixing. This is an important goal for future research.

References

Altmann, M. (1993) 'Reinterpreting network measures for models of disease transmission', *Soc. Net.* **15**, 1–17.

Anderson, R.M., Gupta, S. and Ng, W. (1990) 'The Significance of sexual partner contact networks for the transmission dynamics of HIV', *JAIDS* **3**, 417–429.

Berkowitz, S.D. (1982) *An Introduction to Structural Analysis: the Network Approach to Social Research*, Butterworth, Toronto.

Blanchard, P., Bolz, G. and Krueger, T. (1988) 'Mathematical modelling on random graphs of the spread of sexually transmitted diseases with emphasis on the HIV infection'. In *Dynamics and Stochastic Processes – Theory and Applications, Lisbon*, Springer-Verlag, Berlin.

Blythe, S., Castillo-Chavez, C., Palmer, J. and Cheng, M. (1991) 'Towards a unified theory of mixing and pair formation', *Math. Biosci.* **107**, 349–407.

Burt, R.S. and Minor, M.J. (1983) *Applied Network Analysis*, Sage, Beverly Hills, CA.

Castillo-Chavez, C. and Blythe, S.P. (1989) 'Mixing framework for social/sexual behavior' In *Mathematical and Statistical Approaches to AIDS Epidemiology*, C. Castillo-Chavez (ed.), Springer-Verlag, Berlin, 275–288.

Catania, J.A., Coates, T.J., Kegels, S. and Fullilove, M.T. (1992) 'Condom use in multi-ethnic neighborhoods of San Francisco: The population-based AMEN (AIDS in Multi-Ethnic Neighborhoods) Study', *AJPH* **82**, 287–7.

Centers for Disease Control (1991a) HIV/AIDS Surveillance Report. January: 1–22.

Centers for Disease Control (1991b) *National HIV Serosurveillance Summary.* Rockville, MD: Centers for Disease Control, Sage, Beverly Hills, CA

Davis, J.A. and Smith, T.W. (1992) *The NORC General Social Survey*, Newbury Park, California.

Ekstrand, M.L. and Coates, T.J. (1990) 'Maintenance of safer sexual behaviors and predictors of risky sex: the San Francisco mens's health study', *AJPH* **80**, 973–77.

Fischl, M., Dickinson, G., Scott, G., Klimas, N., Fletcher, M.A. and Parks, W. (1987) 'Evaluation of heterosexual partners, children, and household contacts of adults with AIDS', *JAMA* **257**, 640–44.

Frank, O. and Strauss, D. (1986) 'Markov Graphs', *JASA* **81**, 832–842.

Gupta, S. and Anderson, R. (1989) 'Networks of sexual contacts: implications for the pattern of spread of HIV', *AIDS* **3**, 807–817.

Haraldsdottir, S., Gupta, S. and Anderson, R. (1992) 'Preliminary studies of sexual networks in a male homosexual community in Iceland', *JAIDS* **5**, 374–381.

Harary, F., Norman, R.Z. and Cartwright, D. (1965) *Structural Models: An Introduction to the Theory of Directed Graphs*, Wiley, New York.

Hays, R.B., Kegeles, S.M. and Coates, T.J. (1990) 'High HIV risk-taking among young gay men', *AIDS* **4**, 901–907.

Hethcote, H. and Yorke, J.A. (1984) *Gonorrhea Transmission Dynamics and Control*, Springer-Verlag, Berlin.

Holland, P. and Leinhardt, S. (1970) 'A method for detecting structure in sociometric data', *AJS* **70**, 492–513.

Hyman, J. and Stanley, E. (1988) 'Using mathematical models to understand the AIDS epidemic', *Math. Biosci.* **90**, 415–473.

Jacquez, J.A., Simon, C.P. and Koopman, J. (1989) 'Structured Mixing: Heterogeneous mixing by the definition of activity groups' In *Mathematical and Statistical Approaches to AIDS Epidemiology*, C. Castillo-Chavez (ed.), Springer-Verlag, Berlin, 301–315.

Koopman, J., Simon, C.P., Jacquez, J. and Park, T. (1989) 'Selective contact within structured mixing groups; with an application to the analysis of HIV transmission risk from oral and anal sex' In *Mathematical and Statistical Approaches to AIDS Epidemiology*, C. Castillo-Chavez (ed.), Springer-Verlag, Berlin, 316–349.

Kretzschmar, M., Reinking, D.P., van Zessen, G., Brouwers, H. and Jager, J.C. (1993) 'Network models: from paradigm to mathematical tool'. To appear in *Modeling the AIDS Epidemic*, E. H. Kaplan and M. Brandeau (eds.).

Laumann, E.O. (1973) *Bonds of Pluralism: The Form and Subsance of Urban Social Networks*, Wiley, New York.

Leinhardt, S. (1977) *Social Networks: A Developing Paradigm*, Academic Press, New York.

Longini, I.M., Clark, W.S., Haber, M. and Horsburgh, R. (1989) 'The stages of HIV infection: waiting times and infection transmission probabilities' In *Mathematical and Statistical Approaches to AIDS Epidemiology*, C. Castillo-Chavez (ed.), Springer–Verlag, Berlin, 111–136.

Marsden, P.V. (1981) 'Models and methods for characterizing the structural parameters of groups', *Soc. Networks*, **3**, 1–27.

Martin, J.L. and Dean, L. (1990) 'Development of a community sample of gay men for an epidemiologic study of AIDS', *Am. Beh. Sci.* **33**, 546–561.

Mollison, D. and Barbour, A.D. (1989) 'Epidemics and random graphs'. In *Stochastic Processes in Epidemic Theory*, J. P. Gabriel, C. Lefèvre and P. Picard (eds.), Springer Verlag, Berlin, 86–89.

Morris, M. (1991) 'A log-linear modeling framework for selective mixing', *Math. Biosci.* **107**, 349–377.

Morris, M. (1995) 'Behavior change and non-homogeneous mixing'. In *Infectious Diseases of Humans*, V. Isham and G. Medley (eds.), Cambridge University Press, Cambridge, to appear.

Morris, M. and Dean, L. (1994) 'The effect of behavior change on long-term HIV prevalence among homosexual men', *Amer. J. Epidemiol.* **140**, 217–232.

Pattison, P. (1993) *Algebraic Models for Social Networks*, Cambridge University Press, Cambridge.

Peterman, T., Stoneburner, R., Allen, J. Jaffe, H. and Curran, J. (1988) 'Risk of HIV transmission from heterosexual adults with transfusion associated infections', *JAMA* **259**, 55–58.

Pollard, A.H. (1948) 'The measurement of reproductivity', *J. Inst. Act.* **74**, 288–305.

Rapoport, A. (1952) 'Ignition phenomena in random nets', *Bull. Math. Biophysics* **13**, 85–91.

Rapoport, A. (1957) 'Contribution to the theory of random and biased nets', *Bull. Math. Biophysics* **19**, 257–277.

Rapoport, A. (1980) 'A probabilistic approach to networks', *Soc. Networks* **2**, 1–18.

Sattenspiel, L. (1987) 'Population structure and the spread of disease', *Human Biology* **59**, 411–438.

Schoen, R. (1982) 'Generalizing the life table model to incorporate interactions between the sexes'. In *Multidimensional Mathematical Demography*, K. C. Land and A. Rogers (eds.), Academic Press, New York, 385–443.

Smith, T.W. (1991) 'Adult sexual behavior in 1989: Number of partners, frequency of intercourse and risk of AIDS', *Family Planning Perspectives* **23**, 102–107.

Smith, T.W. (1992) 'A methodological analysis of the sexual behavior question on the General Social Surveys', *J. Off. Stat.* **8**, 309–325.

Strauss, D. and Ikeda, M. (1990) 'Pseudolikelihood estimation for social networks', *JASA* **85**, 204–12.

Taylor, J., Kuo, J.-M. and Detels, R. (1991) 'Is the incubation period of AIDS lengthening?', *JAIDS* **4**, 69–75.

United States Bureau of the Census (1991) 'Household and family characteristics: March 1991, Table 14'. In *Current Population Reports*, Series P-20, (ed). U.S. Government Printing Office, Washington, DC, 146.

Wasserman, S. and Faust, K. (1994) *Social Network Analysis: Methods and Applications*, Cambridge University Press, Cambridge.

Wiley, J., Herschkorn, S. and Padian, N.S. (1989) 'Heterogeneity in the probability of HIV transmission per sexual contact: the case of male-to- female transmission in penile-vaginal intercourse', *Stat. Med.* **8**, 93–102.

The Effect of Antigenic Diversity on Endemic Prevalence

Sunetra Gupta
Katharine Trenholme
Martin Cox
Roy Anderson
Karen Day

Summary

The rapid rise with age in exposure to *Plasmodium falciparum* malaria has generally been ascribed to its high transmissibility. In this chapter, we propose that this interpretation is only valid for infections that induce lifelong immunity, and thus cannot be applied to malaria. The delay in development of protective immunity to malaria permits a rapid increase in exposure with age for low values of the basic reproductive rate (transmissibility) that are consistent with epidemiological observations, and particularly with realistic measures of the duration of infectiousness. The long period required to develop protective immunity to malaria can be explained by the antigenic diversity of the parasite. We present data on patterns of seroconversion to 5 antigenically distinct isolates of *P. falciparum* in a holoendemic malarious area, showing that exposure to any one serotype rises slowly with age. This indicates that malaria can be seen as a basket of mildly transmissible antigenic types, each of which may induce lifelong serotype-specific immunity. The basic reproductive rate of malaria, as calculated from this data appears to be between 6 and 7, which is an order of magnitude lower than typical previous estimates.

1 Introduction

Plasmodium falciparum malaria is one of the major causes of child mortality and morbidity in tropical and sub-tropical regions. The number of yearly reported cases is in the range of 200 million with more than 2 million deaths (Struchler 1984). The success of global malaria eradication programmes has been limited by the development of drug resistance in the parasite and of resistance to insecticides in the mosquito vector (Bruce-Chwatt 1988). The design of vaccines against malaria is complicated by the complex interaction of the parasite with the immune system of the host, as well as the non-linear dynamical consequences of the relationship between diminishing exposure to infection and the development and maintenance of natural immunity at the population level (Anderson, May and Gupta 1989, Halloran, Struchiner and Spielman 1989, Struchiner, Halloran and Spielman 1989). However, by far the most important impediment to vaccination has been the perceived high transmissibility, or basic reproductive rate (R_0), of the parasite (Anderson and May 1991). Such high values typically derive from the analysis of the rapid rise with age in the proportion of individuals that have been exposed to *P. falciparum* infection. In this paper, we propose that such an interpretation is valid only for infections that induce lifelong immunity, and therefore cannot be applied to malaria, as immunity to the latter appears only to develop after a long period of exposure. Using age-structured mathematical models, we explore the effects of a delay in the development of immunity on the age-exposure profile of an endemic infectious agent within a given host population.

It has been suggested that the long period required to develop immunity to malaria is a consequence of the antigenic diversity of the malaria parasite (Day and Marsh 1990). The molecular characterisation of the *P. falciparum* genome has revealed that many of the natural immunogens are polymorphic (Anders and Smythe 1989). Genetic diversity of *P. falciparum* has been demonstrated in the field by differences in drug resistance, chromosome size and isoenzymes, and also by serological differences in antigens (Kemp *et al.* 1990, Forsyth *et al.* 1989, Conway and McBride 1991). In this chapter, we discuss the impact of antigenic diversity of the age-profile of malaria, and attempt to calculate its basic reproductive rate by using patterns of seroconversion to five antigenically distinct isolates in a hyperendemic malarious area (Madang region of Papua New Guinea).

2   The basic reproductive rate of malaria

By definition, the number of infections in a community can only grow if every infected individual can infect at least one other person. In a totally suscepti-ble population, this information is provided by a combination of parameters influencing parasite transmission, known as the basic reproductive rate. The basic reproductive rate of malaria may be given as:

$$R_0 = m\alpha^2 b L_M D c \qquad (2.1)$$

where m is the number of mosquitoes per human host, α is the mosquito biting rate (which is raised to the second power as two biting events must take place to complete the cycle), b denotes the probability that an infective mosquito bite will produce an infection in the host, L_M is the average lifespan of the mosquito, D is the average duration of infectiousness in the human host, and c is the probability an infectious 'feed' will lead to sporozoite production in the vector.

This expression is a modification of the R_0 associated with the Ross-Macdonald model for malaria (reviewed by Aron and May 1982). In the latter, an infective feed is assumed always to cause an infection in the mosquito (i.e. $c = 1$) and the duration of infectiousness, D, is assumed to be coterminus with the duration of infection. The basic reproductive rate may be much reduced by taking into account the distinction between infection and infectiousness as the duration of infectiousness may be considerably shorter than the duration of infection. The measurement of the duration of infectiousness is complicated by uncertainties regarding the biology of the sexual stages of the parasite (reviewed in Gupta 1992). Furthermore, 'the association between gametocytaemia and infectiousness is not perfect' (Nedelman 1988) as certain criteria must be fulfilled before gametocytes can successfully infect and fertilize within a mosquito. The average duration of infectiousness in the human host may thus be of the order of a few weeks in contrast to several months of parasitaemia. Epidemiological support for this hypothesis may be obtained by comparing the prevalence of parasitaemia and gametocytaemia in field surveys. For instance, the Garki Project (Molineaux and Gramiccia 1980) note that the average prevalence of *P. falciparum* parasites is about 80% in the wet season, while the proportion of individuals positive for gametocytes is less than 20%, implying that the duration of gametocytaemia (which may be longer than the duration of infectiousness) is 1/4 the average duration of parasitaemia.

3 Age-exposure curves and the basic reproductive rate

An age-exposure graph represents the proportion of individuals in different age groups that have been exposed to a particular disease agent. In the case of many common viral and bacterial infections, these profiles may be constructed from serological surveys for the presence or absence of specific antibodies (Anderson and May 1991). It can be shown that if these infections induce lifelong immunity, the average age, A, at which an individual typically acquires an infection is inversely related to its basic reproductive rate. Conversely, the basic reproductive rate, R_0 may be obtained from an age-exposure profile, using the simple relationship:

$$R_0 = L/A \qquad (3.1)$$

where L is the average lifespan of the host (Anderson and May 1991). As clearly indicated by (3.1), the average age at infection is low (1-2) for highly transmissible diseases such as measles, and higher (9-10) for less transmissible diseases such as rubella. It should be mentioned that large variations may exist in the basic reproductive rates and concomitant average ages at infection for the same disease between different communities (reviewed in Anderson and May 1991).

4   Age-exposure profiles for malaria

Age-exposure profiles for *P. falciparum* malaria (henceforth, *Pf*) may be obtained by serological methods such as passive indirect haemagglutination (IHA), indirect fluorescent antibody tests (IFA) and tests involving the detection of precipitating antibodies (Precipitin test). Serological surveys conducted using these three methods in the Garki project unequivocally indicate that the proportion of infants positive for *Pf* antibodies rises sharply by age after an initial decline associated with the loss of maternal antibodies, so that over 80% of children are exposed to *Pf* by the age of one year. If the same relationship were to exist between the basic reproductive rate and the average age at infection as defined for infections inducing lifelong immunity in (3.1), one might directly postulate that the basic reproductive rate of *Pf* was extremely high, with values of the order of 60-80.

The principal difference between a malaria transmission system and the microparasitic disease systems for which (3.1) holds, is the lack of development of lifelong immunity upon infection with the malaria parasite. To explore whether this difference in establishment of immunity could alter the the age-exposure profile of malaria, we may employ an age-structured mathematical model for malaria transmission involving overlapping categories of exposed, x, and 'immune', z, hosts. Unexposed hosts are assumed to acquire infection from infectious (= infected, for simplicity) mosquitoes, present in proportion y in the vector population. Once exposed, an individual remains in the 'exposed' for life; hence the rate of loss of exposed individuals is identical to the community death rate, Thus, following the Ross-Macdonald model:

$$\frac{\delta x}{\delta a} + \frac{\delta x}{\delta t} = m\alpha b(1 - x)y - \mu x \qquad (4.1)$$

Similarly 'non-immunes' acquire infection from an infectious mosquito, and become immune. Immunity is lost at a rate r. Thus:

$$\frac{\delta z}{\delta a} + \frac{\delta z}{\delta t} = m\alpha b(1 - z)y - hz \qquad (4.2)$$

The proportion, y, of infectious mosquitoes, grows with contact with infectious hosts. The proportion of hosts infectious at any given time is assumed to

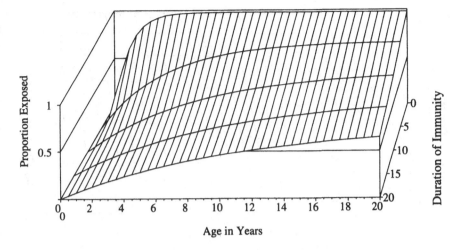

Figure 1: The age–prevalence of exposure, plotted as a function of the average duration of immunity in the population, H $(= 1/h)$, for a basic reproductive rate of 2.

be at instantaneous equilibrium, as loss of infectiousness, at a rate σ, occurs on a much faster timescale than immunity loss. Since the event of infection confers both immunity and infectiousness, the gain terms are identical to both immune and infectious compartments. The proportion infectious may thus be given as $m\alpha b(1 - Z)/\sigma$, where Z is the total proportion of the population immune. Again, following the Ross-Macdonald model:

$$\frac{dy}{dt} = \alpha(1 - y)\frac{m\alpha b(1 - Z)y}{\sigma} - \mu_m y$$

$$= \frac{m\alpha^2 b}{\sigma}(1 - y)y\left(-\int z(a)l(a)da\right) - \mu_m y \qquad (4.3)$$

Age exposure profiles at endemic equilibrium may be extracted from this framework by setting the time derivatives to zero, and finding solutions to the resultant set of ordinary differential equations.

Figure 1 shows the results of such an exercise in terms of the proportions exposed of each age, plotted as a function of the average duration of immunity in the population, $H (= 1/h)$. The surface confirms that a low population average duration of immunity can cause proportions exposed to rise sharply with age, even when the basic reproductive rate of the infection is low. The basic reproductive rate used in Figure 1 is 2; we provide for comparison in Figure 2, the age exposure profiles for a range of basic reproductive rates in the case where infection induces lifelong immunity ($h = \mu$). The steepness of age exposure profiles commonly encountered for malaria thus are not necessarily indicative of a high basic reproductive rate for the disease, but may instead

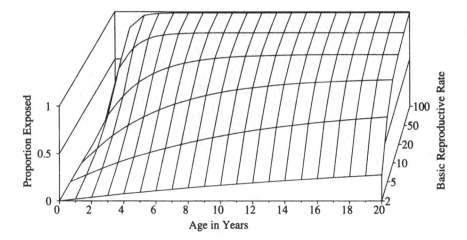

Figure 2: The age exposure profiles for a range of basic reproductive rates in the case where infection induces lifelong immunity (i.e. if $h = \mu$).

be a consequence of the low average duration of immunity in the population.

The average age at first infection (or exposure) where immunity endures for an average of $H \ (= 1/h)$ years, can be shown to be, to a good approximation,

$$A_H = H/R_0 \tag{4.4}$$

More generally, for Type II survivorship, $A = 1/\lambda^*$ yields

$$A_H = \frac{H + Dc\gamma}{R_0 - 1} \tag{4.5}$$

$$A = \frac{L + Dc\gamma}{R_0 - 1} \tag{4.6}$$

where $\gamma \ (= \alpha L_M)$ is the average number of times a mosquito bites during its lifetime. If both immunity and infectiousness are coterminus with the duration of infection then the former expression may be written as: $A = D(1 + \gamma)/(R_0 - 1)$, (Dietz 1988).

Despite rapid advances in the molecular characterisation of the parasite, and mechanisms of host response, the development and maintenance of protective immunity to *Pf* malaria is still very poorly understood. Young children in rural Africa may experience anywhere between 1 to 5 clinical attacks of malaria per year (Greenwood, Marsh and Snow 1991). It appears that older subjects do develop a functional but non-sterilising immunity that manifests itself in a reduction of clinical episodes. However, a substantial reduction in parasite rates (proportion of individuals with asexual malaria parasites) is only observed in adults. Parasite rates tend to peak in children of around 10 years of age, and slowly decline to low but significant levels in adults (Marsh 1992). The duration of immunity to further infection is thus very low in the age group 0–15 (as to be non-existent even), increasing slowly to higher levels in adults. As a result, the mean duration of protective immunity across all age classes, H, may much lower than the average lifespan of an individual, L. It can be shown that the ratio of the proportion of the total population exposed in the case where average duration of immunity is H, X_H, to the proportion exposed in the case where immunity is lifelong, X_L, is:

$$X_H/X_L = 1 - (1 - H/L)(1/R_0) \qquad (4.7)$$

The difference in total proportions exposed as a consequence of low levels of protective immunity is thus more apparent at low values of R_0. This is intuitively plausible, since the relative contribution of the absence of immediate protective immunity to the risk of exposure, mediated by higher levels of infection, is lower when the risk of exposure is very high, even with lifelong immunity, as a result of high R_0.

5   The effect of antigenic diversity on the age-exposure profile of malaria

It has been postulated that the delay in the development of protective immunity to *Pf* malaria may be a consequence of the antigenic diversity of the parasite, as it has commonly been observed that immunity develops only after exposure to various different antigenic types or 'strains' (Day and Marsh 1990). This collective immunity may simply be the aggregation of strain-specific responses, or alternatively may be due to the reinforcement of strain-transcending immunity through multiple exposure (Marsh and Howard 1986). If 'malaria' is indeed a basket of strains, each inducing some degree of protective immunity, we may expect to see a disjunction between the age-exposure profile of each strain and the age-exposure to 'malaria', where the latter is defined as the experience of any one of several strains. Indeed, in the limit where each strain confers lifelong immunity, exposure may rise very slowly with age for any particular strain, and yet rise rapidly with age for the disease construct of '*Pf* malaria'. Figure 3 presents a set of preliminary data for the rise in exposure by age to 5 *P. falciparum* isolates, differing in parasite-induced erythrocyte surface antigens (PIESA), serologically distinguishable by antibody mediated parasite infected cell agglutination (PICA) tests. The data was collected in the Madang region of Papua New Guinea, where year-round malaria transmission causes over 80% of children to be exposed to malaria by the age of 1 year. Figure 3 indicates however that the proportion exposed to any one particular isolate rises only slowly with time, and that less than 25%

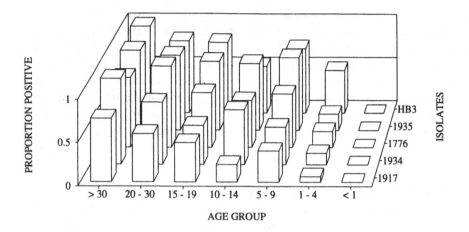

Figure 3: A set of data for the rise in exposure by age to 5 P. falciparum isolates, differing in parasite-induced erythrocyte surface antigens (PIESA).

of children will have typically seen the corresponding 'strain' or antigenic type by the age of 4 years. The HB3 isolate appears to be an exception which could be interpreted as a result of higher R_0, but is more likely to be explained by cross-reactivity patterns. Each strain thus exhibits an age-specific pattern of exposure that is consistent with the hypothesis that strain-specific immunity be endure for long periods. Exposure to the surface antigen associated with a single wild isolate in rural Gambians (Marsh *et al.* 1989) shows a similar age profile. Interestingly, this was the only immune factor that showed a consistent protective effect against clinical malaria, among a range of host immune responses to asexual blood stages examined for protective effects by Marsh and colleagues.

The average age of infection with any one of '*n*' different strains, where each essentially confers lifetime protection, is given by

$$A_n = \frac{L}{\sum R_{0i}} \tag{5.1}$$

where R_{0i} is the basic reproductive rate of strain i (Gupta *et al.* 1994). Comparing with (3.1), we see that 'malaria', as a composite of a variety of strains, behaves in the same manner as an infection inducing lifelong immunity with a high R_0, where the latter is an aggregate of the basic reproductive rates of the constituent strains. It should not be inferred however that 'malaria' defined in this manner has a high basic reproductive rate, since this definition also precludes the establishment of lifelong immunity upon a single exposure.

Figure 4 expresses the same data set as that of Figure 3 in terms of pro-

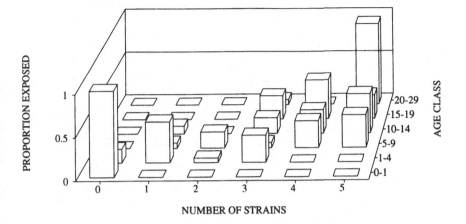

Figure 4: The data set in terms of proportions of each age class that have seen exactly 'n' serotypes or 'strains', as indicated on the axes.

portions of each age class that have seen exactly 'n' strains, as indicated on the axes. The pattern reveals that only in the adult classes will the majority of individuals have seen all five strains. Children under 5 years of age are likely have seen less than three strains.

The predicted proportion of individuals of age a that will have seen exactly 'n' strains out of 5, may be calculated simply as

$$^5C_n x(a)^n (1 - x(a))^{5-n},$$

given complete independence of strain transmission and assuming that basic reproductive rates are essentially similar between strains. If infection confers lifelong immunity, we may write

$$x(a) = 1 - e^{-(L/R_0)a} \qquad (5.2)$$

The matrix of proportions in age class that have seen exactly 'n' (more or less identical) strains may thus be calculated for a given value of R_0. Figure 5 demonstrates the results of this simple mathematical exercise for basic reproductive rates of:

- (a) 1.5,

- (b) 7 and

- (c) 10.

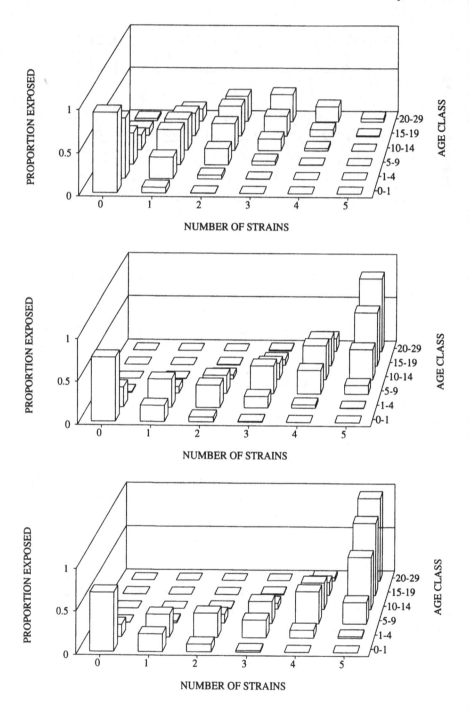

Figure 5: The predicted proportion of individuals of age a that will have seen exactly 'n' serotypes OR 'strains' out of 5, for average R_0 values of (a) 1.5, (b) 7, (c) 10.

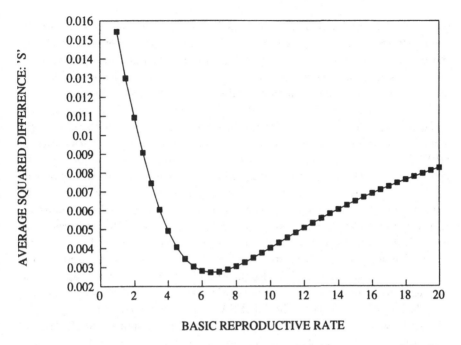

BASIC REPRODUCTIVE RATE

Figure 6: How an inverse measure of the 'goodness of fit' expresses a minimum around R_0 values of 6-7.

The correspondence at a basic reproductive rate of 7 with the pattern exhibited by the data is transparent. To determine whether there was a trend with R_0 in the correspondence of the distribution generated by the model with the data, we employed a simple measure: $S = \sum(O - E)^2$, of the 'goodness of fit'. Figure 6 demonstrates a remarkably smooth relationship between the quantity 'S' and the basic reproductive rate, with a clear minimum around 6-7. We believe that this result, although based on a small sample of individuals, unequivocally indicates that the basic reproductive rate of malaria is much lower than previous estimates. The argument that strain-specific immunity may not develop upon single exposure will tend to reduce the average value of R_0 even further, as L will be replaced in (5.2) by H, and a corresponding reduction of a factor H/L will be required in R_0 to maintain the same age-exposure profile.

6 Discussion

We have shown that a low average age of infection with *P. falciparum* does not reflect high transmissibility of the parasite, but may instead be an indication of the circulation of many distinct antigenic types or strains of the parasite, each with moderate to low transmissibility. In such circumstances, immunity to 'malaria' (where the later is defined as the experience of one or more strains) may appear short lived, when in reality immunity to a specific strain is lifelong and reinfection occurs as a result of exposure to different strains. Age-structured epidemiological data on patterns of exposure to different serotypes of *P. falciparum* strongly indicates that experience of one antigenic type does not influence the likelihood of infection with other antigenic types examined in the Papua New Guinea setting. The surface antigens (PIESA) described in this study have recently been shown to undergo antigenic variation (Roberts *et al.* 1992), which is thought to play an important role in immune evasion so as to prolong the duration of a single infection (of particular importance in parasite persistence in areas of marked seasonality in transmission). This may at first sight appear to complicate the interpretation of our field data. It seems unlikely however that seroconversion to any of the five antigenic types in our study occurs as a consequence of clonal antigenic variation, since in vitro studies (Roberts *et al.* 1992) reveal very rapid rates of emergence of new antigenic variants that are inconsistent with the slow accumulation of experience of the 5 PIESA serotypes as recorded in Fig. 3. It seems likely that antigenic diversity, as reflected in the multitude of 'strains' constituting malaria, is of significance in ensuring parasite persistence within the host population, while antigenic variation through switching of agglutination phenotypes during clonal expansion within the host is of significance in extending the duration of infection (and hence the infectious period) in order to increase the likelihood of transmission from a single host.

Whilst we favour antigenic diversity as the cause of a short average duration of immunity in the population, these epidemiological patterns may equally be generated by repeated exposure to poorly immunogenic but conserved determinants of immunity. In either case, our analyses reveal that the transmissibility of malaria has been grossly overestimated.

The most significant practical implication of this result is that, at these low values of R_0, malaria will be easier to control through vaccination strategies directed at conserved ('strain-transcending') aspects of the host-parasite immune interaction. Conversely, antigenic diversity may limit the efficacy of a vaccine, and may encourage the selection of more virulent parasite types. A strain-specific vaccine, by reducing parasite heterogeneity, may increase the stability of the transmission system, particularly at low values of R_0 (Gupta 1992). In order to exploit the low transmissibility of malaria, it is necessary therefore to invest in the design of a vaccine that circumvents the antigenic diversity of the parasite.

Finally, we would like to point out that our conclusions regarding the relationship between age-exposure profiles and duration of immunity have a very general application in that any infection that does not induce a lifelong protective immune response, such as the common STDs, will conform to this paradigm.

References

Anders, R.F. and Smythe, J. (1989) 'Polymorphic antigens in *Plasmodium falciparum*', *Blood* **74**, 1865–1875.

Anderson, R.M. and May, R.M. (1991) *Infectious diseases of humans: dynamics and control* Oxford University Press, Oxford.

Anderson, R.M., May, R.M. and Gupta, S. (1988) 'Non-linear phenomena in host-parasite interactions', *Parasitology* **99**, S59–S79.

Aron, J.L. and May, R.M. (1982) 'The population dynamics of malaria'. In *Population dynamics of infectious diseases: theory and applications*, R.M. Anderson (ed.), Chapman and Hall, London, 139–179.

Bruce-Chwatt, L.J. (1988) *Essential Malariology* William Heinemann Medical Books Ltd., London.

Conway, D.J. and McBride, J.S. (1991) 'Population genetics of Plasmodium falciparum within a malaria hyperendemic area', *Parasitology* **103**, 7–16.

Day, K.P. and Marsh, K. (1990) 'Naturally acquired immunity to malaria', *Parasitol. Today* **7**, A68.

Dietz, K. (1988) In *Principles and Practice of Malariology*, W.H. Wernsdorfer and I. McGregor (eds.), Churchill Livingstone, London, 913–998.

Forsyth, K.P., Anders, R.F., Cattani, J. and Alpers, M.A. (1989) 'Small area variation in prevalence of an S-antigen serotype of *Plasmodium falciparum* in villages of Madang, Papua New Guinea', *Am. J. Trop. Med. Hyg.* **40**, 344–350.

Greenwood, B.M., Marsh, K. and Snow, R.W. (1991) 'Why do some children develop severe malaria?', *Parasitol. Today* **7**, 277–281.

Gupta, S. (1992) *Heterogeneity and the transmission dynamics of infectious diseases*, PhD thesis, University of London.

Gupta, S, Trenholme, K., Anderson, R.M. and Day, K.P. (1994) 'Antigenic diversity and the transmission dynamics of *Plasmodium falciparum*', *Science* **263**, 961–963.

Halloran, M.E., Struchiner, C.J. and Spielman, A. (1989) 'Modelling malaria vaccines II: Population effects of stage-specific malaria vaccines dependent on natural boosting', *Math. Biosci.* **94**, 115–149.

Kemp, D.J., Cowman, A.F. and Walliker, D. (1990) 'Genetic diversity in *Plasmodium falciparum*', *Adv. in Parasitology* **29**, 75–149.

Marsh, K. (1992) 'Malaria – a neglected disease?', *Parasitology* **104**, S53–S69.

Marsh, K. and Howard, R.J. (1986) 'Antigens induced on erythrocytes by *P. falciparum* expression of diverse and conserved determinants', *Science* **231**, 150–152.

Marsh, K, Hayes, R.H., Otoo, L., Carson, D.C. and Greenwood, B.M. (1989) 'Antibodies to blood stage antigens of *Plasmodium falciparum* in rural Gambians and their relationship to protection against infection', *Trans. R. Soc. Trop. Med. Hyg.* **83**, 293–303.

Molineaux, L. and Gramiccia, G. (1980) *The Garki Project* World Health Organisation, Geneva.

Nedelman, J. (1984) 'Inoculation and recovery rates in the malaria model of Dietz, Molineaux and Thomas', *Math. Biosci.* **69**, 209–233.

Roberts, D.J., Craig, A.G., Berendt, A.R., Pinches, R., Nash, G., Marsh, K. and Newbold, C.I. (1992) 'Rapid switching to multiple antigenic and adhesive phenotypes in malaria', *Nature* **357**, 689–692.

Struchiner, C.J., Halloran, M.E. and Spielman, A. (1989) 'Modelling malaria vaccines I: New uses for old ideas', *Math. Biosci.* **94**, 87–113.

Struchler, D. (1984) 'Malaria prophylaxis in travelers: the current position', *Experimentia* **40**, 1357–1362.

Part 5
Data Analysis: Estimation and Prediction

Statistical Challenges of Epidemic Data

Niels Becker

1 Introduction

The analysis of infectious disease data presents new statistical challenges, because standard methods such as likelihood inferences are often too complicated to implement. The complexities arise because the infection process is only observed partially. This introduces many integrals into the likelihood function which cannot be simplified.

Statisticians have used several ways to overcome these difficulties. One way is to restrict the analysis to data on the outbreaks in households, assuming these to be independent. For small groups, like households, likelihood based inference remains feasible. The assumption that the outbreaks within households evolve independently is a worry. It is generally true that the rate of transmission between a susceptible individual and an infectious individual is much higher when they are from the same household. Nevertheless, the chance that a susceptible from an infected household is infected from outside can be just as high as being infected from within the household, when there are many infectives outside households. In other words, the accumulated force of infection acting on a susceptible from outside might be just as large as the accumulated force of infection acting from within the household. Methods for the analysis of data from independent outbreaks in households are well documented, see Bailey (1975) and Becker (1989), and we do not review these methods here.

Another way of coping with difficult likelihood methods is to make assumptions or approximations which enable the times of infection and the durations of infectious periods to be deduced, in which case a comprehensive likelihood analysis becomes feasible. This method is reviewed in Section 2.

A third approach is to use non-likelihood methods of inference. One such approach is the simulated method of moments, which takes advantage of results from the rich theory of martingales to derive estimating equations. It has found considerable success in the epidemic context and is discussed in Section 3.

A further approach is to use a simplified model for the analysis. The 'trick here is to simplify the model in a way so that the analysis remains relevant to the objectives of the study. Two illustrations of this approach are given in Section 4.

339

2   Deduction of the realised infection process

Inference for epidemic data would be, apart from the modelling, a standard statistical problem if only we could observe most of the infection process. We illustrate this with a simple example.

Suppose it is known how many individuals are susceptible and the times when infections occur, as well as the latent and infectious periods of all infected individuals, are observable. We don't need to know who is infected by whom. Under the assumption of homogeneous mixing the likelihood function is given by

$$L(\alpha, \beta, \gamma) = \left[\prod_i f_X(x_i; \alpha)\right] \left[\prod_i f_Y(y_i; \gamma)\right] \beta^{N_\tau} \exp\left(-\beta \int_0^\tau I_t S_t \, dt\right), \quad (2.1)$$

where

f_X is the density function of the latent period indexed by parameter α,

f_Y is the density function of the infectious period indexed by parameter γ,

β is the disease transmission rate,

N_t is the total number infected by time t,

I_t is the number of infectives at time t,

S_t is the number of susceptibles at time t, and

τ is the time when the epidemic ends.

The separable nature of the likelihood function permits separate inferences about the parameters α, β and γ. For example, the maximum likelihood estimate of β is

$$\hat{\beta} = N_\tau \Big/ \int_0^\tau I_t S_t \, dt, \quad \text{with} \quad \text{s.e.}(\hat{\beta}) = \hat{\beta}\Big/\sqrt{N_\tau}.$$

It is interesting that the solution to the underlying stochastic epidemic model is not available, but statistical inference, which relies on the stochastic model, is feasible when the infection process is observed in detail.

Note that the likelihood term concerned with the transmission parameter β is like that for a Poisson parameter, suggesting that a comprehensive log-linear regression analysis of disease transmission is available when data are observed in such detail. It is tempting to try to deduce this level of detail from the available data, so as to take advantage of this comprehensive method of analysis.

In practice one is usually aware of infectives only when they show symptoms, but it is sometimes possible to deduce, at least approximately, the times when infections occurred and when infected individuals are infectious. For example, the measles rash erupts about 14 days after infection, with relatively little variation, and it is reasonable to assume that individuals are infectious during the observable prodromal period, i.e. the period prior to the eruption of the rash during which other symptoms of illness are displayed. This specification is sufficient to make the analysis suggested above available.

Assume now that details of the realised infection process can be deduced. We describe a regression analysis which focusses on the transmission rate and heterogeneity therein.

Infection occurs over continuous time, however data are usually collected from day to day, or week to week. It is therefore convenient to perform the analysis in terms of time units $dt = 1$ day, say. This is an appropriate time unit for many diseases, including measles, chickenpox and influenza. For infections with slow progression to disease, such as HIV, a month or a quarter might be more appropriate. The transition from continuous time to discrete time is straightforward. The number infected, in a homogeneously mixing community, during time increment dt around time t is dN_t, which has a Poisson distribution with mean $\beta I_t S_t\, dt$. Observations on the dN_t's give the same likelihood term as in (1). For the discrete-time approximation dN_t is taken as the number infected on day t and $dt = 1$.

A more general model, which can be thought of as an approximation to nonhomogeneous mixing, is to take the mean as $\mu_t = \beta_0 I_t^{\beta_1} S_t^{\beta_2}$, where dt has been taken as 1. Then

$$\ln(\mu_t) = \ln(\beta_0) + \beta_1 \ln(I_t) + \beta_2 \ln(S_t),$$

indicating a log-linear model in the parameters $\ln(\beta_0)$, β_1 and β_2 with Poisson error. This is a common statistical model which may be fitted to data by readily available software such as GLIM. An analysis based on this model is illustrated by Becker (1989, Section 6.4).

The advantages of this approach are realised when we have data on covariates such as age, sex, vaccination status and household sizes. For the clarity of concepts it is useful to go back a step and remember that the Poisson distribution is arrived at by considering infections in time increments as independent Bernoulli trials. More specifically, we consider for each individual on each day whether or not they are infected. Then the

$$K_t^{(i)} \equiv \begin{cases} 1, & \text{if susceptible } i \text{ escapes infection on day } t \\ 0, & \text{otherwise} \end{cases}$$

are treated as independent variables with

$$K_t^{(i)} \quad \sim \quad \text{Binomial}\,[1, \exp(-\eta_t^{(i)})],$$

where $\eta_t^{(i)}$ is the force of infection acting on susceptible i on day t. Strictly speaking, $\eta_t^{(i)}$ should be $\int_{\text{day } t} \eta_x^{(i)}\, dx$, but as there is usually little change in the infection intensity during a day and only daily data are likely to be available, it is appropriate to use $\eta_t^{(i)}$.

The covariate information can be incorporated by expressing the force of infection acting on susceptible i as

$$\eta_t^{(i)} = \sum_j \beta_{ij} I_t^{(ij)},$$

where $I_t^{(ij)}$ is the number of infectives of type j to which individual i is exposed on day t. Here 'type' is determined by age, sex, vaccination status, etc. The β parameters contain the subscript i since these rates may depend on the characteristics such as age, sex and vaccination status of susceptible i.

We then have a log-linear model for binomial data, which can be fitted to data with a user-defined model in GLIM. In applications it is more convenient to analyse the data with a logistic link-function in GLIM and this is the recommended method for determining which factors significantly improve the fit of the model. Once a parsimonious model is arrived at, and interest is focussed on the estimates of the parameters, it is better to fit the log-linear model with binomial error as this preserves the direct interpretation of the β's as transmission rates.

This method of analysis is illustrated with an application to common cold data by Becker (1989, Chapter 6), where earlier references are cited, and an application to measles data by Becker and Wang (1993). These applications illustrate that the approach provides a comprehensive analysis capable of determining sources of heterogeneity in the transmission of infectious diseases and of addressing questions of epidemiological importance. Specifically, the measles application finds that the infectiousness of measles prior to the prodromal period is negligible.

3   A simulated method of moments

Complicated likelihoods can sometimes be avoided by using alternative approaches to inference. For example, for some parameters it is possible to construct a known function f of D, the observed data of an epidemic, and θ, the parameter of interest, such that $\mathrm{E}\, f(D, \theta) = 0$. Functions with this property are called estimating functions, because $\hat{\theta}$, the solution of $f(D, \theta) = 0$ provides an estimate of θ. The approach is similar to the method of moments. In the epidemic context results from the rich theory of martingales have been useful to construct such estimating functions and associated variances. We give an outline of this approach, but first introduce the parameter of interest.

3.1 The infection potential

The infectivity, or infectiousness, function λ_u quantifies how infectious the individual is u time units after being infected. Typically, λ stays at zero for some time, the latent period, before rising to a plateau and finally declining to zero. The infectivity function for HIV, on the other hand, is thought to have a high value for a three to six month period just after infection, followed by a long period when it is near zero before rising again as the individual approaches AIDS diagnosis.

A common assumption about the infectivity function is

$$\lambda_u = \begin{cases} \beta, & X \leq u \leq X + Y, \\ 0, & \text{otherwise}, \end{cases} \tag{3.1}$$

where X and Y are the durations of the latent and infectious period, respectively. We use this infectivity function to introduce the mean infection potential, which is our parameter of interest. The random quantity

$$\Theta_i = \int_0^\infty \lambda_u^{(i)} \, du = \beta Y_i \, .$$

is called the *infection potential* of infective i because it is of the form
(transmission rate) × (period for which it operates).

Our parameter of interest is

$$\theta = \mathrm{E}(\Theta) = \beta \, \mathrm{E}(Y),$$

the mean infection potential.

Here we just want to illustrate ideas, so we make the simplifying assumption that all infected individuals have the same deterministic infectivity function λ_u. Then the probability of a susceptible being infected, when exposed to a single infective for the duration of her infectious period, is $p = 1 - e^{-\theta}$. This relationship is useful since p has a very direct epidemiological interpretation.

3.2 Martingale methods

Assume that all individuals are equally susceptible to infection, and let g_u denote the force of infection acting on each susceptible at time u. Then

$$N_t - \int_0^t g_u S_u \, du \tag{3.2}$$

is a zero mean martingale. The force of infection has a complicated expression given by

$$g_u = \sum_{i=1}^n \left[\int_{s=0}^u \lambda_{u-s} \, dK_s^{(i)} \right] I_u^{(i)}.$$

Here $K_s^{(i)}$ indicates whether individual i has been infected by time s, and its role in the expression is to start the infectivity function at the time when individual i is infected. The term $I_u^{(i)}$ indicates whether individual i is still not removed. The complicated nature of the expression for g_u is of little concern to us.

Assume that infectives are removed upon discovery of symptoms. Let the time from infection until discovery of symptoms have hazard function γ_u, and let R_t denote the number of removals by time t. Then

$$R_t - \int_0^t h_u \, du \qquad (3.3)$$

is a zero mean martingale, where h_u, the removal intensity acting on the infective population, has expression

$$h_u = \sum_{i=1}^n \left[\int_{s=0}^u \gamma_{u-s} \, dK_s^{(i)} \right] I_u^{(i)}.$$

This expression is like that for g_u, except that λ is replaced by γ.

On the basis that both infectiousness and the risk of discovery, with removal, are driven by the level of illness we now make the assumption that

$$\lambda_u = \theta \gamma_u \quad \text{for all } u. \qquad (3.4)$$

The infection potential for an infective is random, because her time of removal is random. Under the proportionality assumption (3.4) it can be shown that the mean infection potential is given by

$$\mathrm{E} \left[\int_0^Y \lambda_u \, du \right] = \theta.$$

Let S_{u-} denote the number of susceptibles just prior to time u. By integrating $1/S_{u-}$ with respect to the martingale (3.2) and substituting (3.4), we obtain the zero mean martingale

$$\int_0^t \frac{dN_u}{S_{u-}} - \theta \int_0^t h_u \, du. \qquad (3.5)$$

Strictly speaking, this martingale should be stopped when there are no susceptibles left, but we do not worry about the finer details here.

Finally, when we subtract θ times martingale (3.3) from (3.5) we obtain the zero mean martingale

$$\int_0^t \frac{dN_u}{S_{u-}} - \theta R_t. \qquad (3.6)$$

The complicated term h_u, involving the unspecified infectivity function, has been eliminated. The estimate is obtained by equating (3.6) at time τ, the end of the epidemic, to zero, its mean, giving

$$\hat{\theta} = \sum_{j=S_\tau+1}^{S_0} \frac{1}{j} \bigg/ R_\tau .$$

The estimate depends only on the initial number of susceptibles, the initial number of infectives and the final number of cases.

For large epidemics the estimate can be written as

$$\hat{\theta} = \frac{-\ln(1 - R_\tau/S_0)}{R_\tau},$$

which is essentially the estimate obtained from the deterministic Susceptible-Infective-Removal (SIR) model (see Bailey 1975, Section 6.2). However, the martingale approach is also able to provide a standard error for our estimate. By following the procedure given in Becker (1989, Chapter 7) under the present assumptions we arrive at

$$\text{s.e.}(\hat{\theta}) = \frac{1}{\sqrt{R_\tau}} \left[\sum_{j=S_\tau+1}^{S_0} \frac{1}{j^2} + \hat{\theta}^2 R_\tau \right]^{\frac{1}{2}} .$$

For large epidemics, central limit theorems enable the construction of confidence intervals and hypothesis testing.

The same derivation applies, with the same results, even when the infectivity function for each infective is chosen at random, as long as the proportionality assumption (3.4) holds for each infective. These delightfully simple results for inference are in stark contrast to the probability distribution for the size of the epidemic, which is inaccessible under such general assumptions.

The model described above contains the commonly studied SIR model, with an exponentially distributed infectious period, as a very particular case.

Tutorial introductions to the requisite martingale methods are given by Becker (1989, Chapter 7), in the context of epidemic models, and by Becker (1993), in the simpler context of data on survival times. A more rigorous review is given by Andersen and Borgan (1985). Applications to inference about the infection potential, differences in infection potentials, relative susceptibility and nonparametric transmission rates are reviewed by Becker (1993). Recent applications to the estimation of vaccine efficacy are given by Haber *et al.* (1991) and Longini *et al.* (1993). Yip (1991) applies the approach to make inference about parameters of a fatal disease model.

4   Models with suitable simplifications

When the preferred transmission model makes the likelihood function inaccessible it is tempting to use simpler models. We should take this path with some reluctance for infectious disease data, because the transmission model captures the mechanism that generates the data, which brings with it a number of advantages. First, the parameters have direct epidemiological interpretations. Secondly, analyses are likely to be more efficient when based on transmission models, as these models provide a soundly based description of parts of the infection process which are not observed. One should try to retain these advantages when contemplating simpler models. We illustrate the point with a couple of examples.

4.1   Example 1: Epidemics in a community of households

Suppose all individuals in a sample of households are tested serologically for susceptibility to a disease at time t_1, before the start of the epidemic season, and tested again at time t_2, the end of the epidemic season, to see who was infected during the time interval (t_1, t_2). This type of study is very important, because it can be designed and conducted with care, and leads to reliable data. Infection is established by laboratory tests and so data does not suffer from misclassifications due to subclinical infections.

Longini and Koopman (1982) propose a simplified model for the analysis of such data. We now describe one way of looking at their model and point out why it is a suitable simplification.

For this discussion we adopt the infectivity function given by (3.1). The force of infection acting on a given susceptible at time t is

$$\beta_w I_t^{(w)} + \beta_b I_t^{(b)} = (\beta_w - \beta_b) I_t^{(w)} + \beta_b I_t \,, \tag{4.1}$$

where w and b indicate 'within-household' and 'between-household', and $I_t = I_t^{(w)} + I_t^{(b)}$ is the total number of infectives in the community. A stochastic model with such assumptions is unlikely to give an accessible likelihood function and a simplifying assumption is called for. The final term in equation (4.1) is neither household nor individual specific and may be taken as a community transmission rate acting on all susceptibles. The probability that a susceptible escapes infection when exposed to the community transmission rate only, over (t_1, t_2), is

$$q_b = \mathrm{e}^{-\int_{t_1}^{t_2} \beta_b I_u \, du} \,.$$

It is, strictly speaking, a random and unknown quantity. A useful simplification is to interpret q_b as a parameter to be estimated from the data. The model used by Longini and Koopman is expressed in terms of q_b and q_w, the probability that a susceptible escapes infection when exposed to a single infective residing in her household for the infective's entire infectious period. The likelihood function corresponding to this simplified model does not have an explicit expression either, but its computation is possible and maximum likelihood estimation is feasible.

Although the model is an approximation to the state of nature and we have replaced an unobserved part of the epidemic by a parameter to be estimated, the nature of the approximation is such that one is now estimating the within-household infection parameter with an allowance for possible infection from outside. In other words, the parameter q_w has retained its interpretation. However, the estimate of the parameter q_b needs to be interpreted with care. Its interpretation is linked to the size of this particular epidemic, so that comparisons of estimates of q_b for different epidemics have limited value. Becker (1992) considers parameter estimation for this problem by using martingale methods.

4.2 Example 2: Reconstructing the HIV epidemic

The long incubation period of HIV infection makes it possible to assess the extent of the epidemic during its course. There is interest in projections of AIDS incidences and in reconstructing the HIV epidemic curve with the hope of discovering trends. The lengthy development of the epidemic, coupled with the serious consequences of HIV infection, brings new difficulties to the analysis of data from this epidemic. Possible behaviour changes during the course of the epidemic and multiple modes of transmission make models complex, and simplifications are needed to make progress.

We consider a model in discrete time, with a month as the unit of time. Choose a time origin at some time prior to the introduction of HIV into the community. Let N_t denote the number of individuals infected in month t. The number of individuals diagnosed with AIDS in month t is R_t, which plays the role of the removal process. We have that

$$E(R_t|N_1, \ldots, N_t) = \sum_{u=1}^{t} N_u p_{t-u} , \qquad (4.2)$$

where p_d is the probability that the duration of the incubation period is d months. We should really allow p_d to depend on calendar time as well, since therapy became available during the course of the epidemic and affected this distribution, but we do not need these complexities to make our point. Taking expectations in (4.2) gives

$$\mu_t = \sum_{u=1}^{t} \nu_u p_{t-u} ,$$

where $\mu_t = \mathrm{E}(R_t)$ and $\nu_u = \mathrm{E}(N_u)$.

The p_d are assumed known, from estimation based on large cohort studies, and observations $r_1, \ldots, r_T$ are available on $R_1, \ldots, R_T$, where T is the most recent time for which the observation on R_t is considered reliable. It is desired to make inferences about the realised, but unobserved values $N_1, \ldots, N_T$. The multiple modes of transmission and possible behaviour changes make it difficult to suggest a suitable manageable *a priori* transmission model for the $N_1, \ldots, N_T$, or even a suitable form for the $\nu_1, \ldots, \nu_T$. This has resulted in the simplified approach of assuming that the $N_1, \ldots, N_T$ are generated by a nonhomogeneous Poisson process. This assumption implies that $R_1, \ldots, R_T$ are independent Poisson variates and we are able to write down the likelihood function given by

$$\prod_{t=1}^{T} \left(\sum_{i=1}^{t} \nu_i p_{t-i} \right)^{r_t} \exp\left(- \sum_{i=1}^{t} \nu_i p_{t-i} \right).$$

The $\nu_1, \ldots, \nu_T$ are now estimated, and taken to be the reconstruction of the HIV epidemic curve, either by assuming some parametric family of curves for them (see Brookmeyer and Gail (1988) for example) or by nonparametric maximum likelihood estimation with smoothing (see Becker *et al.*, (1991), for example).

The point is that we have again simplified the problem by replacing an unobserved part of the infection process by parameters to be estimated. Here the substitution is so severe that no aspect of transmission has been retained in the model. However, the mean of the nonhomogeneous Poisson process has complete flexibility so that one can feel comforted that it is able to reproduce the shape of the epidemic curve. We can not feel so comfortable about its ability to give the right measure of precision for the estimate, since the precision is likely to be influenced by the dependence in the infection data, which has been sacrificed by this simplification of the model. The question of precision deserves further investigation.

References

Andersen, P.K. and Borgan, O. (1985) 'Counting process models for life history data', *Scand. J. Statist.* **12**, 97–158.

Bailey, N.T.J. (1975) *The Mathematical Theory of Infectious Diseases and its Applications*, Griffin, London.

Becker, N.G. (1989) *Analysis of Infectious Disease Data*, Chapman and Hall, London.

Becker, N.G. (1992) 'Analysis of infectious disease from a sample of households', *IMS Lecture Notes* **18**, 27–40.

Becker, N.G. (1993) 'Martingale methods for the analysis of epidemic data', *Statist. Meth. Med. Res.* **2**, 93–112.

Becker, N.G., Watson, L.F. and Carlin, J.B. (1991) 'A method of non-parametric back-projection and its application to AIDS data', *Statist. in Med.* **10**, 1527–1542.

Becker, N.G. and Wang, D.Q. (1993) 'Severe outbreak of measles in an isolated German village, 1861: II. Analysis of transmission rates'. Research Report 92/21, Department of Statistics, La Trobe University.

Brookmeyer, R. and Gail, M.H. (1988) 'A method for obtaining short-term projections and lower bounds on the size of the AIDS epidemic', *J. Amer. Statist. Assoc.* **83**, 301–308.

Haber, M., Longini, I.M. and Halloran, M.E. (1991) 'Estimation of vaccine efficacy in outbreaks of acute infectious diseases', *Statist. in Med.* **10**, 1573–1584.

Longini, I.M., Halloran, M.E. and Haber, M. (1993) 'Estimation of vaccine efficacy from epidemics of acute infectious agents under vaccine-related heterogeneity. *Math. Biosci.* **117**, 271–281.

Longini, I.M. and Koopman, J.S. (1982) 'Household and community transmission parameters from final distributions of infections in households', *Biometrics* **38**, 115–126.

Yip, P. (1991) 'Inference for a fatal disease', *Appl. Math. and Comp.* **41**, 89–97.

Primary Components of Epidemic Models

Andrew Cairns

1 Introduction

Recent years have seen the use of increasingly complex models for epidemic growth. For example, the emergence of the AIDS epidemic has resulted in the development of models including a variety of features: non-exponential or staged incubation periods; variable infectiousness; varying levels of promiscuity; and increasingly complex contact structures (for example, Anderson *et al.* 1988, 1989, Bailey 1988, Blythe and Anderson 1988a,b, Bongaarts 1989, Cairns 1990a,b, 1991, Dietz 1988, Hethcote and Yorke 1984, Jacquez *et al.* 1988, Koopman *et al.* 1988, May and Anderson 1984, Wilkie 1989). All of these developments are necessary to increase our understanding of the mechanics of transmission.

Very often, though, this complexity is not matched by the level of detail in the available data. This makes it very difficult to carry out the process of model fitting without pooling data from a number of sources. For example, in relation to the AIDS epidemic we have AIDS incidence data as the primary source to which we can add data from seroprevalence studies, and studies into social behaviour. Such an approach is, however, very time consuming.

This paper presents an alternative approach to model fitting and projection, making use of the notion of a *Primary Component*. A Primary Component is function of the basic parameters which dictates epidemic dynamics (the classic example being the basic reproductive ratio, R_0). This paper shows that a complex model with many parameters may only have a small number of Primary Components. By their nature, if we know the values of the small number of Primary Components then we will be able to predict how the epidemic will progress to a high degree of accuracy. In terms of fitting a model to, say, incidence data this means that instead of estimating the full range of basic parameters, we only need to concentrate on estimating a small number of Primary Components.

Section 2 will introduce the general concepts by considering a very simple model for epidemic spread, and then discussing problems encountered in attempting to fit a model for the spread of AIDS.

Sections 3 to 5 will outline the principles underlying Primary Components and discuss how our choice of Primary Components is principally objective

350

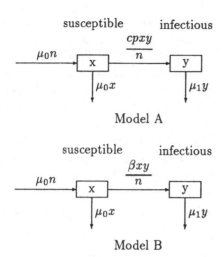

Model A

Model B

Figure 1: Two simple models for epidemic spread

and data oriented. For example, our choice may depend on the level of detail required in a projection.

Section 6 will illustrate the process of a Primary Component analysis with reference to a (simple) model for the spread of HIV and AIDS. Two sets of data will be considered – AIDS incidence data only; and AIDS incidence data combined with data on the incidence of new infections – which will illustrate the effect on our choice of Primary Components of the level of detail in the data.

Section 7 will describe various stages involved in the process of model fitting and projection. This is based on estimation of the Primary Components only, and also covers the important topic of estimating confidence limits for both the values of the Primary Components and the projection of the epidemic.

2   Background

Consider models A and B for epidemic growth (Figure 1).

The only difference between these two models is that where model A has the two parameters c (the contact rate) and p, model B has the single parameter β. The reason for this is that the formulation used in model A gives us, in a simplistic way, a more detailed understanding of the mechanics of transmission. If, on the other hand, we are interested only in looking at epidemic dynamics then (provided $\beta = cp$) the two models will give the same results. So in this sense one parameter in model A is redundant.

This reduction in the number of parameters is similar to approaches described by Nåsell (1985) and Bailey and Duppenthaler (1980). Nåsell, who considers equilibrium incidence of malaria, uses dimensional analysis to strip out a number of unnecessary parameters. Bailey and Duppenthaler present a detailed and systematic approach to sensitivity analysis by considering the full set of basic parameters. By incorporating the uncertainty associated with each parameter they assess which parameters have the most influence on the level of incidence at a particular point in time.

This then introduces the first theme of the current paper: that, in the context of epidemic dynamics, it may only be necessary to know a reduced set of parameters or components.

Consider next the equations which describe the dynamics of model B:

$$\frac{dx}{dt} = \mu_0 n - \mu_0 x - \frac{\beta x y}{n} \tag{2.1}$$

$$\frac{dy}{dt} = \frac{\beta x y}{n} - \mu_1 y \tag{2.2}$$

Suppose the value of β is known to be equal to 0.1. What can be said about the epidemic? The answer is, of course, 'very little': the epidemic could die out or it could take off and be quite substantial. We need to know more than β.

This provides motivation for the second theme: that it can often be appropriate to reparametrize a model in a more meaningful way. For example, in model B we may use some combination of:

$\tau_0 = \frac{1}{\mu_0}$, the mean lifetime in the absence of infection (2.3)

$\tau_1 = \frac{1}{\mu_1}$, the mean duration of infectiousness (2.4)

$R_0 = \beta \tau_1$, the Basic Reproductive Ratio: the mean number of (2.5)
secondary cases of infection caused by one primary infective
in the early stages of the epidemic

$\theta = \beta - \mu_1$
$= \frac{R_0 - 1}{\tau_1}$, the initial growth rate (2.6)

In particular, knowing θ or R_0 immediately tells us something about how the epidemic will progress: θ tells us about the early dynamics; while R_0 tells us about the peak and the equilibrium.

The present work was motivated by the author's work on a model for the spread of HIV and AIDS (Cairns 1991). As with many such models it was relatively complex, involving more than 10 parameters and incorporating variable infectiousness (for example, Blythe and Anderson 1988a, Anderson *et al.* 1989), a staged incubation period (Longini *et al.* 1988, 1989) and varying levels of promiscuity (Anderson *et al.* 1989, Blythe and Anderson 1988b, Jacquez *et al.* 1988, Koopman *et al.* 1988). The objective of the exercise was to obtain a projection of the epidemic within a reasonable timescale and keeping down the amount of computing time as far as possible.

As with many diseases HIV and AIDS is characterized by a lack of detail in the data. Perhaps the best or most reliable we have for the UK as a whole is the incidence of AIDS diagnosis. This presented a significant problem: that of how to fit a complex model to a crude data set? It was found that a wide range of parameter values would fit the data equally well: that is, the likelihood surface was found to be relatively flat.

Countering this problem, though, it was observed that many of the parameter sets fitting the data were in fact unrealistic. As an extreme example, incubation periods down to one year may fit the data when, in fact, we know this to be of the order of 10 years. It was also noted that despite the wide range of acceptable parameter values, the range of projections obtained from them was relatively narrow.

The tentative conclusion that can be drawn from this is that it may be possible to save considerable time by concentrating effort on estimating a small number of key components rather than the full set of basic parameters.

3   Primary Components

In order to facilitate the conclusions of Section 2 it is necessary to introduce the concept of *Primary Components*: functions of the basic parameters which dictate epidemic dynamics (Mollison 1984). Besides this basic description or definition there are additional desirable requirements which act as a guide in our selection of the best set of Primary Components.

(i) The set of Primary Components should be as small as possible. (ii) Each Primary Component must be simple to interpret. (iii) Each Primary Component should influence either short term or long term dynamics but not both.

Requirement (i) ties in with the objective of minimizing the time spent in fitting a model to a set of data.

Requirement (ii) follows from from the remarks made in Section 2 on the repara-metrization of a model. For example, R_0, the reproductive ratio, is a commonly used Primary Component with a simple interpretation; whereas β is not. One further justification for this requirement is that it makes it easier to transmit our conclusions from the exercise to non-experts or laymen. In fact (i) and (ii) can conflict, for it may be that the set of Primary Components could be reduced further but at the cost of leaving a set in which one or more of the Primary Components no longer had a simple interpretation. In such circumstances it may be undesirable to proceed with this final shrinkage of the set in order to retain the ease of interpretation.

Requirement (iii) is a useful condition from the point of view that it eases comparison of simulations using different parameter sets.

In fact (ii) is the principal reason why the process is not replaced by the more rigorously founded statistical theory of Principal Component Analysis. This would produce a set of orthogonal components in order of their magnitude of influence on the likelihood function (and hence on the dynamics of the epidemic). So, while a Principal Component Analysis might produce a theoretically best set of Primary Components, the result would both be at the cost of interpretability and also of restricting the influence of a component to either short or long term dynamics.

Complementing the set of Primary Components we have the set of secondary parameters. The characteristics of this set is that provided the Primary Components remain fixed then we can vary the secondary parameters without significantly altering the dynamics of the epidemic. In terms of model fitting this means that if we can identify the values of the Primary Components then it is not of significance whether we know the values of the secondary parameters or not. Knowledge of the secondary parameters will not improve the fit of the model.

If, on the other hand, we do find that we can vary the secondary parameters within a *realistic range* and significantly alter the dynamics, then this indicates that the set of Primary Components is in some way incomplete or inadequate.

Keeping the notion of a realistic range firmly in mind is an important part of the process. For example, if we know the mean incubation period, τ, lies in the range 6 to 10 months then our conclusions may be different from knowing that the range is much wider, say 2 to 20 months. In the former case varying τ may not have a significant effect on epidemic dynamics, whereas in the latter we may have crossed over the vague division between insignificant and significant variation.

Consider now a typical epidemic curve (Figure 2). This has three principal features: initial growth; the peak; and the equilibrium level of infection.

Looking again at model B we can identify two Primary Components: θ the initial, underlying exponential growth rate; and R_0 the reproductive ratio. If we can fix θ then increasing R_0 will increase both the peak and the equilibrium while leaving the early dynamics largely untouched. On the other hand varying θ while R_0 remains fixed has the effect of varying early dynamics but not significantly altering the size of the peak or the equilibrium. What we cannot do, because of the simplicity of the model, is to fix both early dynamics and the peak while having different equilibrium levels. This sort of

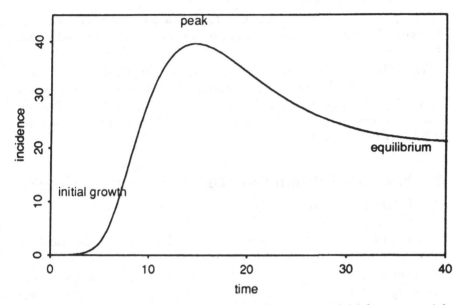

Figure 2: Principal features of an epidemic curve: initial, exponential growth; peak size; equilibrium.

situation requires a more complex model with two or more long term Primary Components.

4 Model analysis

We now effectively have two approaches to model analysis.

The standard or more traditional approach tends (with some notable exceptions) to vary one or two parameters at a time with the inevitable effect that both short and long term dynamics also change. It is easy to conclude from this that all parameters are key ingredients in the model and that they all need to be estimated. In fact the observed changes in dynamics will be due to variation of the small number of Primary Components. For example, variation of medium and long term dynamics is commonly due to changes in the value of R_0.

The alternative approach discussed here takes a more flexible stance. The idea is to consider a model as a whole rather than to focus in on one or two parameters at a time. We then aim to build up a set of Primary Components and, just as importantly, to be able to vary some parameters without materially affecting the dynamics of the model.

This gives us quite a contrast: the standard approach aims to maximize differences between simulations; while the alternative aims to minimize such differences.

The difference between this approach and that described by Bailey and Duppenthaler (1980) is that here we consider the full set of dynamics rather than a single point in time and, whereas Bailey and Duppenthaler look at the basic parameters as independent entities, here we look at a smaller number of Primary Components.

5 Factors influencing the choice of Primary Components

A number of interactive factors need to be taken into account when choosing a set of Primary Components.

The first, and most important, factor is to consider what the purpose of modelling is. What are the aims and objectives? Is it just to estimate the total size of an epidemic or is it to assess the impact over time on specific subgroups? Estimating the total size could require only one Primary Component whereas subgroup analysis over time may require three or four Primary Components.

Second, how detailed is the set of data that we wish to fit the model to. If there is insufficient data then it may not be possible to adequately estimate all of the preferred choice of Primary Components. A consequence of this is that it may not be possible to meet the objective with any great degree of accuracy unless additional data is made available. For example, analysis by subgroup may not be possible if the data set only gives details for the population as a whole.

Third, we need to ask ourselves what is a 'realistic' range of secondary parameters? The example, in Section 3 illustrated this by considering the degree of uncertainty in the length of the incubation period. Such an assessment will be based on other investigations into the spread and development of the disease. Greater uncertainty may mean that a parameter previously classed as 'secondary' may now have a potential impact on the results of a projection. So the set of Primary Components may need to be redefined or even increased in size.

A closely related fourth factor is the required level of accuracy in a projection. For example, is it acceptable to estimate incidence in 10 years' time as, say, 100 ± 10 when a more accurate analysis would come up with an answer of 98.8 ± 10.2? The more accurate we require a projection to be the more likely it is that we will require additional Primary Components. The reason is that the required level of accuracy determines the definition of 'insignificant variation of dynamics' in the context of secondary parameters. Thus a greater degree of accuracy in the projection means that for some secondary parameters the 'realistic' range may need to be restricted somewhat to avoid having to redefine the set of Primary Components.

6 A simple model for the spread of HIV and AIDS

This section now illustrates the process of a Primary Component Analysis by reference to a simple model for the spread of HIV and AIDS. In particular the model assumes homogeneous mixing and is not, therefore, intended for serious application to the real epidemic! (It is in fact a simplification of the models analysed by Jacquez *et al.* (1988), Anderson *et al.* (1989) and Cairns (1991).) Its purpose here is to show how we can take a model (here with eight basic epidemic parameters) and identify a small number of Primary Components. Recent studies (Longini *et al.* 1991, 1992) also point to six rather than three pre-AIDS infection stages as giving a more accurate representation of the development of HIV.

The equations governing the dynamics of the model are

$$\frac{dx}{dt} = \mu n - \mu x - \Lambda x \tag{6.1}$$

$$\frac{dy_1}{dt} = \Lambda x - (\gamma_1 + \mu)y_1 \tag{6.2}$$

$$\frac{dy_2}{dt} = \gamma_1 y_1 - (\gamma_2 + \mu)y_2 \tag{6.3}$$

$$\frac{dy_3}{dt} = \gamma_2 y_2 - (\gamma_3 + \mu)y_3 \tag{6.4}$$

$$\frac{dy_4}{dt} = \gamma_3 y_3 - (\gamma_4 + \mu)y_4 \tag{6.5}$$

where

$$n = \text{disease free, stable population size} \tag{6.6}$$

$$\Lambda = \frac{M \sum \beta_k y_k}{n} \tag{6.7}$$

$$= \text{infection intensity on one susceptible}$$

$$M = \text{mean number of partners per year} \tag{6.8}$$

$$\beta_k = \text{probability of infection per partner}$$
$$\text{in stage } k \text{ of infection} \tag{6.9}$$

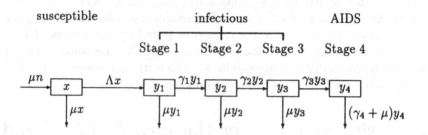

Figure 3: A model for the spread of AIDS

We set $\beta_2 = 0$ as stage 2 corresponds to infecteds who are asymptomatic and non-infectious.

We also define

$$
\begin{aligned}
\tau_k &= \text{mean time spent in stage } k \text{ of infection} \\
&= (\gamma_k + \mu)^{-1} && (6.10) \\
p_k &= \text{probability that a new infective reaches stage} \\
&\quad\; k \text{ of infection} \\
&= \prod_{j=1}^{k-1} \frac{\gamma_j}{(\gamma_j + \mu)} && k = 2,3,4 && (6.11)
\end{aligned}
$$

The model can be represented as in Figure 3.

As with many epidemic models the expected size of the epidemic initially grows like $e^{\theta t}$. It is shown in Cairns (1990a, 1991) that θ is the largest solution of

$$
D(\theta)\beta_1 + E(\theta)\beta_3 + F(\theta)\beta_4 = G(\theta) \qquad (6.12)
$$

where D, E, F and G are given by

$$
\begin{aligned}
D(\theta) &= M(\gamma_2 + \mu + \theta)(\gamma_3 + \mu + \theta)(\gamma_4 + \mu + \theta) && (6.13) \\
E(\theta) &= M\gamma_1\gamma_2(\gamma_4 + \mu + \theta) && (6.14) \\
F(\theta) &= M\gamma_1\gamma_2\gamma_3 && (6.15) \\
G(\theta) &= (\gamma_1 + \mu + \theta)(\gamma_2 + \mu + \theta)(\gamma_3 + \mu + \theta)(\gamma_4 + \mu + \theta) && (6.16)
\end{aligned}
$$

A formula for the basic reproductive ratio can also be derived (Cairns 1990a, 1991):

$$
R_0 = M(\beta_1\tau_1 + p_3\beta_3\tau_3 + p_4\beta_4\tau_4) \qquad (6.17)
$$

Given values for the basic parameters we may derive values for θ (numerically) and R_0.

However, the Primary Component approach suggests that we should do the reverse. The aim is to minimize changes between simulations, and one of the best ways of doing this is to fix θ, thereby 'fixing' the early stages of the epidemic. We also can also fix R_0 and any other potential Primary Components and use these these as constraints in setting the values of the basic parameters (for example, $M\beta_1$, $M\beta_3$, $M\beta_4$ being derived from equations (6.12) and (6.17)).

Any analysis requires a first 'guess' at a set of Primary Components. For this model the clear choices are θ and R_0.

There is one obvious secondary parameter M which is always paired with one of the β_k. This is similar to the reduction from model A to model B in Section 2.

Parameters that we are not sure about are: $\alpha = \beta_4/\beta_3$ (not an immediately obvious choice, but it has a clear meaning and fixing θ, R_0 and α then uniquely determines the β_k); and the τ_k $(k = 1,2,3,4)$. (Here we consider only the epidemic parameters. It may be felt that n, a population parameter, also needs to be included in an analysis).

The first experiment (working with a time unit of one month) fixed θ, R_0 and α and allowed the τ_k to vary ($\theta = 0.06$, $R_0 = 8$ and $\alpha = \beta_4/\beta_3 = 2$). With (τ_k) equal to $(4, 50, 60, 24)$ (consistent with Longini *et al.* 1988, 1989), $n = 10000$ and $M = 2.5$ we find that $\beta_1 = 0.094$, $\beta_3 = 0.038$ and $\beta_4 = 0.076$.

In Figure 4, curves (a) and (b) give typical examples. Since θ is fixed initial dynamics are well matched but the two curves have different peak and equilibrium incidence of AIDS. We can conclude from this that R_0 *on its own* as a long term Primary Component is not appropriate.

What we do not know is whether a single but different Primary Component will be sufficient or whether we will need more than one long term Primary Component: this will require further investigation. A useful step is to look at equilibrium incidence: if we wish to fix long term dynamics then we must fix the equilibrium. It straightforward to show that equilibrium incidence of AIDS is given by

$$a_e = \gamma_3 y_3 = \mu n p_4 \left(1 - \frac{1}{R_0}\right) \qquad (6.18)$$

Experiment 2 fixed the equilibrium incidence of AIDS but allowed R_0 and the τ_k to vary (subject to this constraint). Figure 4 again gives a typical comparison (curves (a) and (c)). Although the epidemic curves now converge to the same equilibrium they can still have different peak sizes. This means

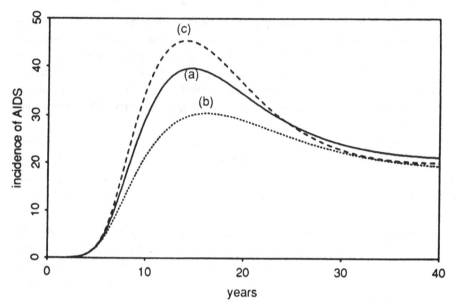

Figure 4: Experiment 1: curves (a) and (b) have θ and R_0 fixed but different τ_k. Experiment 2: curves (a) and (c) have θ and equilibrium incidence of AIDS, a_e, fixed.

that at least one more Primary Component will be required, and the formula for equilibrium incidence of AIDS suggests using p_4 and R_0.

Experiment 3 fixed θ, R_0, α and p_4 and varied the τ_k by up to $\pm 20\%$ (consistent with Longini *et al.* 1989). The constraint of having p_4 fixed, however, means that there are only three degrees of freedom in setting the τ_k, so here τ_1, τ_2 and τ_4 were varied and the value of τ_3 determined by the values of τ_1, τ_2 and p_4. This constraint also ties in with unpublished results associated with the work of Longini *et al.* (1989) who found small negative covariances between the transition intensities (Longini, personal communication).

Selected results are plotted in Figure 5. The solid curve represents the central parameters – $(\tau_k) = (4, 50, 55, 24)$ – while the dotted curves are two of the most extreme. The maximum deviations from the central curve are about $\pm 2\%$ to 3% which was felt for many situations to be quite tolerable. So this means that τ_1, τ_2 and τ_4 can be taken as secondary parameters.

Finally it was necessary to consider whether $\alpha = \beta_4/\beta_3$ is a secondary parameter or not. So Experiment 4 fixed θ, R_0 and the τ_k (hence p_4) and varied α by up to 50% about its central value of 2 (reflecting the greater

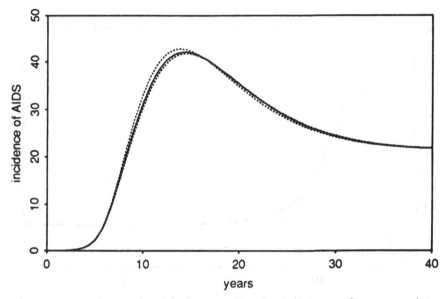

Figure 5: Incidence of AIDS. θ, R_0 and p_4 fixed (Primary Components), α fixed and τ_1, τ_2 and τ_4 varying by up to $\pm 20\%$. The worst cases are plotted.

uncertainty in this ratio). Dynamics were found to vary by less than $\pm 1\%$ so α is also a secondary parameter.

So from 8 basic epidemic parameters M, τ_1, τ_2, τ_3, τ_4 (or $\gamma_1, \gamma_2, \gamma_3, \gamma_4$) β_1, β_3 and β_4 we have found three Primary Components: θ, the initial growth rate; R_0, the basic reproductive ratio; and p_4 the proportion of new infectives who will be diagnosed as having AIDS before dying. We also have five secondary parameters: M; τ_1, τ_2, τ_4; and $\alpha = \beta_4/\beta_3$.

It was noted in Section 2 that the process of model fitting commonly results in a relatively flat likelihood surface. We can now qualify that observation. Where the Primary Components remain fixed the likelihood surface is flat. If, on the other hand, we allow the Primary Components to vary then we will find a well defined peak.

7   The inclusion of infection data

The analysis described in Section 6 considered the case where AIDS incidence data represented the only reliable source of data. It may be, however, that

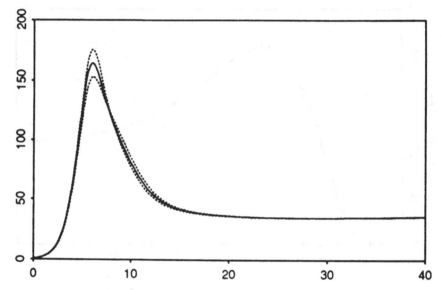

Figure 6: Incidence of new infection. θ, R_0 and p_4 fixed (Primary Components), α fixed and τ_1, τ_2 and τ_4 varying by up to $\pm 20\%$. The worst cases are plotted.

further data relating to the incidence of new infection is available (for example, Bailey 1988; Koopman, private communication). A Primary Component analysis must now look at both AIDS and infection curves simultaneously.

From the analysis of Section 6 it is sufficient that θ, R_0 and p_4 are fixed for us to be able to determine the AIDS incidence curve to within a small margin of error.

Figure 6 shows how the incidence of new infection varies if θ, R_0 and p_4 are fixed and τ_1, τ_2 and τ_4 allowed to vary by $\pm 20\%$ about their central values. Differences between curves peak at around $\pm 4\%$. These differences include short durations, where, although the infection curves all have the same rate of exponential growth, the different parameter values mean that different infection curves start at different levels subject to the AIDS incidence curves being properly matched at short durations.

These differences may not be felt to be significant, in which case θ, R_0 and p_4 remain sufficient as the set of Primary Components.

If the differences are considered to be unsatisfactory then two possibilities for a fourth Primary Component have been identified.

The first is

$$p_4(\theta) = \frac{\gamma_1\gamma_2\gamma_3}{(\gamma_1 + \mu + \theta)(\gamma_2 + \mu + \theta)(\gamma_3 + \mu + \theta)} \tag{7.1}$$

It can be shown that the underlying exponential AIDS and infection incidence curves stay in the ratio $p_4(\theta)$ to 1. Thus fixing both θ and $p_4(\theta)$ will fix both the infection and AIDS incidence curves. Fixing R_0 and p_4 in addition reduces medium term differences between incidence curves around the peak to more acceptable levels.

The variations in Figure 6 are of the order of only 3% to 4% at the worst points on the curve. The reason for these low values can now be clarified by considering $p_4(\theta)$. Allowing the τ_k to vary by $\pm20\%$ could produce changes of similar magnitude in $p_4(\theta)$. However, the constraint that p_4 is fixed limits the range of variation of $p_4(\theta)$ to around $\pm4\%$.

The second possibility for a fourth Primary Component (but theoretically less justified than $p_4(\theta)$) is the waiting time spent in stage 2 of infection, τ_2. This still leaves the possibility of small variations in the short term dynamics ($\pm4\%$) but gives less variation around the peak.

8   Model fitting and projection

Suppose we have observed quarterly incidence of AIDS $A_1, A_2, ..., A_T$. The purpose of model fitting and projection is to estimate parameter values by fitting, for example, the deterministic epidemic curve to the observed data and then projecting the best fitting curve.

We split the set of parameters, ϕ, into three subsets: ϕ_P, the Primary Components; ϕ_S, the secondary parameters; and ϕ_N, the initial conditions (nuisance parameters). The set of parameters ϕ leads to a deterministic AIDS incidence curve $a_1, a_2, ..., a_T$. The log-likelihood, assuming Poisson errors, is

$$l(\phi) = \sum_{t=1}^{T}(A_t \log a_t - a_t) + \text{constant} \tag{8.1}$$

(for example, see Bailey and Estreicher 1986; Cairns 1991).

It is just as easy to develop functions for other distributions: for example, the negative binomial distribution, with $Var(A_t) > E(A_t) = a_t$.

The traditional approach to model fitting requires optimization over all parameters giving the true maximum likelihood (ML)

$$\hat{l} = l(\hat{\phi}_P, \hat{\phi}_S, \hat{\phi}_N) = \sup_{\phi} l(\phi) \tag{8.2}$$

In Sections 2 and 6 it was discussed how the nature of the likelihood surface could give rise to a misleading maximum likelihood estimator $\hat{\phi}$: the maximum likelihood estimates of the secondary parameters could be far from the true values. However, the maximum likelihood estimates of the Primary Components will be reasonable.

Rather than maximize over the full set of basic parameters, then, it is proposed that the likelihood function be maximized over the Primary Components only. If this is combined with the use of *realistic* secondary parameters it will give rise to a projection which is very close to the true maximum likelihood projection. This is because varying the secondary parameters hardly has any effect on the dynamics and hence on the likelihood, whereas varying the Primary Components will alter the dynamics and lower the likelihood.

Define $\bar{\phi}_N(\phi_P)$ to be the set of initial conditions which maximizes $l(\phi)$ given ϕ_P and ϕ_S, and let $\tilde{\phi}_P$ be the Primary Component Maximum Likelihood Estimate (PCMLE): that is

$$\tilde{l} = l(\tilde{\phi}_P, \phi_S, \bar{\phi}_N(\phi_P)) = \sup_{\phi_P} l(\phi_P, \phi_S, \bar{\phi}_N(\phi_P)) \tag{8.3}$$

Then the general reasoning behind Primary Components and Secondary Parameters means that $\tilde{l} \approx \hat{l}$, $\tilde{\phi}_P \approx \hat{\phi}_P$ and that the PCML projection will be very close to the true ML projection. That is, it is sufficient to estimate the Primary Components rather than to estimate the full set of basic parameters.

A $100(1-\alpha)\%$ confidence region (or support region) for ϕ_P, using standard likelihood ratio techniques, is

$$C(k_\nu) = \left\{ \phi_P : \tilde{l} - l(\phi_P, \phi_S, \bar{\phi}_N(\phi_P)) < k_\nu \right\} \tag{8.4}$$

for some constant k_ν, where ν is the number of Primary Components. Using large sample approximations (for example, see Silvey 1970) k_ν is 0.5 times the $100(1-\alpha)\%$ point of the χ^2_ν distribution. For example, if $\alpha = 0.05$ and $\nu = 3$ then $k_\nu = 3.91$.

Alternatively we can construct a confidence interval for a single Primary Component, say R_0, by projecting $C(k_1)$ onto the R_0 axis, where $k_1 = \frac{1}{2}\chi^2_{1,0.95}$.

Similarly we can obtain a confidence interval for the expected incidence of AIDS in each quarter t in the future. This is

$$P_t = \left\{ a_t(\phi) : \phi_P \in C(k_1), \phi_N = \bar{\phi}_N(\phi_P) \right\} \tag{8.5}$$

This construction mimics the method of Cox and Medley (1989), but where they use an empirical curve, here a full model is used.

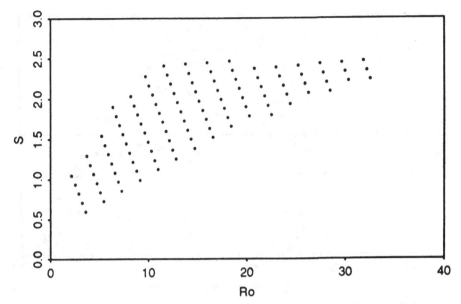

Figure 7: Lattice approximation to the confidence region for two Primary Components R_0 and S (see Cairns 1991).

In practice the confidence regions and intervals cannot be computed exactly. Instead we set up a suitable lattice $\mathcal{L}$ of points in the ϕ_P space (see Cox and Medley 1989, Cairns 1991). We then take $C'(k) = C(k) \cap \mathcal{L}$, and estimate the true $C(k)$ by eye or by applying some numerical techniques. This construction of $C'k$ is illustrated in Figure 7, for two Primary Components (the size of the region reflecting the fact that only early incidence data was used to estimate two long term Primary Components).

Similarly, we approximate the confidence interval P_t by

$$P_t' = \left\{ a_t(\phi) : \phi_P \in C(k_1) \cap \mathcal{L}, \phi_N = \bar{\phi}_N(\phi_P) \right\} \tag{8.6}$$

$$= \left\{ a_t(\phi) : \phi_P \in C'(k_1), \phi_N = \bar{\phi}_N(\phi_P) \right\} \tag{8.7}$$

Construction of P_t' is illustrated in Figure 8. Each point in the graph represents the projected quarterly incidence of AIDS versus log-likelihood (+ constant) for one point on the lattice. Points with a log-likelihood more than $k_1 = 1.92$ from the maximum are excluded and the endpoints of P_t' are then taken as the minimum and maximum of those left remaining.

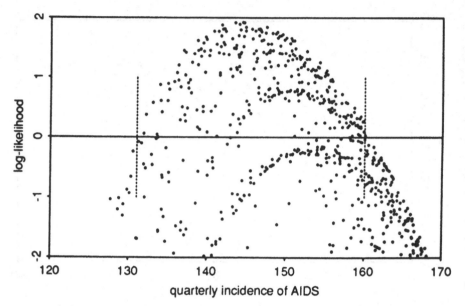

Figure 8: Construction of a 95% confidence interval for a_t. Each point represents projected incidence against log-likelihood (+constant) for one point on the lattice. The limits for the confidence interval are taken as the most extreme of those points plotted with a log-likelihood of within $\frac{1}{2}\chi^2_{1,1-\alpha}$ of the maximum (1.92 for $\alpha = 0.05$).

The full set of confidence intervals is shown in Figure 9. The jagged curve shows the actual incidence of AIDS over time (one simulation of a stochastic model). The smooth curve represents the PCML projection based on the first 15 years of incidence data and the upper and lower dotted curves represent typical 95% confidence limits for the *expected* incidence at time t.

With only early incidence data confidence intervals for future incidence may be very wide, reflecting the uncertainty in the estimated values of the long term Primary Components. With more data up to the peak and beyond, this uncertainty becomes much reduced and the confidence intervals become much narrower.

9   Discussion

The Primary Component approach may appear to suggest that more detailed analyses of specific aspects of a model become redundant. This is not necessarily the case though. For example, it is felt that an accurate description of

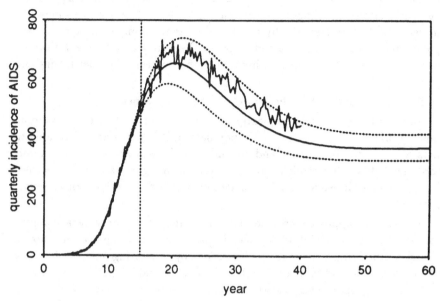

Figure 9: Confidence bounds for projection for $T = 15$: maximum likelihood projection (solid, smooth curve); upper and lower 95% confidence bounds (dotted curves). Actual realisation shown beyond $T = 15$ for comparison.

the first stage of infection (its duration, τ_1, and level of infectiousness, β_1) is an essential step in progressing towards making a reasonable projection. This is not inconsistent with the Primary Component approach.

First, stage 1 of infection has a strong influence on the initial growth rate, θ, and on R_0: both Primary Components. (The importance of β_1 in relation to R_0 depends on the significance of β_1 in relation to β_3 and β_4. Recent studies are beginning to suggest that the probability of infection *per contact* in stage 1 may be much higher than in stages 3 and 4. Such differences might lead to an alternative and possibly larger set of Primary Components.) The Primary Component approach estimates β_1 and τ_1 indirectly, whereas other analyses take a more direct approach by following a cohort of individuals infected or at risk from HIV infection. It should be noted, however, that the analysis of Cairns (1990b, 1991) found that a high degree of accuracy in estimates of basic parameters (here β_1 and τ_1) would be required before significant improvements in the accuracy of a projection could be achieved.

Second, independent investigations into the values of specific parameters is a vital part of the process of a Primary Component analysis. It is important to know what we mean by a realistic range is for each secondary parameter, and such knowledge comes from carrying out independent investigations. An investigation which successfully narrows the range of one or more secondary parameters could result in a reduction in the number of Primary Components thereby speeding up and improving the process of model fitting and projection.

Primary Component analysis has two important aspects.

First, although model complexity is an important part of understanding how an infection spreads through a population, it is necessary to be able to look at a model as a whole and to understand what are the most important elements of that model. Primary Components give us just such a view by identifying the small number of factors which dictate how an epidemic progresses.

Second, the approach provides us with a means of applying a complex model to a relatively simple dataset. In particular, this paper argues how a model can be fitted to a set of incidence data by estimating only the Primary Components. In addition, a valuable side-effect is that we have a simple way of quantifying the level of uncertainty in a projection.

An important conclusion from simulation studies is that with only early incidence data (as in the AIDS epidemic) we cannot place much reliance on any single projection made.

The method described here has not considered the possibility of behavioural changes or changes in the treatment of individuals infected with HIV. This is a problem considered by Becker and Egerton (1994) and it will be interesting to see whether or not the methods described here can be applied successfully to such situations.

10   Further work

There are a number of areas which will merit further development or investigation.

(a) Investigate the accuracy of the projections and the confidence intervals by carrying out some Monte-Carlo studies. For example, simulate 100 epidemics, fit the model 100 times and produce 100 PCML projections and confidence intervals.

(b) We need to look at the effect model choice has on the process of projection. What if the model is too simple? What if the model contains some wrong assumptions or structure? How do these problems affect the accuracy of a projection or is the method relatively robust: that is, is the projection relatively insensitive to the choice of model?

(c) How can we make better use of the intrinsic variability of the data? For example, successive months may not be independent as the model and likelihood here assume. Instead, a high number of cases this month may mean there will be fewer new cases next month. Initial steps have been made in this area: for example, Sugihara and May (1990) who model measles data as a chaotic time series and Cairns (1991, 1992) who uses the variability of the data as stochastic feedback.

Acknowledgements

I would like to thank Jim Koopman, Ira Longini, Ingemar Nåsell and a referee for their helpful remarks during the preparation of this paper.

References

Anderson, R.M., Blythe, S.P., Gupta, S. and Konings, E. (1989) 'The transmission dynamics of the human immunodeficiency virus type 1 in the male homosexual community in the United Kingdom: the influence of changes in sexual behaviour', *Phil. Trans. R. Soc. Lond. B* **325**, 45–98.

Anderson, R.M., May, R.M. and McLean, A.R. (1988) 'Possible demographic consequences of AIDS in developing countries', *Nature* **332**, 228–234.

Bailey, N.T.J. (1988) 'Simplified modelling of the population dynamics of HIV/AIDS', *J. R. Statist. Soc.A* **151**, 31–43.

Bailey, N.T.J. and Duppenthaler, J. (1980) 'Sensitivity analysis in the modelling of infectious disease dynamics', *J. Math. Biol.* **10**, 113–131.

Bailey, N.T.J. and Estreicher, J. (1986) 'Epidemic prediction and public health control with special reference to influenza and AIDS', *Proc. 1st World Congress of Bernoulli Society* (Tashkent, Sept. 1986) Utrecht, VNU Science Press.

Becker, N.G. and Egerton, L.R. (1994) 'A transmission model for HIV with application to the Australian epidemic', *Math. Biosci.* **119**, 317–319.

Blythe, S.P. and Anderson, R.M. (1988a) 'Variable infectiousness in HIV transmission models', *IMA J. Math. Med. Biol.* **5**, 181–200.

Blythe, S.P. and Anderson, R.M. (1988b) 'Heterogeneous sexual activity models of HIV transmission male homosexual populations', *IMA J. Math. Med. Biol.* **5**, 237–60.

Bongaarts, J. (1989) 'A model of the spread of HIV infection and the demographic impact of AIDS', *Stat. Med.* **8**, 103–20.

Cairns, A.J.G. (1990a) 'Epidemics in heterogeneous populations II: Non-exponential incubation periods and variable infectiousness', *IMA J. Math. Med. Biol.* **7**, 219–230.

Cairns, A.J.G. (1990b) *Epidemics in heterogeneous populations: Spread, estimation and control* PhD Thesis, Dept. of Actuarial Mathematics and Statistics, Heriot-Watt University, UK.

Cairns, A.J.G. (1991) 'Model fitting and projection of the AIDS epidemic', *Math. Biosci.* **107**, 451–489.

Cairns, A.J.G. (1992) 'Epidemic estimation with removal time data', *The Theory of Probability and its Applications* **37**, 374–377 (in Russian).

Cox, D.R. and Medley, G.F. (1989) 'A process of events with notification delay and the forecasting of AIDS', *Phil. Trans. R. Soc. Lond. B* **325**, 135–45.

Dietz, K. (1988) 'On the transmission dynamics of HIV', *Math. Biosci.* **90**, 397–414.

Hethcote, H.W. and Yorke, J.A. (1984) *Gonorrhea Transmission Dynamics and Control*, Lecture Notes in Biomathematics **56**. Springer, Heidelberg.

Jacquez, J.A. *et al.* (1988) 'Modelling and analyzing HIV transmission: the effect of contact patterns', *Math. Biosci.* **92**, 119–99.

Koopman, J., Simon, C. and Jacquez, J. (1988) 'Sexual partner selectiveness: Effects on homosexual transmission dynamics', *J. AIDS* **1**, 486–504.

Longini, I.M. *et al.* (1989) 'Statistical analysis of the stages of HIV infection using a Markov model', *Stat. Med.* **8**, 831–843.

Longini, I.M., Clarke, W.S., Haber, M. and Horsburgh, R. (1989) 'The stages of HIV infection: Waiting times and infection transmission probabilities'. In *Mathematical and Statistical Approaches to AIDS Epidemiology*, C. Castillo-Chavez (ed.), Lecture Notes in Biomathematics **83**, 111–137, Springer, Berlin.

Longini, I.M., Clark, W.S., Gardner, L.I. and Brundage, J.F. (1991) 'The dynamics of $CD4^+$ T-Lymphocyte decline in HIV infected individuals: a Markov modelling approach', *J. AIDS* **4**, 1141–1147.

Longini, I.M., Byers, R.H., Hessol, N.A. and Tan, W.Y. (1992) 'Estimating the stage-specific numbers of HIV infection using a Markov model and back calculation', *Stat. Med.* **11**, 831–843.

May, R.M. and Anderson, R.M. (1984) 'Spatial heterogeneity and the design of immunization programs', *Math. Biosci.* **72**, 83–111.

Mollison, D. (1984) 'Simplifying simple epidemic models', *Nature* **310**, 224–25.

Nåsell, I. (1985) *Hybrid Models of Tropical Infections*, Lecture Notes in Biomathematics **59**. Springer, Berlin.

Silvey, S.D. (1970) *Statistical Inference.* Chapman and Hall, London.

Wilkie, A.D. (1989) 'Population projections for AIDS using an actuarial model', *Phil. Trans. R. Soc. Lond. B* **325**, 99–112.

Estimation and Prediction
in Tropical Disease Control:
the Example of Onchocerciasis

Hans Remme
Soumbey Alley
Anton Plaisier

Summary

The identification of the most cost-effective and sustainable control strategies
is important for all diseases, but particularly so for the tropical diseases because of the dramatic economic and development problems of the countries
where these diseases are endemic. This requires, however, reliable predictions
of the long term impact of alternative control strategies, while the implementation, evaluation and timely adjustment of these control strategies requires
a sound quantitative understanding of the epidemiological trends to be expected during the control period. Epidemiological modelling can be helpful
in this respect by providing the necessary quantitative framework (Remme
1992).

The development and quantification of epidemiological models for tropical
diseases is not a simple matter. The epidemiology of these diseases is very
complex as it depends on the dynamic interaction of at least three populations, i.e. the parasites, the human hosts and the vectors. Another complication, though a fortunate one, is the recent development of new control
tools for which the long term impact is not yet known (WHO 1991). These
include new drugs, such as ivermectin for onchocerciasis, praziquantel for
schistosomiasis and MDT for leprosy, and new biologicals for vector control
in onchocerciasis and lymphatic filariasis. Vaccines for malaria, leishmaniasis
and schistosomiasis are under various stages of development, as are a number
of immunodiagnostic tools.

There are several examples of successful and practical applications of epidemiological modelling in disease control. For the tropical diseases, the best
example is found in the Onchocerciasis Control Programme in West Africa
(OCP). In this article we describe the gradual introduction of applied epidemiological modelling in the OCP, the various models developed of increasing

complexity, the estimation of the major parameters in these models and the use of modelling in evaluation of control and in predicting the impact of alternative control strategies available to the control programme. Finally we will shortly discuss the main factors which have contributed to the effectiveness of modelling in the OCP and refer to similar initiatives for epidemiological modelling of other tropical diseases.

1 Onchocerciasis and the Onchocerciasis Control Programme (OCP) in West Africa

Onchocerciasis is a major parasitic disease which is endemic in large parts of Africa and in isolated foci in Central and South America and in Yemen. It has been estimated that as many as 18 million people are infected with the parasite, the filarial nematode *Onchocerca volvulus*, and more than 99% of those infected live in Africa (WHO 1987a). The adult worm produces millions of microfilariae which migrate into the skin of the human host. The parasite is transmitted by a blackfly which ingests microfilariae during a bloodmeal on man. In the fly, some of these microfilariae develop into infective larvae which may be transmitted to another person during a subsequent bloodmeal to develop into new adult worms. The microfilariae are the main cause of the clinical manifestations of the disease which include dermal, lymphatic and systemic complications. However, the most severe complications are onchocercal lesions of the eye which may ultimately lead to total blindness. It is estimated that 340,000 people are blind as a result of onchocerciasis. The majority of the onchocercal blind are found in the West and Central African savanna belt where the disease is most severe. There, onchocerciasis is not only a major public health problem, but often also an obstacle to socio-economic development. Fear of the disease has led to the depopulation of relatively fertile river valleys where the vector of the disease, *Simulium damnosum s.l.*, has its breeding sites and where transmission is most intense (Remme and Zongo 1989).

The possibilities for onchocerciasis control are limited. Until recently chemotherapy was not an option because the existing drugs for the treatment of onchocerciasis produced very serious adverse reactions which prevented their utilization on a mass scale (WHO 1987a). The only alternative was vector control through the application of larvicides to the rivers where the breeding sites of the vector are found. During the 1950s vector control was applied successfully in certain isolated foci in East Africa where the vector *Simulium neavei s.s.* was completely eliminated (Roberts *et al.* 1967). But experiences in West Africa had shown that isolated vector control was not appropriate because of the wide distribution of the infection and the active migratory behaviour of the West African savanna vectors of the *Simulium damnosum* complex. The only possible approach was larviciding of all breeding sites over an extensive area and during a long period of time. This was the approach chosen for the Onchocerciasis Control Programme in West Africa (OCP) when it was launched in 1975 in the Volta river basin area which, at that time, was the most severely affected region in the world.

The strategy of the OCP was to interrupt transmission through vector control, and to keep it interrupted until the parasite reservoir in the human hosts had died naturally and fallen to such a low level that there would be no recrudescence of the disease when vector control is stopped and the vector is allowed to return (WHO 1987a). Based on very limited information from the East African control programmes on the longevity of onchocerciasis infection in man, the Programme was initially planned to last for a period of 20 years.

2 Force-of-infection model: interpretation of epidemiological trends

During the first 8 years of larviciding from 1975 to 1983, vector control was quite successful in most of the Programme area according to the results of the entomological evaluation which indicated that transmission had been brought down to insignificant levels. However, the epidemiological evaluation had not been able to demonstrate a major epidemiological change during all these years of control.

Epidemiological surveys had been undertaken at intervals of 3-4 years in more than 150 indicator villages which represented all the major river basins in the original Programme area. Each survey had included skin snip examinations for the presence and intensity of *O.volvulus* microfilariae (Prost and Prod'hon 1978). The routine analysis of these data had, after 8 years of control, not yet provided clear evidence of interruption of transmission or of an important decline in the parasite reservoir. No children below the age of 5 years were found to be infected, but not many infections would have been expected in this age group even if there had been no control. The standardized prevalence of microfilariae in the skin snip, which was at that time the current epidemiological index, had shown only a limited decline during the first eight years of control (Kirkwood *et al.* 1983). To most observers these results appeared to be unsatisfactory and the question was raised if vector control really had interrupted transmission and if reinfection was not still occurring at an undetected but nevertheless significant level. Others, who were willing to take the entomological evaluation data as evidence of interruption of transmission, were worried about the slow decline in the prevalence of infection and became concerned about the required duration of vector control and the cumulative costs involved in the expensive aerial larviciding operations. For long term planning and financing of the Programme it was therefore urgent to arrive at a better understanding of the epidemiological impact of vector control and to make credible predictions of the expected trends in onchocerciasis infection during the remaining control period.

A new analytical methodology was introduced which took the dynamics of the parasite and of the human population into account. The basis of this work was the development of a simple force-of-infection model for onchocerciasis, and its application for a study of the age-specific epidemiological trends during a period of vector control (Remme *et al.* 1986). The most important factors included in the model are the longevity of an infection, the aspect of super-infection, age-specific exposure, and the intensity of transmission during the pre-control period. An onchocerciasis infection was defined as 'the infection of an individual by infective larvae and the subsequent development of one adult female worm which produces microfilariae to the extent that they can be detected in the skin'. This definition allowed for the modelling of superinfection, i.e. multiple, separate infections which occur in parallel in the same individual. The duration of an infection depends on the survival of the adult worm which lives relatively well-protected in subcutaneous nodules and it is believed that the death of adult worms is mainly due to the natural process of ageing. Therefore, a constant survival rate was purposely not used in the model as this would imply an exponential distribution of the longevity of infection, with the majority of worms living only a short period but with a small proportion of worms surviving unrealistically long. As shown with an earlier model for onchocerciasis (Dietz 1982) this would have resulted in predictions of the trends in onchocerciasis infection after interruption of transmission which are at variance with those observed in East Africa. Instead, in this first simple model, the longevity of infection was taken constant, consisting of a pre-patent period with a duration of σ and a patent period with a duration of τ. The force-of-infection $\beta(x)$ is a function of the relative exposure at age x and the annual level of transmission in the community. The level of transmission varies greatly between communities, resulting in great differences in the force-of-infection, and therefore in endemicity levels. In the model this was taken into account but it was assumed that for a given community, the annual level of transmission and the force-of-infection did not vary over time during the pre-control period.

The force-of-infection model for onchocerciasis specifies among others that above the age of $\sigma + \tau$ the expected pre-control prevalence of infection at age x, $F(x)$, is given by:

$$F(x) = 1 - \exp\{-\int_{x-\sigma-\tau}^{x-\sigma} \beta(t)dt\}, \quad x > \sigma + \tau. \qquad (2.1)$$

On the basis of anecdotal information on age-specific exposure, mainly provided by the staff of the epidemiological field teams, it seemed reasonable to assume that the exposure to the vector, and therefore to infection, increases with age till the age of 10 years. From then onward, both male and female children accompany their parents in their daily activities outside the village compound and near the river banks, and they become fully exposed to the bites of *S. damnosum* s.l. In the force-of-infection model therefore it is assumed that over the age of 10 years $\beta(x) = \beta$. As a result, the formula for the prevalence of patent infection simplifies for the older age groups as follows:

$$F(x) = 1 - \exp(-\beta\tau) \quad x > 10 + \sigma + \tau \tag{2.2}$$

while the number of patent infections per person follows a Poisson distribution with mean $\beta\tau$. Thus over the age of $10 + \sigma + \tau$ years both the prevalence and the number of patent infections per person are independent of the actual age.

A simple extension of this force-of-infection model gives equally simple formulas for the prevalence and number of patent of infections after y years of interruption of transmission as a result of vector control. Let $F(x,y)$ be the probability of having at least one patent infection and $P_k(x,y)$ the probability of having k patent infections at age x after y years of successful vector control. It can be shown that:

$$\begin{aligned} F(x,y) &= 1 - \exp\{-\int_{y-\sigma-\tau}^{0} \beta dt\} \quad x > 10 + \sigma + \tau, \sigma < y < \sigma + \tau, \\ &= 1 - \exp\{-\beta(\sigma + \tau - y)\} \end{aligned} \tag{2.3}$$

and

$$\begin{aligned} P_k(x,y) &= \frac{\{\beta(\sigma + \tau - y)\}^k \exp\{-\beta(\sigma + \tau - y)\}}{k!} \\ & x > 10 + \sigma + \tau, \quad \sigma < y < \sigma + \tau \end{aligned} \tag{2.4}$$

based on the Poisson arrival of infections. For the population above the age of $10 + \sigma + \tau$ years, neither the prevalence of infection nor the distribution of the number of infections depends on the actual age, but only on the pre-control force-of-infection, on the length of the pre-patent and patent periods, and on the duration of control. The mean number of infections is equal to $\beta(\sigma + \tau - y)$, and is thus a linear function of the duration of control, which decreases from a level determined by the pre-control force-of-infection to zero after $\sigma + \tau$ years of control. Therefore, though the actual trend in the mean number of infections per person depends on the pre-control intensity of transmission, and therefore on the level of endemicity, the relative trend is the same for all endemicity levels.

The epidemiological trends predicted by this simple model were fitted and tested against the observed trends in the prevalence and mean load of microfilariae in skin snips taken from a cohort population from 23 villages in an

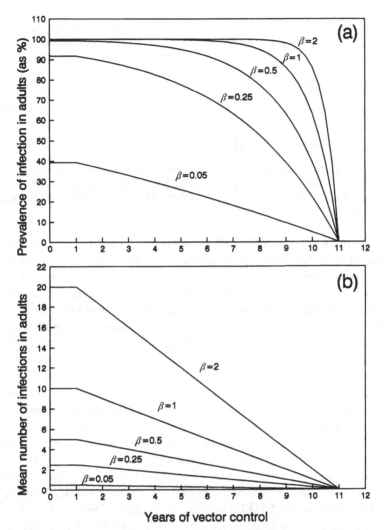

Figure 1: The trends predicted by the force-of-infection model in (a) the prevalence of infection in adults and (b) the mean number of infections per adult during a period of vector control.

area with 8 years of successful vector control. The fitting resulted in a crude (but first ever) estimate for τ of 10 years, while σ was taken equal to 1 year on the basis of scanty information in the literature. The predicted trends for the prevalence and mean mf loads in adults are given in Figure 1.

The model predictions had important implications for the epidemiological evaluation of the impact of vector control. They showed that epidemiological trends during the control period are not uniform but depend on the initial en-

Village	Endemicity level		Estimated Numbers of adult female O.volvulus per person aged 20 years or more		
	Standardized prevalence of mf (as %)	CMFL (as mf/snip)	Arithmetic mean	Geometric mean	95th percentile
Folonzo	71.5	30	7.3	5.9	15
Tiercoura	77.6	71	16.7	10.5	46

Table 1. Estimates of the pre-control worm burden per person above the age of 20 years in two villages with different endemicity levels. The estimates were obtained by fitting ONCHOSIM (see Section 4) to the skin snip data for villages with 12 years of vector control.

demicity level of the population and vary between age groups. The prevalence of infection is too insensitive to be useful for the evaluation in hyperendemic villages during most of the control period (Figure 1a). The most sensitive and meaningful statistic for a comparative analysis and for the assessment of epidemiological changes would be the mean number of infections, or the mean number of productive female worms per person above the age of 20 years (Figure 1b). The number of adult worms cannot be measured directly. However, the microfilarial load in the skin provides an indirect measure of this, assuming that there are no major density dependent mechanisms operating within the human hosts which regulate microfilarial production and survival. This reasoning led to the introduction of a new epidemiological index, the Community Microfilarial Load (CMFL) which is the geometric mean microfilarial load per skin snip among the population above the age of 20 years (Remme et al. 1986), see Table 1. Within and outside the OCP, the CMFL has now become the preferred index of endemicity of onchocerciasis, partly because it could later be demonstrated that the risk of onchocercal blindness is linearly related to the CMFL (Remme et al. 1989). The use of the CMFL in the epidemiological evaluation enabled also a much better appreciation of the significant epidemiological impact of 8 years of vector control in the OCP, and it could be shown that in 90% of the original Programme area, vector control had already achieved a reduction in the parasite reservoir of more than 70% (WHO 1987b).

3   Host-parasite model: prediction of trends during vector control

Once the new analytical methodology had provided the epidemiological evidence of the effectiveness of the first 8 years of vector control, the focus of attention shifted toward the epidemiological trends to be expected in subsequent years. Of particular interest were predictions of the ultimate decline in the prevalence of infection as this would indicate how many years of vector control would be required. The force-of-infection model, with the assumption of a constant longevity of infection, was clearly not appropriate for such predictions and it became necessary to develop a more sophisticated model which would take the variability in the duration of infection into account. Furthermore, for the interpretation of the observed epidemiological trends in different parts of the Programme area it became increasingly important to have predictions of the trends to be expected in the distribution of microfilarial loads in different age groups, and not only in the prevalence and mean mf load in adults.

In order to respond to those needs, the so-called "Host-Parasite" model was developed (Remme *et al.* 1990). This is a stochastic computer simulation model which uses the technique of microsimulation (Habbema *et al.*, in press). It involves the simulation of the life histories of all individual human hosts living in a community, and of the individual life histories of all adult parasites harboured by these human hosts. The lifehistories are generated from probability distributions for which the parameters were estimated using demographic information, results from specific parasitological studies (Karam *et al.* 1987) and fitting of the model to the epidemiological evaluation data for selected reference villages in the OCP. The major parameters of the host-parasite model which govern the epidemiological trends are the pre-control force-of-infection (which determines the endemicity level), exposure heterogeneity between individuals, the longevity of the adult worm and worm-age specific mf production. Model output shows the predicted trends in the distribution and summary statistics of skin mf loads by age and sex during the vector control period.

The host-parasite model provided much more realistic predictions of the epidemiological trends during the later years of control. The first predictions with this model were made in 1985, after 10 years of control, and indicated that the prevalence of infection would fall to levels close to zero after 14-15 years of interruption of transmission. The epidemiological data collected during subsequent years confirmed this prediction and generally showed a good agreement between the predicted and observed trends (see Figure 2 for an example of the predicted and observed trends in mf distribution in a hyperendemic village). This good agreement supports the basic assumptions underlying the host-parasite model, including the hypothesis that the reproductive lifespan of the adult female worm is the main determinant of the epidemiological trends during a period of vector control, and the absence of a major density dependent mechanism in the human host which regulates mf production. It also indicates that the quantification of the model was based on realistic estimates of the most important parasitological parameters. These

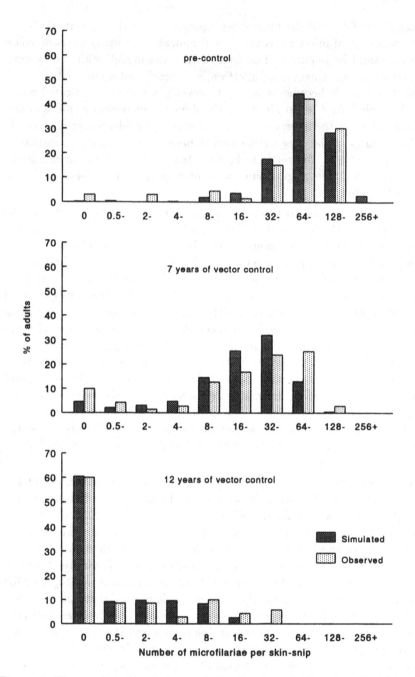

Figure 2: The predicted and observed distribution of skin microfilarial loads among adults in the village of Tiercoura, Burkina Faso, after different periods of vector control.

included an estimate of 10.4 years for the average duration of infection, which corresponds to a mean reproductive lifespan of *O.volvulus* of 9-9.5 years, and an estimated upper limit of 15 years for 95% of infections. These estimates represent only one possible quantification of the model, and a detailed sensitivity analysis, which used a longer series of epidemiological data, was later undertaken to determine the complete range of parameter values which are consistent with the observed epidemiological trends (Plaisier *et al.* 1991a).

For several years the host-parasite model became the principal epidemiological tool for the interpretation of the epidemiological evaluation data collected in dozens of indicator villages. Two examples of the routine application of the model for this purpose are given in Figures 3a and 3b, the first showing a typical example of a satisfactory epidemiological trend in a well controlled area, the second giving the results for a village in a focus where there had been local breakdowns in vector control.

4 ONCHOSIM: a microsimulation model for onchocerciasis transmission and control

When the duration of vector control approached 12 years, and the prevalence of infection started to show the predicted accelerating decline throughout the central Programme area, it became urgent to answer the next major question: when could the expensive larviciding operations be stopped without running a unacceptable risk of recrudescence of infection and disease. To answer this question, it became necessary to develop again another, and this time a much more complicated, model which described the full transmission cycle. The result was ONCHOSIM (Plaisier *et al.* 1990), a comprehensive transmission model which allows the simultaneous simulation of a human and parasite population, the dynamics of the vector population and of interventions based on larviciding and/or chemotherapy (see Figure 4).

The basic structure of ONCHOSIM was designed during a meeting at OCP headquarters in January 1987, which was attended by representatives from all technical units of the OCP and by several external experts. The meeting identified the most important operational questions for which a model should be developed. It also recommended that, in order to ensure a sufficiently flexible model which could easily be adapted according to new scientific insights or new operational needs, the same technique of stochastic microsimulation be used as in the host-parasite model.

A detailed description of ONCHOSIM is provided in Plaisier *et al.* (1990) and in Habbema *et al.* (in press).

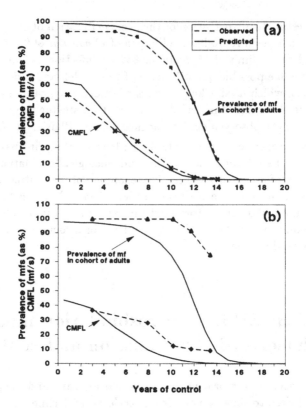

Figure 3: The predicted and observed trend in the prevalence of microfilaria in skin snips (mfs) and in the Community Microfilarial Load (CMFL) during the vector control period. Figure 3a is for the village of Tiercoura, Burkina Faso, and gives a typical example of a trend in an area with satisfactory control. Figure 3b is for the village of Nakong, Ghana, from a focus for which there have been localized breakdowns in control.

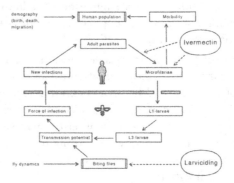

Figure 4: A schematic representation of the ONCHOSIM microsimulation model for onchocerciasis transmission and control.

5   Examples of the use of ONCHOSIM in the prospective evaluation of control

Since 1989, ONCHOSIM has been used routinely for the prospective evaluation of control strategies based on vector control, large scale ivermectin treatment and combinations of these two methods. This has involved the simulation of onchocerciasis transmission and infection in the human population in endemic foci, and of the epidemiological impact of control, over a period of decades. A typical simulation begins some hundred years before the start of control in order to generate a stable human population with respect to age, onchocerciasis infection and blindness, followed by the simulation of some 50-75 years after the start of control.

In this section we will show the results for five indices, i.e. the (in reality unknown) prevalence of mature female worms, the prevalence of microfilariae in the skin snips (assuming two skin snips per person), the Community Microfilarial Load (CMFL), the Annual Transmission Potential (ATP, Walsh *et al.* 1978) and the prevalence of onchocercal blindness. The results are presented in graphs which show the relative changes in these indices, taking for each index the pre-control value as 100%.

5.1   Vector control

The impact of successful vector control   Figure 5 shows the predicted impact of 15 years of successful vector control. The trends in the five indices are very similar to those observed in the central OCP area where vector control has been very successful. Vector control results in the virtual interruption of transmission and the ATP drops to zero after the start of control. The CMFL shows the near linear decline, already predicted by the force-of-infection model, and falls to values close to zero after 10-12 years of control. The prevalence of adult worms and the prevalence of mf in the skin snip decrease initially slower but show subsequently an accelerated decline towards insignificant levels after 15 years of control. The prevalence of blindness hardly changes during the first 5 years of control when there is still some incidence of blindness in cases with high mf loads. After this period the prevalence of blindness decreases slowly as a result of mortality among the blind. After 15 years of control the local reservoir of the parasite has fallen so low that there is no longer any incidence of infection when the vector is allowed to return but when there is no reintroduction of the parasite.

Recrudescence after pre-mature interruption of vector control   The long term objective of the OCP is to ensure that there will be no recrudescence of infection and disease. However, it was never very clear what was

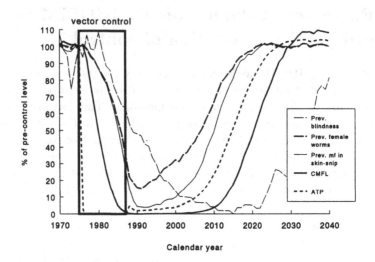

Figure 5: The predicted epidemiological trends during 15 years of successful vector control.

to be expected in case of recrudescence. Modelling has been very useful in clarifying this issue, and Figure 6 shows the results of a simulation of recrudescence if vector control is interrupted too early. The fact that recrudescence is taking place will initially not be obvious. The prevalence of mf continues to decrease for several years. New infections occur immediately after the return of the vector, as is shown by the increase in the prevalence of adult female worms, but during the first years after cessation of vector control it will be difficult to detect the recrudescence of infection by entomological methods and cross-sectional skin snip surveys. However, after a period of several years of apparent calm, the prevalence of mf will show an accelerating increase and return to the pre-control value if no intervention is undertaken. The other indices will increase in a similar fashion but with a delay of 5 to 30 years. The increase in prevalence will cause an accelerated rise in the ATP, and this will result in a higher incidence of (super)infection and an increase in the CMFL. Once the CMFL has reached the pre-control level the parasitological situation will have returned to an equilibrium situation. It will take several more years before there has been a complete recrudescence of onchocercal blindness.

Required duration of vector control   A large series of simulations has been run to determine the risk of recrudescence in relation to the duration of vector control after taking the uncertainty in the quantification of the most sensitive parameters into account. Simulations of successful vector control indicate that recrudescence is likely if larviciding is stopped after 12 years of control. The breakpoint appears to be a control period of 13 years. The par-

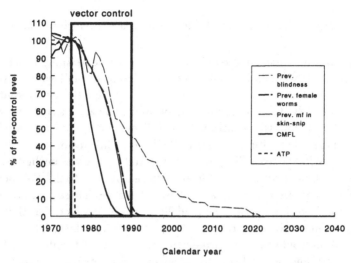

Figure 6: The predicted epidemiological trends after an insufficient period of vector control (12 years in this simulation) and subsequent recrudescence of onchocerciasis infection and disease.

asite reservoir died out in a large number of simulations of 13 years of control but in most simulations with very high biting rates and unfavourable assumptions on the probability of mating and the initial slope of the L1-uptake function, there was recrudescence of infection (Plaisier *et al.* 1991b). In simulations with 14 years of successful vector control there was only recrudescence in some simulations with combinations of extreme assumptions.

In case of incomplete vector control the required duration of larviciding is longer and depends on the effectiveness of control. A reduction in the vector density of some 98% has nearly the same impact as complete interruption of transmission. But a reduction of 90% would require a continuation of vector control for 25 years before a situation without risk of recrudescence has been reached.

Entomological evaluation after cessation of vector control On the basis of these model predictions, the OCP concluded that 14 years of successful vector control were required in each Programme area but that subsequently vector control could be stopped in a given area if the following criteria were met: (i) according to the entomological evaluation there had been no significant transmission during the 14 years of control, (ii) the epidemiological trends in all indicator villages in the area were consistent with the model predictions, and (iii) no children born since the start of control had become infected. In areas where all these criteria were met, the vector was allowed to return. Nevertheless, in order to validate whether the decision to stop had been correct, special entomological studies were undertaken of vector infectivity levels during the first two years after cessation of vector control.

A difficulty in these entomological studies was to determine which vector infectivity levels were to be considered as insignificant and which levels reflected an unacceptable risk of transmission. This question was studied in a number of ONCHOSIM simulations of epidemiological situations with a medium to very low risk of recrudescence. These simulations indicated that, if the number of flies with L3 larvae in the head (F3h) was in the order or 0.9 to 1.3 flies per 1000 parous flies, the risk of recrudescence was negligible. However, in simulations where vector infectivity reached 1.4 to 2.2 F3h per 1000 parous flies, there were several cases of recrudescence. These results were the basis for the following operational guidelines: if the observed infectivity level would be significantly lower than 1 F3h per 1000 parous flies, the entomological evaluation would have confirmed the correctness of the decision to stop vector control, and no further entomological evaluation would be required at the site in question. If vector infectivity would be significantly higher than 2 F3h per 1000 parous flies, the risk of recrudescence would be unacceptable and vector control should be started again. In the range between 1 and 2 F3h per 1000 parous flies it would be difficult to take a decision on the basis of the model predictions alone, and in such situations additional information on the specific local situation should be taken into account. These guidelines were used to develop sequential decision charts for the entomological evaluation. Figure 7 shows such a chart in which the data have been plotted for Nabere, one of the post-control evaluation points in the central OCP area. For the purpose of comparison the pre-control data for the focus of Asubende in Ghana have been added to this figure. Todate, the post-control data have confirmed the correctness to stop larviciding in 10 out of 11 foci studied.

5.2   Chemotherapy based control

In 1982, seven years after the start of vector control, a promising development in the field of chemotherapy of onchocerciasis occurred when Aziz and his collaborators reported from a small clinical trial that ivermectin was an effective microfilaricide which was much better tolerated than the previous microfilaricide of choice, diethylcarbamazine (Aziz et al. 1982). Though this report was initially received with scepticism, subsequent clinical trials confirmed the conclusion and the manufacturer of the drug informed the OCP in 1986 that it had started procedures for registration of ivermectin for the treatment of human onchocerciasis. At that stage it became urgent for the Programme to decide if it was going to use ivermectin in the control of onchocerciasis, and if so, how.

The answer to this question was not straightforward. The OCP was a time

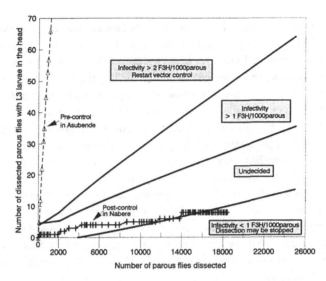

Figure 7: A decision chart for the post-vector control entomological evaluation of vector infectivity levels. The results are shown for the evaluation in the village of Nabere along the river Bougouriba, Burkina Faso, where over 18,000 flies were dissected during the first year after cessation of vector control. For comparison purposes the pre-control results are plotted for the village of Asubende, Ghana.

limited programme which was achieving its objective through the interruption of transmission by vector control exclusively. A question of major operational importance, therefore, was to what extent ivermectin mass treatment could contribute to transmission control, whether on its own or in combination with vector control.

The study of this new question required another model development and ONCHOSIM was expanded with a submodel which allowed the simulation of ivermectin treatment and its effect on the parasite in the human host. This submodel has been quantified using the results from a community trial in Asubende, Ghana (Remme *et al.* 1989), which has yielded one of the most extensive longitudinal skin snip data sets after repeated ivermectin treatment. Initially, ivermectin was modelled principally as a microfilaricide but preliminary observations on a possible effect of treatment on mf production by the adult worm have also been taken into account. In the first model quantification a female worm does not produce mf during a period of 3 months after ivermectin treatment of the human host, while it was assumed that every ivermectin treatment reduced the maximum reproductive capacity of the female worm by 10%. The treatment coverage, compliance and exclusion criteria have also been quantified using the results of the Asubende trial.

Impact of large scale ivermectin treatment on transmission and disease The predicted impact of 25 years of annual large scale ivermectin treatment is shown in Figure 8. In this simulation it has been assumed that the treatment coverage does not decrease during the full 25 year period, an assumption which was initially considered rather unrealistic but which has become more acceptable over time when ivermectin treatment has proven to be highly popular and treatment compliance did not decline during the first 5 years of mass-treatment. Figure 8 shows that every mass treatment results in an immediate drop in prevalence of skin mf and in the CMFL. During the subsequent 12 months both indices increase again as a result of mf repopulation. After the first treatments the prevalence returns nearly to the pre-treatment level but the CMFL stays below 40% of its initial value. The treatment has reduced transmission during the first post-treatment year by more than 50%. All these predictions are very similar to those which have been observed during the first three years of the community trial of ivermectin in Asubende (Figure 9).

The reduction in transmission and in the incidence of infection has a cumulative effect over time and results in a steady reduction in the intensity of onchocerciasis transmission. However, the long term impact on the parasite reservoir is not sufficient to prevent the immediate and rapid recrudescence of the intensity of infection and disease when annual treatment is stopped after 25 years. Many other simulations of scenarios based on annual or six-monthly ivermectin treatment in non-controlled areas gave the same type of results. It seems therefore that large scale ivermectin treatment cannot achieve the progressive reduction and final elimination of a parasite reservoir in an endemic area. In the absence of other methods of intervention or a major cumulative effect on the adult worm, ivermectin treatment will have to be continued for a very long period of several decades at least.

Though large scale ivermectin treatment does not appear to be appropriate for interruption of transmission in endemic areas in Africa, it is likely to be very effective for disease control as long as a sufficient coverage can be maintained. Comparative simulations of the incidence of blindness during control by larviciding versus control by ivermectin treatment clearly shows the greater impact on disease with ivermectin treatment during the first 5-8 years of control. After this period the two methods are comparable from the point of view of disease control.

The incidence of blindness has been modelled in a simplistic way as a function of mf accumulation by the human host during his life time. This enabled a sufficiently accurate simulation of the impact of vector control. However, results from ophthalmological follow-up surveys during the community trials of ivermectin suggest that ivermectin treatment may result in regression of early stage ocular lesions. The current model may therefore even underesti-

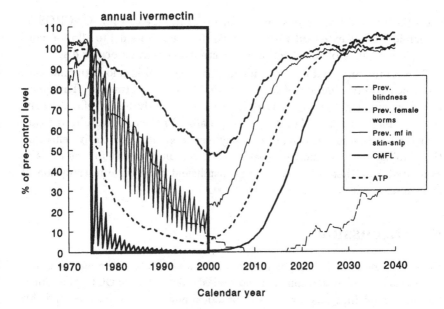

Figure 8: The predicted impact of 25 years of annual ivermectin treatment in a hyperendemic onchocerciasis focus.

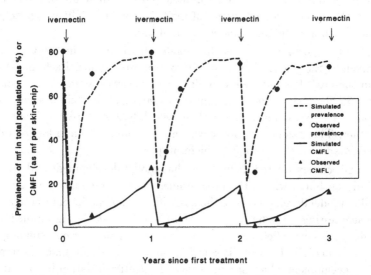

Figure 9: The predicted trend in the prevalence of microfilariae in the total population and in the CMFL during the first three years with annual ivermectin treatment in the onchocerciasis focus of Asubende, Ghana, and the observed results obtained during 9 epidemiological surveys undertaken during this period.

mate the potential of ivermectin treatment for disease control. ONCHOSIM is therefore being extended with an ocular disease sub-model to allow a more realistic modelling of the effect of ivermectin treatment on ocular disease.

The community trial in Asubende has now resulted in a longitudinal data set which covers a period of 6 years with 5 annual treatments. The quantification of chemotherapy in ONCHOSIM is currently being refined by fitting the model to these latest follow-up data. Preliminary results indicate that repeated ivermectin treatment may have a greater cumulative effect on the viability or reproductive capacity of the adult worm than was initially estimated, but that the effect is still insufficient to achieve interruption of transmission with annual ivermectin treatment alone.

6 Discussion

Epidemiological modelling has played an important role in the planning, implementation and evaluation of onchocerciasis control in the OCP. The contribution of modelling has been a very practical and constructive one, and this has been recognized by the staff of the different technical and management units of the control programme. Such a general recognition of the practical value of modelling is certainly not common and it is therefore of interest to reflect on the special characteristics of modelling in the OCP which helped to make it such a useful and widely accepted tool.

The most important factor is that model development in the OCP has been driven by the practical needs of the control programme. Each modelling phase in the OCP has followed a similar cycle, always starting with a major practical problem which the Programme was facing in the field of evaluation or operational decision making; a problem which had to be resolved, one way or the other. The standard response was the development of a tailored model, designed to address the specific problem in question.

A second, closely related, factor was that model development and testing was solidly anchored within the programme. Programme staff were actively involved in model development, in the quantification of model parameters and in extensive testing of the model using data from the control programme itself. Such a direct link with field research and control is critical for epidemiological modelling. Too often, however, it is lacking and there remain many examples of model development which are undertaken in relative isolation from control. We strongly believe that much more efforts should be undertaken to try to link epidemiological modelling to field research and control, as previously recommended by Bradley (1982), and that modellers in particular should take more initiative in this respect.

The third is that the OCP is a large and flexible control programme which is open to the findings of operational research and willing to adapt its strategy where needed. Furthermore, the Programme has large and comprehensive databases on the entomological, parasitological, demographic and clinical aspects of onchocerciasis and its control, and this greatly facilitated model quantification and testing.

The fourth factor is that modelling was never static but always evolving. This will continue in the future. One new focus of modelling is the development of a simple epidemiological surveillance system which can be sustained by the participating countries themselves after the cessation of OCP (Habbema *et al.* 1992). Another is the refinement of the quantification of the effect of repeated ivermectin treatment, an issue also of great interest to countries outside the OCP. The long term impact of ivermectin treatment on the parasite reservoir is likely to be greater in other endemic areas, such as in Central America, where the local vector species are less effective at low skin mf loads than the West African savanna vector. Currently this issue is of particular relevance for control in the Americas where the aim is to eliminate onchocerciasis. A future modelling focus will be the control of onchocercal skin disease in the many endemic areas where the local parasite strains are not very pathogenic to the eye.

The success with epidemiological modelling in onchocerciasis research and control has led to similar initiatives for other tropical diseases. The first was lymphatic filariasis, a disease caused by other filarial parasites which have a lifecycle similar to *O. volvulus*. Following the recommendations of a meeting on epidemiological modelling for research and control of lymphatic filariasis, which was held in 1990 in Geneva, a project has been started to develop for this disease a microsimulation model similar to ONCHOSIM. This model will be quantified and tested in a multidisciplinary filariasis research project in Recife, Brazil. The ultimate aim of this model is to help design more cost-effective control strategies for this disease which will enable the reactivation of control in the many endemic countries where filariasis control is stagnating or nonexistent.

Leprosy epidemiologists and controllers have also reviewed the state of the art in epidemiological modelling, including the approaches used in onchocerciasis (anon. 1992). They recommended the further development of simulation models for the prediction of future epidemiological trends in leprosy following the introduction of control strategies based on multi-drug therapy, which are very effective in reducing case loads, but for which the impact on transmission and on the incidence of new cases is not yet known. An international project has now been launched to develop such a model, initially for the epidemiological and control situation in South India.

Finally, the experience with modelling in the OCP has revived interest in epidemiological modelling for schistosomiasis control. A meeting on this topic was held in Geneva in October 1992 and brought together experts in schistosomiasis epidemiology and control, and experts in epidemiological modelling (WHO 1992). It was concluded that epidemiological modelling has the potential to become an equally important, practical tool for the planning and evaluation of schistosomiasis research and control, as it has become for onchocerciasis, and further development and application of epidemiological modelling of schistosomiasis was strongly encouraged. However, it was considered essential that this would involve a dynamic collaboration between modelers and field researchers. The meeting stated that "the importance of such collaboration cannot be over-emphasized and the fruitful interaction between modelers and epidemiologists during the meeting provided a very positive example in this respect".

The time seems ripe for more multi-disciplinary modelling initiatives which focus on practical questions of tropical disease control in endemic countries. The example of onchocerciasis shows that such initiatives may greatly contribute to the control of these diseases.

References

Anonymous (1992) 'International meeting on the epidemiology of leprosy in relation to control: major conclusions and recommendations', *Leprosy Review* **63**, 123–124.

Aziz, M.A., Diallo, S., Diop, I.M., Lariviere, M. and Porta, M. (1982) 'Efficacy and tolerance of ivermectin in human onchocerciasis', *Lancet*, ii, 171–173.

Bradley, D.J. (1982) 'Epidemiological models: theory and reality'. In *The population dynamics of infectious diseases: theory and applications*, R.M. Anderson, (ed.) Chapman and Hall, London, 213–24.

Dietz, K. (1982) 'The population dynamics of onchocerciasis'. In *The population dynamics of infectious diseases: theory and applications*, R.M. Anderson, (ed.) Chapman and Hall, London, 213–241.

Habbema, J.D.F., De Vlas, S.J., Plaisier, A.P., and van Oortmarssen G.J. (1995a) 'The microsimulation approach to epidemiological modelling of helminth infections, with special reference to schistosomiasis', *Amer. J. Tropical Med. and Hyg.*, in press.

Habbema, J.D.F., van Oortmarssen, G.J. and Plaisier, A.P. (1995b) 'The ONCHOSIM model and its use in decision support for river blindness control'. In *Models for Human Infectious Diseases: Their Structure and Relation to Data*, V. Isham and G. Medley (eds.) Cambridge University Press, Cambridge, to appear.

Habbema, J.D.F., Plaisier, A.P., Alley, E.S. and Remme, J. (1992) 'Epidemiological modelling for onchocerciasis control', *Parasitology Today* **8**, 99–103.

Karam, M., Schultz-Key, H. and Remme, J. (1987) 'The population dynamics of Onchocerca volvulus after 7 to 8 years of vector control in West Africa', *Acta Tropica* **44**, 445–457.

Kirkwood, B., Smith, P., Marshall, T. and Prost, A. (1983) 'Variations in the prevalence and intensity of microfilarial infections by age, sex, place and time in the area of the Onchocerciasis Control Programme', *Trans. R. Soc. Trop. Med. Hyg.* **77**, 857–861.

Philippon, B. (1977) 'Etude de la transmission d'*Onchocerca volvulus* (Leukart, 1983) par *Simulium damnosum* Theobald 1903, en Afrique Tropicale', *Travaux et Documents de l'ORSTOM* **63**.

Plaisier, A.P., van Oortmarssen, G.J., Habbema, J.D.F., Remme, J. and Alley, E.S. (1990) 'ONCHOSIM, a simulation model for the transmission and control of onchocerciasis', *Comp. Meth. and Programs in Biomed.* **31**, 43–56.

Plaisier, A.P., van Oortmarssen, G.J., Remme, J. and Habbema, J.D.F. (1991a) 'The reproductive lifespan of *Onchocerca volvulus* in West African savanna', *Acta Tropica* **48**, 271–284.

Plaisier, A.P., van Oortmarssen, G.J., Remme, J., Alley, E.S. and Habbema, J.D.F. (1991b). 'The risk and dynamics of onchocerciasis recrudescence after cessation of vector control', *Bull. WHO* **69**, 169–178.

Prost, A. and Prod'hon, J. 'Le diagnostique parasitologique de l'onchocercose, revue critique des methodes en usage', *Médecine Tropical* **38**, 519–532.

Remme, J. (1978) 'Epidemiological modelling for tropical disease control', *Leprosy Review* **63**, 40s–47s.

Remme, J., Ba, O., Dadzie, K.Y. and Karam, M. (1986) 'A force-of-infection model for onchocerciasis and its applications in the epidemiological evaluation of the Onchocerciasis Control Programme in the Volta River Basin area', *Bull. WHO* **64**, 667–681.

Remme, J., Baker, R.H.A., De Sole, G., Dadzie, K.Y., Walsh, J.F., Adams, M.A., Alley, E.S. and Avissey, H.S.K. (1989) 'A community trial of ivermectin in the onchocerciasis focus of Asubende, Ghana. I. Effect on the microfilarial reservoir and the transmission of *Onchocerca volvulus*', *Trop. Med. and Parasitol.* **40**, 367–374.

Remme, J., De Sole, G. and van Oortmarssen, G.J. (1990) 'The predicted and observed decline in the prevalence and intensity of onchocerciasis infection during 14 years of successful vector control', *Bull. WHO* **68**, 331–339.

Remme, J. and Zongo, J.B. (1989) 'Demographic aspects of the epidemiology and control of onchocerciasis in West Africa'. In *Demography and vector-borne diseases*, M. Service (ed.), CRC Press, Boca Raton, 367–386.

Roberts, J.M.D., Neumann, E., Goeckel, C.W. and Highton, R.B. (1967) 'Onchocerciasis in Kenya 9, 11 and 18 years after elimination of the vector', *Bull. WHO* **37**, 195–212.

Walsh, J.F., Davies, J.B., Le Berre, R. and Garms, R. (1978) 'Standardization of criteria for assessing the effect of *simulium* control in onchocerciasis control programmes', *Trans. R. Soc. Trop. Med. Hyg.* **72**, 675–676.

WHO (1987a) 'WHO Expert Committee on Onchocerciasis: third report', *WHO Technical report Series*, No. 752.

WHO (1987b) 'Twelve years of onchocerciasis control in Western Africa', *World Health Statistics Annual* 1987, 19–22.

Some Current Trends in Estimating Vaccine Efficacy

Ira Longini

Elizabeth Halloran

Michael Haber

Summary

We review model-based methods that have been used for estimating vaccine efficacy (VE) from a single wave of an epidemic in a closed population. Then we derive VE estimators from cross-sectional data for the case of endemic infectious diseases in populations with vital dynamics. This is followed by a discussion of methods of estimating VE that include age structure and general distributions of the response to vaccination.

1 Introduction

Epidemic models have been used to derive vaccine efficacy (VE) estimators from data generated by vaccine field trials and observational studies. By using a modeling approach, we can explicitly specify the natural history of the infectious agent, the dynamic individual and population level effects of the vaccine on transmission, and the biological action of the vaccine on the host. Until now, there have been three basic classes of model development: The first class of models consists of SIR (Susceptible-Infected-Removed) epidemic models for a single wave of an epidemic (Haber *et al.* 1991a,b, Longini *et al.* 1993a,b, Svensson 1991). These models have been motivated by field studies that measure vaccine efficacy from outbreak investigations, and thus, do not consider vital dynamics (i.e., births, deaths, age structure, migration). The second class of models included complex models for specific infectious diseases. One example is a model for malaria vaccines (Halloran *et al.* 1989, Struchiner *et al.* 1989, Struchiner *et al.* 1990). This model has been used to develop estimators of VE for vaccines targeted at different stages of host-parasite development under endemic conditions. The third class consisted of general models that do not include the dynamics of particular infectious diseases (Smith *et al.* 1984, Halloran *et al.* 1992, Brunet *et al.* 1993). This approach has been successfully used to develop the conceptual and epidemiologic tools for estimating VE. In many cases, it has been possible to convert the VE model into a multivariable statistical model (Rhodes *et al.* 1995). Such a model has recently been used to study different estimators and study designs for measuring VE from field trials for proposed prophylactic AIDS vaccines (Halloran *et al.* 1994).

In this paper, following a brief introduction to data forms in Section 2, we formulate the mathematical model that will be employed for VE estimation in Section 3. Then, in Section 4, we review some of the progress that has been made in developing VE estimators for the models described by class 1 above and give a few of the multivariable extensions of these models. In Section 5, we concentrate on outlining methods for developing VE estimators for endemic disease situations. Finally, we discuss current and future problems in Section 6.

2   Data forms

For the case of a single wave of an epidemic, we will assume that we have a closed population of unvaccinated and vaccinated persons and that the infection status of these persons can be ascertained. If the epidemic starts at time 0, then we will define the data over a time interval $[0, t]$. If our only information is the cumulative numbers infected in the unvaccinated and vaccinated up to and including time t, then we will refer to such data as 'attack rate data'. On the other hand, if we know the infection onset times, then we will refer to such data as 'event-history data'.

For the case of an endemic infectious disease, we will assume that we have an open population of unvaccinated and vaccinated persons and that the population is in equilibrium with respect to both size and the endemic process. We will then sample the population at some time t, enabling us to ascertain the present and (sometimes) past infection status of these persons. We will refer to data from this process as 'prevalence data'.

3   The basic model

We consider a population of size $n(t)$ at time t, which is partitioned into $m+1$ mutually exclusive (vaccine-related) strata defined by their post-vaccination level of susceptibility, each of size $n_\nu(t)$. Stratum 0 consists of unvaccinated individuals, and thus, the fraction of the population that is vaccinated at time t is $f(t) = 1 - [n_0(t)/n(t)]$, $0 \leq f(t) \leq 1$. Let $n_V(t) = \sum_{\nu=1}^{m} n_\nu(t)$, which is the total number vaccinated at time t. The fraction of the vaccinated in stratum ν at time t is $\alpha_\nu(t) = n_\nu(t)/n_V(t)(\sum_{\nu=1}^{m} \alpha_\nu(t) = 1)$. In models with vital dynamics, the birth and death rates, μ, will be equal in order to establish an equilibrium population size. We will assume that there is negligible disease-related excess mortality. There are $S_\nu(t)$, $I_\nu(t)$, and $R_\nu(t)$, susceptibles, infected and removed individuals, respectively, in stratum ν, at time t, where $S_\nu(t) + I_\nu(t) + R_\nu(t) = n_\nu(t)$ for all t. The total number infected at time t is $I(t) = \sum_{\nu=0}^{m} I_\nu(t)$. Individuals mix homogeneously with contact rate λ (contacts per unit time). The probability that a susceptible in stratum ν is infected by a single contact with a single infective is β_ν, referred to as the 'susceptibility' of a person in stratum ν. We assume that we begin vaccination at time t_0 by vaccinating persons at birth and that vaccine-induced immunity does not wane. The parameter $\theta_\nu = \beta_\nu/\beta_0$ is the relative susceptibility of vaccinated persons in stratum ν compared to the susceptibility of unvaccinated persons. We let $\alpha_\nu = \alpha_\nu(t_0)$, and then the summary relative susceptibility is $\bar{\theta} = \sum_{\nu=1}^{m} \alpha_\nu\theta_\nu$. We assume that the level of infectiousness of infected persons does not vary by vaccination strata. In order to make our models conform with the standard types of SIR and SIS epidemiological models, we will assume that infectives recover at a constant rate, γ, per unit of time.

The set of differential equations describing the epidemic process, for $\nu = 0, ..., m$, is

$$dS_\nu(t)/dt = -\lambda\, \beta_\nu S_\nu(t)I(t)/n(t) + \mu[n_\nu - S_\nu(t)], \qquad (3.1)$$
$$dI_\nu(t)/dt = \lambda\, \beta_\nu S_\nu(t)I(t)/n(t) - (\gamma + \mu)I_\nu(t), \qquad (3.2)$$
$$dR_\nu(t)/dt = \gamma\, I_\nu(t) - \mu R_\nu(t), \qquad (3.3)$$

with initial conditions

$$S_\nu(t_0) = n_\nu(t_0), \quad R_\nu(t_0) = 0, \quad \nu = 0, ..., m; \quad I_\nu(t_0) > 0, \qquad (3.4)$$

for at least one ν,

More specific values for $I_\nu(t_0)$ are given below.

The stratum-specific VE is

$$VE(\theta_\nu) = 1 - \theta_\nu, \qquad (3.5)$$

and the summary VE under heterogeneity is

$$VE(\bar{\theta}) = 1 - \bar{\theta}. \qquad (3.6)$$

Various vaccine distributions are specified by setting the $\alpha's$ and $\beta's$ to their appropriate values (Halloran *et al.* 1992). The $\beta's$ and thus, the $\theta's$ could be random variables following some distribution (Greenwood and Yule 1915, Brunet *et al.* 1993, Svensson 1991).

In this paper, we will consider two simple vaccine distributions. The first is the leaky vaccine distribution ($m = 1$), so

$$VE(\theta) = 1 - \theta, \qquad (3.7)$$

where θ is the relative susceptibility. The second is the all-or-none vaccine distribution ($m = 2$, $\beta_0 = \beta_1$, $\beta_2 = 0$) so $\bar{\theta} = \alpha_1$. The parameter of interest is $\bar{\theta} = \alpha_1 = 1 - \alpha_2$. Then the VE is

$$VE(\bar{\theta}) = \alpha, \tag{3.8}$$

where $\alpha = \alpha_2$.

4   Past results

Most past models have been applied to single outbreaks. In this case, we set $\mu = 0$ in (3.1)–(3.3), and we consider a single wave of an epidemic, where vaccination takes place at time t_0 which is also the starting time of the epidemic. Then $n_\nu(t) = n_\nu$ and $\alpha_\nu(t) = \alpha_\nu$, for all t. The epidemic starts with with the introduction of a single unvaccinated infective, i.e., $I_0(t_0) = 1$, $I_\nu(t_0) = 0$, $\nu = 1, ..., m$. We will first deal with attack rate data. Assuming no loss to follow-up, we define the attack rate by time t as

$$AR_\nu(t) = 1 - [S_\nu(t)/n_\nu]. \tag{4.1}$$

We substitute (3.3) into (3.1), integrate from 0 to t and then evaluate at (4.1), which yields

$$\beta_\nu = -\frac{\gamma}{\lambda n R(t)}\log_e[1 - AR_\nu(t)]. \tag{4.2}$$

For a leaky vaccine distribution, we evaluate (4.2) at (3.7), yielding the VE estimator

$$\hat{V}E(\theta) = 1 - [\log_e(1 - \hat{A}R_1(t))/\log_e(1 - \hat{A}R_0(t))], \tag{4.3}$$

where the $\hat{A}R_\nu(t)$ are estimates from the observed epidemic. The estimated attack rates are binomial proportions. From standard likelihood theory

$$\hat{A}R_\nu(t) \xrightarrow{D} N\{AR_\nu(t), AR_\nu(t)[1 - AR_\nu(t)]/n_\nu\}, \quad \text{as } n_\nu \longrightarrow \infty, \tag{4.4}$$

where $N\{\mu, \sigma^2\}$ indicates a normal distribution with mean, μ, and variance, σ^2. Note that, given $R(t)$, $AR_0(t)$ and $AR_1(t)$ are independent. Applying the method of statistical differentials (delta method – see Chapter 12 in Agresti 1990) to (4.3) and evaluating at (4.4) yields

$$\hat{V}E(\theta) \xrightarrow{D} N\{VE(\theta), [AR_1(t)/n_1 + \theta^2 AR_0(t)/n_0][\log_e(1 - AR_0(t))]^{-2}\}, \tag{4.5}$$

as $n_\nu \longrightarrow \infty$ and, where $I(t)$ is sufficiently large.

Expression (4.5) is used to construct hypothesis tests and confidence intervals on $VE(\theta)$.

From (4.2, 4.3) we can write

$$S_1(t)/n_1 = [S_0(t)/n_0]^\theta, \qquad (4.6)$$

which demonstrates that we have a proportional hazards assumption (Cox and Oakes 1984) for the leaky vaccine distribution (Smith *et al.* 1984, Brunet *et al.* 1993). If we let $\phi = \log_e(\theta)$, then we can estimate ϕ using the standard proportional hazards model from either attack rate or event-history data. This is useful when we need to include covariates in the analysis.

For an all-or-none vaccine distribution, we evaluate (4.2) at (3.8), yielding

$$AR_0(t) = AR_1(t), \qquad (4.7)$$

but $AR_1(t)$ is not observable. However, the attack rate in the vaccinated, $AR_V(t)$, is observable. Substituting $AR_V(t)$ and (3.8) into (4.7) yields the estimator for $VE(\alpha)$, which is

$$\hat{V}E(\alpha) = \hat{\alpha} = 1 - [\hat{A}R_V(t)/\hat{A}R_0(t)]. \qquad (4.8)$$

Let $a = \log_e(1 - \alpha)$, then

$$\hat{a} = \log_e \hat{A}R_V(t) - \log_e \hat{A}R_0(t). \qquad (4.9)$$

We apply the same methods to (4.9) as we applied to derive (4.3), (4.4), to get

$$\hat{a} \xrightarrow{\text{D}} N\{a, [(1 - AR_V(t))/(n_V AR_V(t))] + [(1 - AR_0(t))/(n_0 AR_0(t))]\}, \quad (4.10)$$

as $n_\nu \longrightarrow \infty$, and $I(t)$ is sufficiently large. Expression (4.10) is used to construct hypothesis tests and confidence intervals on $VE(\alpha)$.

In order to set up the estimation of VE with covariates for an all-or-none vaccine distribution, we can use a logistic function reparameterization of the attack rates,

$$AR_0(t) = [1 + \exp(b_0)]^{-1}, \quad AR_V(t) = [1 + \exp(b_0 + b_1)]^{-1}. \qquad (4.11)$$

Then the parameters b_0 and b_1 can be estimated, along with important parameters of the covariates via logistic regression. Thus the estimated VE is

$$\hat{V}E(\alpha) = 1 - [1 + \exp(\hat{b}_0)]/[1 + \exp(\hat{b}_0 + \hat{b}_1)]. \qquad (4.12)$$

5   Endemic diseases

In this case, $\mu > 0$ in (3.1)–(3.3), but, again, $n_\nu(t) = n_\nu$ and $\alpha_\nu(t) = \alpha_\nu$. For a leaky vaccine distribution, the fixed points of the process in the SI plane are given by the set

$$\{S_0(t), S_1(t), I_0(t), I_1(t)\} \longrightarrow \{S_0, S_1, I_0, I_1\}, \text{ as } t \longrightarrow \infty.$$

The two specific fixed points of (3.1)–(3.3) are

$$E_1 = \{n_0, n_1, 0, 0\}, \quad \text{infection free,}$$
$$E_2 = \{S_0, S_1, I_0, I_1\}, \ 0 < I_\nu < n_\nu, \ \nu = 0, 1, \quad \text{endemicity.} \quad (5.1)$$

For the initial conditions, we assume that the vaccination is started when the system is in the endemic equilibrium $\{S_0, 0, I_0, 0\}$ without vaccination. The reproduction number when f of the population is vaccinated is

$$R_f = \lambda[(1 - f)\beta_0 + f \ \beta_1]/[\gamma + \mu].$$

Then, we have the following threshold theorem.

Threshold Theorem *If $R_f \leq 1$, then E_1 is globally asymptotically stable, and if $R_f > 1$, then there is a unique fixed point E_2 that is globally asymptotically stable.*

The theorem has been proved by Simon (1993), and details will be presented elsewhere. If fixed point E_2 is stable, then from (3.2) we obtain the following balance equation

$$I/n = [(\gamma + \mu)I_\nu]/(\lambda\beta_\nu S_\nu), \quad \text{for} \ \nu = 0, 1, \quad (5.2)$$

which is evaluated at (3.5), yielding the VE estimator

$$\hat{V}E(\theta) = 1 - \hat{\theta} = 1 - (\hat{I}_1/\hat{S}_1)/(\hat{I}_0/\hat{S}_0). \quad (5.3)$$

We write the equilibrium proportions in the susceptible, infected, and removed classes as $p_\nu = S_\nu/n_\nu$, $q_\nu = I_\nu/n_\nu$, and $r_\nu = R_\nu/n_\nu$, respectively. Then, the estimated relative susceptibility from (5.3) becomes

$$\hat{\theta} = (\hat{p}_1/\hat{q}_1)/(\hat{p}_0/\hat{q}_0). \quad (5.4)$$

We note that $\hat{p}_\nu$, $\hat{q}_\nu$, and $\hat{r}_\nu$ are multinomial proportions. From standard likelihood theory

$$\hat{p}_\nu \xrightarrow{D} N\{p_\nu, p_\nu(1 - p_\nu)/n_\nu\}, n_\nu \longrightarrow \infty. \quad (5.5)$$

The same holds for $\hat{q}_\nu$. We note that there is conditional independence for the different estimators across ν, but there is dependence within strata given by

$$\text{Cov}(\hat{p}_\nu, \hat{q}_\nu) \cong -p_\nu q_\nu/n_\nu. \quad (5.6)$$

Now let $\hat{\phi} = \log_e(\hat{\theta})$, and we apply the method of statistical differentials to (5.4), evaluating at (5.5), (5.6), yielding

$$\hat{\phi} \xrightarrow{D} N\{\phi, \sigma_\phi^2\}, \quad (5.7)$$

as $n_\nu \longrightarrow \infty$ and I is sufficiently large, where

$$\sigma_\phi^2 = \sum_{\nu=0}^{1} \left[\frac{(1-p_\nu)}{p_\nu} + \frac{(1-q_\nu)}{q_\nu} + 2 \right] \frac{1}{n_\nu}. \tag{5.8}$$

Expressions (5.7) and (5.8) are used to construct hypothesis tests and confidence intervals on $VE(\theta)$.

For an all-or-none vaccine distribution, the fixed points of the process in the SI plane are given by the set

$$\{S_0(t), S_1(t), S_2(t), I_0(t), I_1(t), I_2(t)\} \longrightarrow \{S_0, S_1, S_2, I_0, I_1, I_2\}, \text{ as } t \longrightarrow \infty.$$

The specific fixed points are

$E_1 = \{n_0, n_1, n_2, 0, 0, 0\}$, infection free,

$E_2 = \{S_0, S_1, n_2, I_0, I_1, 0\}$, where $0 < I_\nu < n_\nu$, $\nu = 0, 1$, endemicity. (5.9)

The reproduction number is

$$R_f = \lambda \beta_0 (1 - \alpha\ f)/(\gamma + \mu),$$

and the above threshold theorem applies to this system. If fixed point E_2 is stable, then from (3.2) we obtain the following balance equation

$$I_0/S_0 = I_1/S_1; \tag{5.10}$$

however, S_1 is not observable, but S_V is. Substituting for S_V yields the VE estimator

$$\hat{V}E(\alpha) = \hat{\alpha} = 1 - \{[1 - (\hat{S}_V/n_V)]/[1 - (\hat{S}_0/n_0)]\}. \tag{5.11}$$

We write the equilibrium proportions in the susceptible and ever infected (i.e., current infected plus removed) classes as $p_\nu = S_\nu/n_\nu$, $q_\nu = (I_\nu + R_\nu)/n_\nu$, respectively. Then, the estimator for $1 - \alpha$ becomes

$$1 - \hat{\alpha} = \hat{q}_V/\hat{q}_0. \tag{5.12}$$

At this point, we proceed exactly as we did for the all-or-none vaccine distribution in Section 4, but with

$$\hat{a} = \log_e \hat{q}_V - \log_e \hat{q}_0. \tag{5.13}$$

Then,

$$\hat{a} \xrightarrow{D} N\{a, (q_V/n_V p_V) + (q_0/n_0 p_0)\}, \text{ as } n_\nu \longrightarrow \infty. \tag{5.14}$$

Expression (5.14) is used to construct hypothesis tests and confidence intervals on $VE(\alpha)$.

6 Discussion

In this paper, we have described a two-step approach for estimating VE from field data. The first step is to describe the infection process of interest by the appropriate mathematical or analytic model, which should include specific vaccine distribution parameters and variables that best describe the investigator's knowledge of the biological action of the vaccine on the host. The second step is to devise methods for carrying out inference on these parameters that take advantage of the model structure and the study design.

We have demonstrated derivations of the VE estimators based on the analysis of the deterministic differential equations (3.1)–(3.3) of the infectious disease process. The analytic solutions to these equations provide closed-form estimators for the VE estimators (4.3), (4.8), (5.3), (5.11). We then apply statistical methods, primarily the delta method, to derive the asymptotic probability distributions of these estimators (4.5), (4.10), (5.7), (5.14). Alternative methods can also be used to derive the VE estimators and their distributions. In the case of no vital dynamics (Section 4), the stochastic analogues of the deterministic models can be formulated as continuous-time counting processes. This had been carried out for the case of the leaky vaccine distribution for one vaccine stratum, $m = 1$ (Becker 1982, Becker 1989), and for multiple strata, $m > 1$ (Longini *et al.* 1993b). In these cases, the estimators and their distributions are identical to those provided by the deterministic approach. In addition, Rhodes *et al.* (1995) have used counting process methods to estimate the VE estimators and their distributions (for the leaky vaccine distribution) for quite general data structures, ranging from detailed infection incidence data to attack rate data. Although recent advances have been made in applying counting process methods to epidemiological problems (Keiding 1991), these methods still need to be better adapted to the specific case of estimating VE for an infectious disease.

In this paper, we have described methods for estimating the relative susceptibility (and thus, VE) for the cases of a one vaccination-stratum leaky vaccine distribution (3.7), and a two vaccination-stratum all-or-none vaccine distribution (3.8). Only a single parameter is estimated for each vaccine distribution: θ, for leaky, and α, for all-or-none. In the case of a single wave of an epidemic, this single parameter is estimable from infection attack rates in the vaccinated and unvaccinated. In the case of an endemic infectious disease that is in equilibrium, only infection prevalence data for the vaccinated and unvaccinated (5.3), (5.11) are needed to estimate the VE. However, in more general cases, we are interested in estimating the whole discrete distribution $\{\alpha_\nu \theta_\nu\}$, which may better reflect heterogeneity in the response to the vaccine. In some situations it may be advantageous to let the relative susceptibility vary continuously according to some probability density function $\alpha(\theta)$, where $\int_0^1 \alpha(\theta)d\theta = 1$. This idea was advanced as early as 1915 by Yule and Greenwood (1915), and further discussed in Halloran *et al.* (1992), but has recently been further developed by Brunet *et al.* (1993). However, in order to estimate more complex discrete, $\{\alpha_\nu \theta_\nu\}$, or continuous, $\{\alpha(\theta)\}$, vaccine distributions, more detailed data are needed. Brunet *et al.* (1993) develop methods for estimating the first and second moments of $\{\alpha(\theta)\}$ from infection incidence data. A common source of heterogeneity in infection data is age. For endemic infectious diseases, cross sectional, age-stratified prevalence data are frequently collected at some calendar time, t. For an SIR disease, these data may be of the form $S(a, t)$, $I(a, t)$, and $R(a, t)$, denoting the number of individuals of age a, at time t. Anderson and May (1991) give extensive analytic treatment to dynamic models of this type, see also Dietz (1975). An important general problem to solve is how to extract information about $\{\alpha(\theta)\}$ from the age-structured data. A more specific problem involves extracting such information when the endemic process is in equilibrium. In this case, the data are of the form $S(a)$, I(a), and $R(a)$. By employing extensions of methods developed by Keiding (1991), information about $\{\alpha(\theta)\}$ can (theoretically) be extracted from a single cross-sectional infection survey (Struchiner *et al.* 1995).

Acknowledgements

This research was partially supported by NIH grants 1-R01-AI32042-02, 1-R29-AI31057-03, and by the Isaac Newton Institute for Mathematical Sciences, Cambridge, UK.

References

Anderson, R.M. and May, R.M. (1991) *Infectious Diseases in Humans*, Oxford University Press, Oxford.

Agresti, A. (1990) *Categorical Data Analysis*, Wiley, New York.

Becker, N.G. (1982) 'Estimation in models for the spread of infectious diseases'. In *Proc. XIth Internat. Biometrics Conf.*, I.N.R.A., Versailles, 145–151.

Becker, N.G (1989) *The Analysis of Infectious Disease Data*, Chapman and Hall, New York.

Brunet, R.C., Struchiner, C.J. and Halloran, M.E. (1993) 'On the distribution of vaccine protection under heterogeneous response', *Math. Biosci.* **116**, 111–125.

Cox, D.R. and Oakes, D. (1984) *Analysis of Survival Data*, Chapman and Hall, New York.

Dietz, K. (1975) 'Transmission and control of arbovirus diseases'. In *Epidemiology*, D. Ludwig and K.L. Cooke (eds.), SIAM, Philadelphia, 104–121.

Greenwood, M. and Yule, U.G. (1915) 'The statistics of anti-typhoid and anti-cholera inoculations, and the interpretations of such statistics in general', *Proc. R. Soc. Med.* **8**, 113–194.

Haber, M. Longini, I.M. and Halloran, M.E. (1991a) 'Measures of the effect of vaccination in a randomly mixing population', *Internat. J. Epidemiol.* **20**, 300–310.

Haber, M. Longini, I.M. and Halloran, M.E. (1991b) 'Estimation of vaccine efficacy in outbreaks of acute infectious diseases', *Stat. Med.* **10**, 1573–84.

Halloran, M.E., Struchiner, C.J. and Spielman, A. (1989) 'Modeling malaria vaccines II: Population effects of stage-specific malaria vaccines dependent on natural boosting', *Math. Biosci.* **94**, 115–49.

Halloran, M.E., Haber, M. and Longini, I.M. (1992) 'Interpretation and estimation of vaccine field efficacy under heterogeneity', *Amer. J. Epidemiol.* **136**, 328–43.

Halloran, M.E., Longini, I.M., Struchiner, C.J. *et al.* (1994) 'Exposure efficacy and change in contact rates in evaluating HIV vaccines in the field', *Stat. Med.* **13**, 357–377.

Keiding, N. (1991) 'Age-specific incidence and prevalence: a statistical perspective', *J. R. Statist. Soc. A* **154**, 371–412.

Longini, I.M., Haber, M., Halloran, M.E. and Chen, R.T. (1993a) 'Measuring vaccine efficacy from epidemics of acute infectious agents', *Stat. Med.* **12**, 249–263.

Longini, I.M.,. Halloran, M.E. and Haber, M. (1993b) 'Estimation of vaccine efficacy from epidemics of acute infectious agents under vaccine-related heterogeneity', *Math. Biosci.* **117**, 271–281.

Rhodes, P., Halloran, M.E. and Longini, I.M. (1995) 'Counting process models for infectious disease data: Distinguishing exposure to infection from susceptibility', *Biometrika* (submitted).

Simon, C.P. (1993) *Personal communication.*

Smith, P.G., Rodrigues, L.C. and Fine, P.E.M. (1984) 'Assessment of the protective efficacy of vaccines against common diseases using case-control and cohort studies', *Int. J. Epidemiol.* **13**, 87–93.

Struchiner, C.J., Halloran, M.E. and Spielman, A. (1989) 'Modeling malaria vaccines I: New uses for old ideas', *Math. Biosci.* **94**, 87–113.

Struchiner, C.J., Halloran, M.E., Robins, J.M. and Spielman, A. (1990) 'The behavior of common measures of association used to assess a vaccination program under complex disease transmission patterns – a computer simulation study of malaria vaccines', *Int. J. Epidemiol.* **19**, 187–96.

Struchiner, C.J., Brunet, R., Halloran, M.E. and Azevedo-Neto, R.S. (1995) 'On the use of state-space models for evaluation of health interventions'. In *Mathematics Applied to Biology and Medicine*, J. Demongeot and V. Capasso (eds.), Wuerz, Winnipeg, to appear.

Svensson, A. (1991) 'Analyzing effects of vaccines, *Math. Biosci.* **107**, 407–412.

Operational Modelling of HIV/AIDS to Assist Public Health Control

Norman Bailey

Summary

Scientific studies always involve a degree of quantitative modelling, and often require the collection and analysis of data over long periods. But decision-makers cannot afford to wait, and must try to achieve a rational balance between conflicting claims based on the best scientific and socio-economic information available.

Scientific modelling in an operational situation entails quantitative methods designed to assist executive and administrative authorities – this is the province of operational research (OR), and operational modelling should be an essential ingredient of all public health decision-making and planning.

1 The public health scene

Public health authorities have a relatively short time horizon, and work with highly aggregated data on a macro-level. Conflicts between ethical, social, economic and political factors are very obtrusive and strategy choices are likely to be controversial. Decisions can have far-reaching consequences, and be socially disruptive if bad compromises are made between alternative choices.

Useful scientific support can often provide approximate answers to public health questions like, 'Given the pattern of reported AIDS cases, what is the likely scenario over the next 5 or 10 years?', 'How many HIV positives are likely to be circulating in the population?', or, 'How can we evaluate the success or failure of health campaigns, therapeutic measures, or other actions?'

Next, what data should be used for operational modelling to assist public health decision-making? General scientific research can investigate any models using any feasible parametric values. But decision-makers need models that demonstrably describe local conditions and that must therefore use parameters estimated from local data. These data must be, and be seen to be, reliable. In my view this rules out, in the context of operational modelling, most socio-medical or socio-economic surveys that involve substantial amounts of self-reported behaviour – particularly injecting drug use and sexual contact patterns.

Good public health data, based on physicians' diagnoses of AIDS cases and laboratory investigations, are thus vital. Major risk groups (gay men, injecting drug users, haemophiliacs, transfusion patients, heterosexuals etc.) must still be distinguished, and some categories will overlap. Attention must still be paid to appropriate micro-level studies. Conflicts between different levels of enquiry must be avoided. But simplifications at the macro-level may depend crucially on heterogeneities at micro-levels effectively averaging out – see below in Section 4.7.

2 Core-groups

Earlier studies of gonorrhoea transmission by Hethcote and Yorke (1984) identified core-groups of highly-active high-risk individuals driving the epidemiological process. The preface to this monograph carried statements by two senior administrators at CDC, Atlanta, USA, recognising its importance in (a) eliminating epidemiological misconceptions, and (b) assisting in the development of national control programmes. The core-group approach is a simplification of known realities. Occam's razor requires that simple models be used as first approximations to macro-level public health problems. We shall therefore identify specific major risk-groups, like gay men, for individual study, but shall limit the number of subgroups rather drastically, retaining only the main epidemiological categories.

The first applications to HIV/AIDS were made by Scherrer *et al.* (1988) in a joint analysis of serial HIV prevalence in a cohort and serial AIDS incidence in San Francisco. Only about 70% of the cohort appeared to be at substantial risk. The size N of the presumed high-activity core-group could be estimated directly by comparing the incidence of AIDS in the cohort with the incidence in the city over a fixed period of time. A relatively simple compartmental model enabled main parameters to be estimated (Scherrer *et al.* 1988, Bailey 1991, Bailey 1992). In particular, we found $\hat{N} = 23,300$, which could be compared with the total size of the gay community, reckoned to be between 70,000 and 100,000 in 1986 (Institute of Medicine 1986). See also Section 4 below.

3 Macro-system dynamics for HIV/AIDS

Mathematical models of infectious disease dynamics go back a long way – to the first recorded use by Daniel Bernoulli in 1760 when he investigated the effectiveness of variolation as a protection against smallpox. Note that this pioneer work was the first example of an individual qualified in both medicine and mathematics undertaking the study of a macro-level public health problem.

There are several approaches to a system dynamics analysis of infectious disease spread at a public health level: (1) simple curve-fitting, which can be useful for short-term predictive extrapolations, but cannot provide estimates of present or future HIV levels or answer 'what if?' questions about, e.g. the likely results of proposed changes in public health policy; (2) any attempts at direct measurements of HIV prevalence are usually unsatisfactory because of unrepresentativeness in statistical samples, unknown sizes of risk groups, and problems of non-response; (3) the popular and relatively successful 'back-calculation' method, in which AIDS incidence data plus information about the incubation period are used to reconstruct the past history of infection – difficulties occur because recent infections are not reflected in the AIDS incidence. It seems to me that all of these approaches are less flexible and versatile than the classical compartmental one that has been widely used by a large number of investigators. But the matter is admittedly controversial (see Brookmeyer (1991)).

The classical approach (see review by Bailey (1975)) has been adversely criticised by some writers (e.g. Brookmeyer 1991, Chin and Lwanga 1991) as requiring a great deal of detailed information that is simply not available – at least in reliable terms. While this criticism can be justifiably applied to the attempted application of micro-models to large-scale problems in the real world, it is claimed here that this degree of detail is unnecessary at the macro-level. In fact a preoccupation with fine structure can be counter-productive at the level of decision-making and forward planning.

4   Major technical factors

Before outlining the simplified model structures advocated here for public health applications, particularly in Switzerland, let us refer briefly to a number of important aspects which can be identified by the analysis of public health data.

4.1   Initial core-size

Following Section 2 above we assume the existence, before the introduction of HIV, of an initial high-activity high-risk core-group, approximately stable with the arrival of new recruits being balanced by departures. When HIV is introduced to this group we must distinguish between negatives and positives, with the latter progressing to an eventual AIDS diagnosis.

4.2 High and low-risk subgroups

Sociological field observations suggest that individuals spend only a limited period of time in a high-activity core-group. We must therefore separate the HIV positives into two subgroups: (a) those who are high-activity and high-risk; and (b) those who have left (a) and can be considered as a low- or even no-risk group. Both subgroups yield AIDS cases, though in general we cannot distinguish their origins.

There are some uncertainties, but it turns out that an approximate investigation allows us to use age-at-diagnosis histograms, which are markedly peaked, to derive age-at-infection histograms, also strongly peaked. And, by introducing the idea of an arrival process with negligible departures, followed by a departure process with negligible arrivals, we can estimate the average residence time in the subgroup from the height of the unimodal approximation to the histograms (see Bailey (1993) for mathematical details).

4.3 Incubation periods

Direct measurement of incubation periods with substantial numbers is rarely possible. Moreover, there are hardly ever any good HIV prevalence data to identify the initial HIV epidemic. Fortunately, the San Francisco studies mentioned in Section 2 above, with cohort data giving serial HIV prevalence figures, taken in conjunction with San Francisco city AIDS incidence figures, allowed a good identification of the incubation period in gay males (see Scherrer *et al.* (1988), Bailey (1991), and Bailey (1992)). The best fit was a chi-square distribution with 12 degrees of freedom (i.e. 6 arbitrary stages), scaled to give a mean of 11.70 ± 0.40 years.

This result has been approximately confirmed by other writers (Longini *et al.* 1989, Lemp *et al.* 1990, Satten *et al.* 1992) giving very similar mean values, and one at least (Satten *et al.* 1992) with 6 explicit stages related to clinical measurements. Assuming that the parameters are biologically oriented (as opposed to probably community-specific parameters like transmission rates), we can use these values in analysing data from other countries, e.g. Switzerland, where there are no usable serial HIV data (see Section 7 below).

4.4 Transmission of infection

In many studies we have assumed that the infectivity of an infected individual is uniformly spread over the incubation period. Redfield and Burke (1988) indicated that there are clear signs of high infectivity at the beginning of the incubation period, dropping down as the body begins to cope with the infection, but rising again at the end when the immune system fails. More recently, Koopman *et al.* (1992) have found evidence of a very high risk initially even before circulating antibodies begin to appear.

It is easy to incorporate such ideas in a compartmental model, but it is not yet entirely clear just what should be the quantitative specifications. At the moment it appears that the overall macro-picture is not highly dependent on the precise assumptions, when looking at key items like initial core-size, but there could be important effects on long term predictions. This aspect obviously needs to be investigated in more detail.

4.5   Reporting delays and under-reporting

A reporting delay is the time interval between the date of diagnosis of AIDS by a physician and the date on which the case is entered into the public health database. This delay is mostly of a bureaucratic nature due to the verification of clinical and social details. Much technical research has gone into this subject (Brookmeyer and Liao 1990, Heisterkamp *et al.* 1989, Rosenberg 1990), but for operational models in public health a simpler approach is required. From public health records of AIDS diagnoses we can compile delay distributions classified by date of diagnosis (grouped over appropriate intervals). These distributions are all right-truncated, depending on date of diagnosis and date of enquiry. In Switzerland nearly all curves are J-shaped with high point close to the origin. It is easy to fit a negative exponential distribution, allowing for truncation, and estimating just one new parameter.

Under-reporting means cases that fail to be reported by the usual physicians' channel. Many cases are in fact diagnosed by doctors but only reported in an eventual death certificate. Special surveillance was instituted in Switzerland in mid-1988, and it soon appeared that 20-25% of AIDS cases in the two main risk groups of gay men and IDUs had previously been missed.

Since patients diagnosed and dying before mid-1988 would not be included in the new scheme, a degree of left-truncation is involved. But we can use the above method, again estimating only one new parameter. Note that delays in the death-certificate route involve both a bureaucratic component as well as the patient's survival time.

4.6   AIDS survival time

The part of the HIV/AIDS model dealing with the patients' survival can be largely decoupled from the part covering HIV infection and AIDS incubation. The two parts, though closely linked in one direction, can be analysed separately. In the present study we have concentrated on infection and incubation. But the area involving actual surviving patients for whom much needs to be done by way of clinical care, treatment, and social support, is also a top priority. Increasing numbers of people are beginning to join this category with the identification of HIV positives in advance of full AIDS.

4.7 Heterogeneity and complexity

The importance of heterogeneity and complexity in infectious disease dynamics, and HIV/AIDS in particular, cannot be exaggerated. In practical applications we must avoid over-parameterisation and a loss of identifiability. We can often justifiably expect a lot of small effects to have some overall average resultant which can be accounted for by a single factor or parameter. See Bailey (1975), Section 14.4 and Nåsell (1977).

Scherrer *et al.* (1988) showed that, in a very simplified theoretical study, a single parameter could account for heterogeneity in partnership duration by assuming a negative exponential distribution of the duration. For average durations up to about one month, there was little effective departure from random mixing.

Again, influenza studies in the USSR (Baroyan and Rvachev 1967, Baroyan *et al.* 1973, Baroyan *et al.* 1977) showed that simplifications in the basic epidemiological assumptions still gave a good prediction of the spread from a city focus to other centres. Later investigations in Geneva (Scherrer *et al.* 1985, Bailey and Estreicher 1987) employing further simplifications, confirmed the Soviet work and suggested that averaging out recognised micro-heterogeneities could still lead to valid results at a public health level.

5 Flow-charts and mathematical modelling

Since there is already a large literature on system dynamics, using flow-charts and modelling, it is unnecessary to dwell on details here. For practical applications by public health officials we need an effective conceptual framework that is readily understood. This must entail simple modelling, with only small numbers of parameters to be estimated from good public health data on AIDS diagnoses and reports. *If the models are not understood, at least in principle, they will not be used.* Decision-makers may not want to spend time on mathematical and computer details, but at any rate with compartmental models all technical conclusions are easily put into practical terms couched in everyday epidemiological and public health language. The broad qualitative flow-chart being used here is shown in Figure 1, while the quantitative version with algebraic symbols appears in Figure 2. The latter effectively defines the symbols when compared with Figure 1, but a full list is given below.

Death certificate (DC) route

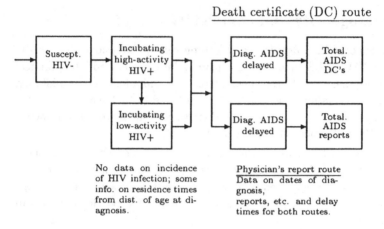

Figure 1: Detailed flow chart related to available public health data

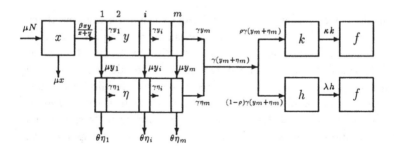

Figure 2: Detailed flow chart defining symbols and showing principal transfer rates

Definition of symbols in Figure 2

- State variables (numbers in compartments)

x	HIV negative susceptibles in core-group
y_i	HIV positives in ith stage of high-activity group
y	Total of all y_is
η_i	HIV positives in ith stage of low-activity group
η	Total of all η_is
h	Diagnosed AIDS cases not yet reported by physicians
u	Diagnosed AIDS cases reported by physicians
k	Diagnosed AIDS cases not yet reported by death certificate
f	Diagnosed AIDS cases reported by death certificate

- Parameters (estimated from data)

a	Initial HIV prevalence
β	Infection transmission rate
N	Initial size of core-group
ρ	Fraction of AIDS cases on death certificate route
γ^{-1}	Average time spent in each incubation period stage
m	Number of stages in incubation period
μ^{-1}	Average time spent in HIV positive high-activity group
θ^{-1}	Average time spent in HIV positive low-activity group
λ^{-1}	Average physicians' reporting delay
κ^{-1}	Average death certificate reporting delay

The corresponding set of differential equations is:

$$\frac{dx}{dt} = -\frac{\beta x y}{x+y} + \mu(N-x); \quad y = \sum_{j=1}^{m} y_j; \quad \eta = \sum_{j=1}^{m} \eta_j;$$

$$\frac{dy_1}{dt} = \frac{\beta x y}{x+y} - (\mu+\gamma)y_1; \quad \frac{d\eta_1}{dt} = \mu y_1 - (\theta+\gamma)\eta_1;$$

$$\frac{dy_i}{dt} = \gamma y_{i-1} - (\mu+\gamma)y_i; \quad \frac{d\eta_i}{dt} = \mu y_i - (\theta+\gamma)\eta_i + \gamma\eta_{i-1}; \quad (5.1)$$

$$\gamma y_m = w; \quad \frac{du}{dt} = \lambda h; \quad \gamma\eta_m = \omega; \quad \frac{df}{dt} = \kappa k;$$

$$\frac{dh}{dt} = (1-\rho)\gamma(y_m+\eta_m) - \lambda h; \quad \frac{dk}{dt} = \rho\gamma(y_m+\eta_m) - \kappa k;$$

where $i = 2, \ldots, m$.

These equations can easily be replaced by the corresponding set of difference equations, with for example $\Delta t = 1$ week or 1 day, which is what we are most likely to use for numerical computation. A few obvious additional mathematical expressions are required to allow for diagnosed cases of AIDS that have not yet been reported due to reporting delays and under-reporting.

6   Parameter estimation and model fitting

Parameter estimation has been carried out by standard maximum-likelihood, using only a few lines of code. Since we do not have a closed expression for the solution of (5.1) we must compute the likelihood function directly for any given set of parameter values. In this application we have chosen to specify the likelihood in terms of AIDS incidence data (mostly based on 6-monthly intervals) regarded as independent Poisson variables whose mean values are determined by (5.1).

Note that the model is in fact 'hybrid' (see Bailey 1993): the process of HIV infection with fairly large numbers is treated deterministically, while allowing for probabilistic variations in the long incubation period phase.

An important practical point is the choice of initial conditions for the numerical solution of (5.1). At an early stage in the HIV epidemic we simply linearised the relevant elements of (5.1) and solved directly. This led to a geometric distribution for the $y_i(0)$, while the $\eta_i(0)$ could be taken as negligible. We need in fact only one new parameter, i.e., a, for the initial prevalence of HIV at $t = 0$.

The chief parameters to be estimated by maximum-likelihood are usually a, β, N and ρ. Other parameters like μ, λ and κ can be calculated independently using appropriate data in the public health records; while θ can also be taken as approximately zero as the main source of removal in the low/no-risk group is the onset of AIDS. The incubation period parameter γ however may have to be taken from other relevant material (as in Sections 4.3 and 7).

7   Applications to Switzerland

Initial studies of Swiss data were started early in 1987. Estimates of coregroup sizes, relative to population size, were based on the San Francisco analysis (see Sections 2 and 3.3 above). But it was discovered early in 1990 that by then there was enough information in the available AIDS incidence date for N to be treated as a parameter to be estimated in the maximum-likelihood computations. It was, however, still necessary to use the San Francisco estimates of the incubation period – as mentioned above in Section 3.3. The approach of Sections 5 and 6 was then followed.

For gay men we obtained $\hat{N} = 2160 \pm 180$ for the initial core-group size at the end of 1978. The proportion of AIDS cases following up death-certificate route was $\hat{\rho} = 0.21 \pm 0.02$. Parameters a and β were not very accurately determined, but a satisfactory model fit was obtained with $\chi^2_{21} = 22.3$. The estimated numbers of HIV positives circulating at the end of 1991 were 1370 in the high-activity group and 520 in the low-activity group, totalling 1890.

The figures for IDUs were $\hat{N} = 1450 \pm 275$, with $\hat{\rho} = 0.26 \pm 0.02$. The HIV positives in the high and low activity groups were 865 and 500, respectively, totalling 1365 at the end of 1991. The goodness-of-fit was $\chi^2_{15} = 19.4$. For further details see Bailey (1993).

Analogous investigations are currently being undertaken for the heterosexual population. But numbers are as yet relatively small, especially as the new more detailed classification into 8 categories according to the *presumed* source of HIV transmission has recently been adopted by the Swiss Federal Office of Public Health. This reveals some interesting and useful patterns but time is required to determine whether the latter are sufficiently reliable to support detailed quantitative modelling.

Further applications to larger European countries, like France and Germany, are in progress. Spot checks show good fits of the modelling described above to situations where larger numbers of observations lead to greatly improved accuracy. Results will be reported elsewhere in due course.

8 Operational research (OR)

The importance of OR to public health decision-making and planning was stressed in the Summary above. While this is not the place to discuss OR in detail, it should be recognised that operational modelling, as reviewed above, is an essential part of the main OR activity. Again, as indicated in Section 1, we are dealing with the broad public health scene at a macro-level, and need relatively simple models, epidemiologically based and using local public health data, in order to provide general guidance in selecting strategy choices. While reasonable accuracy is necessary, and models must be adequately validated, extreme precision is neither required nor, probably, attainable.

The expectation is that approximate future scenarios can be constructed for alternative strategy choices depending on different ways of meeting demands for therapeutic, health-care and preventive services. Practical decision-making will in general require an integration of the epidemiologically based modelling with some form of socio-economic modelling. This means that the usual type of interdisciplinary OR team must be well acquainted with modern scenario analysis applied to public health activities. See, for example, the recent publication in the Netherlands (Ruitenberg 1992). But it must be emphasised that such scenario analyses must be closely geared to epidemiological models that have been fitted to local data (i.e. not merely using plausible parameter values) as strongly urged in this review.

References

Bailey, N.T.J. (1975) *The Mathematical Theory of Infectious Diseases and its Applications*, Griffin, London.

Bailey, N.T.J. (1991) 'The use of operational modelling of HIV/AIDS in a systems approach to public health decision making', *Math. Biosci.* **107**, 413–430.

Bailey, N.T.J. (1992) 'Parameter estimation in the operational modelling of HIV/AIDS'. Chapter 19 of *The Art of Statistical Science*, K.V. Mardia, (ed.) Wiley, New York.

Bailey, N.T.J. (1993) 'An improved hybrid HIV/AIDS model geared to specific public health data and decision-making' , *Math. Biosci.* **117**, 221–237.

Bailey, N.T.J. and Estreicher, J. (1987) 'Epidemic prediction and public health control, with special reference to influenza and AIDS.' In *Proc. 1st World Congress Bernoulli Society*, VNU Science Press, Utrecht. 507–516.

Baroyan, O.V. and Rvachev, L A. (1967) 'Deterministic epidemic models for a territory with a transport network', *Kibernetika* **3**, 67–74.

Baroyan, O.V., Rvachev, L.A., Frank, K.D., Shashkov, V.A. and Basilevski, U.V. (1973) 'Mathematical and computer modelling of influenza epidemics in the USSR', *Vestn. Akad. Med. Nauk.* **28**, 26-30.

Baroyan, O.V., Rvachev, L.A. and Ivannikov, Yu.G. (1977) *Modelling and Prediction of Influenza Epidemics in the USSR*, CVR, Moscow.

Brookmeyer, R. (1991) 'Reconstruction and future trends of the AIDS epidemic in the United States, *Science* **253**, 37–42.'

Brookmeyer, R. and Liao, J. (1990) 'The analysis of delays in disease reporting: methods and results for the acquired immunodeficiency syndrome', *Amer. J. Epidemiol.* **132**, 355–365.

Chin, J. and Lwanga, S.K. (1991) 'Estimation and projection of adult AIDS cases: a simple epidemiological model' *Bull. WHO*, **69**, 399–406.

Heisterkamp, S.H., Jager, J.C., Ruitenberg, E.J., van Druten, J.A.M., and Downs, A.M. (1989) 'Correcting reported AIDS incidence: a statistical approach', *Statist. in Med.* **8**, 963–976.

Hethcote, H.W. and Yorke, J.A. (1984) *Gonorrhea transmission dynamics and control* Lecture Notes in Biomathematics **56**, Springer, Berlin.

Institute of Medicine (NAS) (1986) *Confronting AIDS*, National Academy Press, Washington DC.

Koopman, J.S., Simon, C.P., Jacquez, J.A., Haber, M. and Longini, I.M. (1992) 'HIV transmission probabilities for oral and anal sex by stage of infection'. Poster presented at VIII International Conference on AIDS, Amsterdam.

Lemp, G.F., Payne, S.F., Rutherford, G.W. *et al.* (1990) 'Projections of AIDS morbidity and mortality in San Francisco', *JAMA* **263**, 1497–1501.

Longini, I.M., Clark, W.S., Byers, R.H. *et al.* (1989) 'Statistical analysis of the stages of HIV infection using a Markov model', *Statist. in Med.* **8**, 831–843.

Nåsell, I. (1977) 'On transmission and control of schistosomiasis, with comments on Macdonald's model', *Theor. Pop. Biol.* **12**, 335–365.

Redfield, R.R. and Burke, D.S. (1988) 'HIV infection: the clinical picture', *Scientific American* October, 70–78.

Rosenberg, R.S. (1990) 'A simple correction of AIDS surveillance data for reporting delays', *JAIDS* **3**, 49–54.

Ruitenberg, E.J. (ed.) (1992) *AIDS up to the year 2000*, Kluwer Academic Publishers, Dordrecht-Boston-London.

Satten, G.A., Longini, I.M. and Clark, W.S. (1992) 'Estimating the incidence of HIV infection using cross-sectional marker surveys.' Poster presented at VIII International Conference on AIDS, Amsterdam.

Scherrer, J.-R., Wanner, G., Bailey, N.T.J., Estreicher, J. (1985) 'Continuous-time modelling in biology.' Report to Swiss National Foundation for Scientific Research.

Scherrer, J.-R., Somaini, B., Bailey, N.T.J., Frei, P., Hirschel, B. and Vorkauf, H. (1988) 'The construction of a population dynamics model of AIDS and HIV infection with applications to clinical and public health decision-making'. Report to Swiss National Foundation for Scientific Research.

Problem Areas

This Appendix presents notes from the discussions on areas for future research that concluded the 1993 NATO workshop on Epidemic Models. Thanks are due to all the workshop participants for their contributions; these notes have been compiled and edited by Stephen Ellner, Odo Diekmann, Niels Becker and Denis Mollison.

1 Model Structure

1.1 Phenomena

Several phenomena were identified as challenges to current epidemic modelling paradigms, requiring new model structures to understand their effects on parameter estimation, forecasting, and policy analysis.

Persistence: Disparities between 'fade out' in real and model epidemics, and the need for tractable ways of incorporating edge effects (migration, or contacts with the 'outside world').

Changing behaviour: Changes in mixing patterns and transmission efficiencies, both secular trends and short-term responses to epidemics.

Evolution and genetics: Genetic variability and its effects, on short time scales (e.g. if the most susceptible hosts are infected first) and on the longer time-scale of Darwinian evolution in disease and host populations.

Control: The complexities of control efforts as they are really implemented.

1.2 Model development

The 'short list' of standard epidemic models (SIS, SIR, 'general stochastic epidemic') is too short – but how much more is needed? Do we need a long list of idiosyncratic models devised for each new situation, or can a 'less short list' be found that is good enough for practical purposes and can form a basis for concerted, theoretical efforts? Aspects that need to be addressed on the 'less short list' include the following:

Transmission models:

- *Models from individual behaviour:* Contact and infection are fundamentally consequences of individual behaviour. Models derived from individual behaviours and their consequences may be more parsimonious than phenomenologial models of mixing patterns, and better for modelling changing behaviours. Individual behaviours are also observable, which may facilitate evaluation of alternative models.

417

- *Forcing:* Basic epidemic parameters fluctuate on a wide range of time scales: daily and seasonal scales due to climate, yearly or longer scales due to changes in behaviour, demography ('baby boom' and similar effects, changing age structure), and evolution. The relative merits and interrelationships of alternative model formulations (e.g. explicit age structure vs. time-varying birth rate in an SIR model) need further exploration.

Uncertainty: In applications it is important to know the extent to which uncertainties about the model limit our ability to make forecasts, taking into account both parameter estimation errors and misspecification of the model. Methods for quantifying uncertainty and its consequences are widely used in 'decision analysis' but have not yet seen much use by epidemic modellers. Tools from filtering theory may be useful for estimating unobserved variables and their effects.

Disease and host life cycles: e.g. micro- vs. macroparasites, development of immunity in hosts.

Neighbourhood structure: recognizing the social, spatial, and transportation network aspects of neighbourhood size and 'distance'.

1.3   Analysis of models

Hard-core mathematical analysis is important for establishing the general principles that govern a range of models. The much-maligned R_0 is perhaps the best example: it gives us a general *theory* to understand epidemic initiation and persistence which can be used very generally without reference to a specific model.

Spatial process models appear to be the Next Big Thing. Research topics of direct relevance to epidemiological applications include

- Limit theorems and determining the variety of limits
- Relations with Cellular Automata, stochastic DEs, etc.
- Dealing with corners, holes, and other features of real space

Nonlinear behaviour (or, the Last Big Thing) : with an emphasis on forcing effects, chaos, etc.

Relations between the predictions of stochastic and deterministic models:

- Stochastic counterparts of nonlinear phenomena such as bifurcations, limit cycles, chaos
- Defining persistence criteria for stochastic models and methods for determining when a model epidemic is persistent

Approximations:

- When can deterministic approximations be used for finite populations?
- Varieties of approximations for stochastic models (deterministic and stochastic).
- 'Correction effects': when we knowingly simplify a model (e.g. collapse to 3 age categories), is there some way to 'correct' for this that is close enough for practical use (e.g. multiply some model parameters, or model outputs, by factors that can be determined without analyzing the more complex model?).

Model 'recognition': More generally, as more complex models are elaborated it becomes harder, and more important, to understand the relationships among models, e.g. to recognize when two formulations are equivalent or nearly so, and how to translate between them. This may require much more than a superficial 'taxonomy' of models, since equivalence is not necessarily obvious: see, for instance, Schaalje and van der Vart (1989) on the complicated relationships between two widely used formulations of stage-structured population models with variable stage durations. Identification of good (optimal?) parametrizations might help: which of the many ways to parametrize a complex model will be most useful for minimizing parameter identifiability problems, suggesting limiting cases (handy epsilons), and revealing similarities with other models?

2   Heterogeneity

Two important aspects of heterogeneity, viz.

- the core group effect
- the speed of propagation

are fairly well understood. Here the first is due to the fact that averaging individual properties with respect to population composition may lead to completely wrong results (see Jacquez et al., this volume, and the references therein; see Adler (1992) for a general monotonicity result), whereas the second is relevant when we are close to reducibility, as in the case of spatial spread in a large domain (see Metz and van den Bosch, this volume). What is far less well understood, and therefore important to investigate, is

- the smoothing out of severe fluctuations by providing buffers

Here we have in mind, for instance, the influence of age and spatial structure on measles dynamics (Grenfell et al., this volume), an issue with close connection to the ecological issue of metapopulation dynamics (Gilpin and Hanski 1991) and the damping of prey-predator cycles.

2.1   How to take averages?

The notion of R_0 is based on a demographic steady state. When, for instance, a veterinarian visits a farm every three months to vaccinate, one has a periodic situation and R_0 should be defined as a dominant Floquet multiplier. More generally one may pose the problem of the influence of time inhomogeneity and in particular concentrate on the
* definition and relevance of R_0 in a changing world.

When a small active group is loosely coupled to a large inactive group, the nonlinearity may be relevant in the small group before the epidemic is noticeable in the large group. In general
* loose coupling of widely differing subgroups

poses an interesting and important problem. In addition the
* relation of R_0 to measurable quantities

should be investigated in far more detail in a variety of contexts.

2.2   Space

The world is far from homogeneous and this may have far reaching consequences for the spread of diseases. One may exploit
* deformation

to transform real space into effective space on the basis of migration and transport patterns (see Cliff, and Metz and van den Bosch, both in this volume). In this way geography starts unifying true space and
* social space.

However, the connectedness and manifold or
* graph structure

of social space is not yet well understood.

For wildlife diseases one has to investigate how contact patterns depend on territories, home ranges and habitat quality. The effective density may stay constant when densities change. In general the
* interaction term for the spatial spread of a wildlife disease

needs further scrutiny (also see De Jong *et al.*, this volume). The most important issue of
* critical community size

has various components such as
* the difference of the time scales of demographic turnover and disease transmission,
* a more careful study of demographic stochasticity in the troughs of the susceptible subpopulation,
* (im)migration and effective population size,
* spatial structure and age structure as buffers.

It will be a hard but rewarding task to disentangle the effects of each of these.

2.3 Genetic heterogeneity

The mechanisms and phenomena related to the

- coevolution of host and parasite

are varied and manifold. Certainly

- strains of malaria: superinfection and cross-immunity

is a hot issue as is

- evolution within a single host (interaction with the immune system, the diversity threshold etc.)

but because of its relevance for agriculture we should also look at

- artificial selection by chemotherapy and culling.

2.4 Vaccine

Of the many questions related to vaccination strategies we choose to mention

- effects of contact patterns in measuring vaccine efficacy
- role of isolated populations
- age structure and loss of protection
- spatial heterogeneity in
  - susceptibles (once more critical community size)
  - effort.

2.5 Data

The collection and analysis of data on

- contact patterns: the mixing of subgroups

is highly relevant for an understanding of dynamical aspects of the AIDS epidemic (see e.g. Morris, this volume). Moreover,

- detecting risk factors in the presence of heterogeneity

is a hard task which could possibly be made lighter by a theoretical analysis.

3 Data Analysis and Prediction

3.1 Design

The statistical design of studies involving infectious diseases is considered a most important area of research. Statisticians have much to offer in this regard to ensure that designs, both in form and size, are suitable for the objectives of the study. Specific mention was made of three types of studies. First, what size of households, and how many, are appropriate for studies in which individuals of households are serologically tested at the start and at the end of an epidemic period. Secondly, studies for estimating vaccine efficacy need to be designed so that vaccinated and unvaccinated individuals are equally exposed to the disease. Thirdly, studies for making inference about the form of the infectiousness function from partner data are required.

Designs are needed which avoid ascertainment biases, and also those which help to reduce labour-intensive experimental techniques. Testing of pooled samples of sera, rather than testing each sample individually, is an example of the latter.

3.2   Statistical issues in the analysis of epidemic data

Deterministic models: A large number of individuals explore epidemic data with the use of deterministic models. There is a need to find a generally accepted method or statistical setting which enables the fitting of such models and ways of assessing whether they adequately describe the data.

Heterogeneity: Another important issue in the area of data analysis is the development of ways for making inferences about central parameters of epidemic models which allow for the inherent heterogeneity among individuals. Analogues of the frailty models used in survival analysis are envisaged for unobserved heterogeneity, but analyses which account for heterogeneity among identifiable groups are also needed.

Choice of model: It is considered important to try to incorporate prior knowledge about parameters into the model or the method of data analysis.

Hierarchical models have not received the attention they deserve. In a geographical context this might relate to the suburban, county, state and national levels.

It would be useful to develop methods for distinguishing between stochastic epidemic, nonlinear time-series and chaos models for descriptions of a specific data set.

Choice of parameters: Epidemic models usually involve many parameters; often more than the data can support. However, these parameters are considered necessary to describe the mechanisms that generate the data. For fitting models with too many parameters it is considered desirable to reparametrize to a set of primary parameters, of small dimension, and the secondary parameters which are less crucial in the description of the data. This retains the interpretation of parameters, but a method is needed for determining the set of primary parameters.

Likelihood methods: The likelihood function corresponding to epidemic data is usually very complicated. There seems considerable scope for developing techniques for computing the likelihood function using stochastic simulation methods.

The likelihood function is very difficult to construct for some epidemic models. It may then be appropriate to work with modified likelihoods. These have been very successful for the analysis of survival data.

Non-likelihood methods: Alternative methods of investigation include the simulated method of moments, of which martingale estimating equations are an example, and indirect methods.

The use of parametric versus nonparametric models in this context deserves discussion, with semi-parametric models likely to offer a suitable compromise.

3.3 Some problems in epidemiology and public health

Some specific problems were raised by the group. Several of these relate to the estimation of R_0, the basic reproduction ratio. They include its estimation in the presence of heterogeneity, including the use of regression techniques. The distributional properties of estimators of R_o in a variety of settings need to be derived. The definition of R_0 and its estimation when the density of infection is important is a worthwhile project. A continuing practical problem is the estimation of R_0 when the infection process is in a transient phase, perhaps as a result of a recently initiated vaccination program.

The analysis of markers of the immune system, when these markers are ascertained retrospectively, is an important practical problem of current interest.

With the recent interest in sexually transmissible diseases, induced by the HIV epidemic, there is an increasing need for analyses of data on self-reporting of contacts obtained from individuals who recently tested positive to a disease.

3.4 Prediction

Model assessment: A greater emphasis on objective-oriented prediction is encouraged, and further work on ways of assessing the model adequacy is needed. The issue of when simple substantive models are preferable to more complicated substantive ones needs further research.

Simulation: The development of a simulation 'language', as a tool for the construction of detailed disease transmission models is desirable, as is construction of interactive software for the simulation of epidemics. Effective guidelines for the use of simulation studies to design and analyse intervention, such as vaccination schedules, are required.

3.5 Data sets

Enthusiasm was expressed by some for the collection of epidemic data sets, with documentation, references and acknowledgements. These could be used to encourage research students to develop new methodology and would help to generate further work and interaction in this area.

References

Adler, F. (1992) 'The effects of averaging on the basic reproduction ratio', *Math Biosci.* 111, 89–98.

Cliff, Andrew (1995) 'Incorporating spatial components into models of epidemic spread', this volume.

de Jong, M., Diekmann, O. and Heesterbeek, J.A.P. (1995) 'How does transmission of infection depend on population size?', this volume.

Gilpin, M.E. and Hanski, I. (1991) *Metapopulation Dynamics: Empirical and Theoretical Investigations*, Academic Press.

Grenfell, B.T., Bolker, B. and Kleczkowski, A. (1995) 'Seasonality, demography and the dynamics of measles in developed countries', this volume.

Jacquez, J., Simon, C.P. and Koopman, J. (1995) 'Core groups and R_0s for subgroups in heterogeneous SIS and SI models', this volume.

Metz, J.A.J., and van den Bosch, F. (1995) 'Velocities of epidemic spread', this volume.

Morris, Martina (1995) 'Data driven network models for the spread of disease', this volume.

Schaalje, G.B. and van de Vart, H.R. (1989) 'Relationships among recent models for insect population dynamics with variable rates of development', *J. Math. Biol.* 27, 399–428.